# GET THE STRAIGHT FACTS ON:

•Painkillers such as Anacin, Bufferin, Tylenol, and the newly available Advil and Nuprin

•Micatin—and how it is revolutionizing the treatment of athlete's foot

•Drugs and pregnancy—WHAT YOU DON'T KNOW <u>CAN</u> HURT YOUR BABY

•Children and drug safety

•Diuretics

•The alcohol level of popular mouthwashes

•Smart strategies for choosing over-the-counter (OTC) drugs

## AND MORE!

"An indispensable part of any health consumer's home library."     —*Newsweek*

"Required reading."     —*Vogue*

"Essential."     —*Library Journal*

*Also by Joe Graedon and Teresa Graedon*

JOE GRAEDON'S THE NEW PEOPLE'S PHARMACY:
DRUG BREAKTHROUGHS OF THE '80S

THE PEOPLE'S PHARMACY-2

# Totally New and Revised

# The People's Pharmacy®

# Joe Graedon

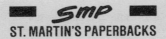
ST. MARTIN'S PAPERBACKS

*This book is dedicated to:*

## BRIAN WEISS
*A true friend who has stood by us through all the chaos, countless crunches, and seemingly constant calamities*

## BILL PINNA
*Who pulled our cookies out of the fire once again*

## PHIL SCHWARTZ
*Whose straightforward approach and willingness to compromise allowed this book to be completed*

## PEOPLE EVERYWHERE
*Who care about their health and who want to learn more about the drugs their doctors prescribe*

THE PEOPLE'S PHARMACY

Copyright © 1985, 1976 by Graedon Enterprises, Inc.

ISBN: 0-312-92962-5

Printed in the United States of America

St. Martin's Paperbacks edition/September 1986

10  9  8  7  6  5

# Notice

The information contained in this book regarding health and medications is the result of careful review by the authors of relevant medical and scientific literature. However, individual reactions to medications and other remedies may vary. Consequently, the authors and publisher strongly urge each reader to consult with his or her physician before starting, stopping, or changing the dose of any medication or treatment and before acting on any of the information contained in this book. The author and publisher disclaim responsibility for any adverse effect or unforeseen consequences resulting from implementing any information mentioned in this book. Any side effect or drug interaction should be reported promptly to a physician.

# Acknowledgments

Several people contributed directly to the completion of this work. Special thanks go to:

**Brian Weiss,** a superb writer who helped make this book a reality

**Dr. David McWaters,** a talented and knowledgeable pharmacist who cheerfully rolled up his sleeves and got into the trenches with us from day one

**Jared Kieling,** whose editorial expertise and professional skill make working with him a pleasure

# Contents

safety and danger of aspirin • The safety and danger of **Indocin** • The safety and danger of **Inderal** • Drug Safety: Protect the bod—it's the only one you've got • Sexual side effects: Doctors' lips are sealed • Buying and storing drugs wisely • Taking your medicine: Harder than you think • **DES:** A tragedy that never should have happened • Getting rid of ineffective drugs • Are the benefits worth the risks?

warning sign of heart disease? • The cholesterol controversy heats up again.

# List of Tables

# Authors' Note

Over the past twelve years an extraordinary number of people have contributed in one way or another to making our People's Pharmacy publications successful. Some provided advice and ideas, while others gave us their love and encouragement. Thank yous to:

Karen Carey
Sid and Helen Graedon
David and Alena Graedon
Betty Lu and Bonnell Frost
Jere Goyan
Dean Edell
Ralph and Lynn Scallion
Marcia and Ricardo Hofer
Tom Ferguson
Gail Schmidt
Kathe Gregory
Phil Lee
Milt Silverman and Mia
  Lydecker
Pedro Cuatrecasas

Cliff Butler
David and Marty Sedwick
Ed and Aleka Leydon
John Barth
Melva Okun
Janet Vultee
Tom Pritchard
Tom Smigel
Roger Williams
Linda Hart
John Doorley
Carolyn Glynn
Pat Barry
Faye Peterson
Susan Moldow

Stan Levy
Carole Dombach
Molly and Frederick
  Bernheim

Chuck and Alice Cambron
David and Carol Hogue
Joanne Hall
Allan Priaulx

# 1

# Introduction

*The People's Pharmacy* started modestly enough. When I was a graduate student in pharmacology, friends, neighbors, relatives, and casual acquaintances often asked me questions about the medicines they were taking. I was shocked to discover that many of these people often didn't even know the names of their medications, let alone how to take them and what side effects to watch out for. It was clear that somewhere the system had broken down. Doctors were prescribing drugs by the truckload, but for the most part they were keeping their patients in the dark about adverse reactions.

My original idea was to scribble down a few guidelines for the folks I had been talking to. As the project grew, my overriding goal became to make people aware of both the benefits and the risks of using medicine and to empower them to make intelligent decisions about their own health care.

The result of that work was the first edition of *The People's Pharmacy,* which to everyone's surprise (especially mine), became a national best-seller and sold over a million copies. A decade has passed, however, and there have been so many changes in the drugs we use that it was clear the time had come to update *The People's Pharmacy.*

Although my wife, Terry, and I have written two additional books over the intervening years—*The People's Pharmacy-2* and *The New People's Pharmacy-3*—these books dealt with different issues. We addressed questions of FDA (Food and Drug Administration) laxity, drug scandals and fraud within the pharmaceutical industry, as well as drug advances during the 1980s. As important as these topics are, it is clear that most of the concerns raised in the original *People's Pharmacy* needed to be updated, since they had not been addressed in our later books. And we have received thousands and thousands of letters from readers over the years indicating that consumers were desperate for more information.

This totally new edition will help people take greater control over their own health care rather than be at the mercy of an indifferent system. With all of the new medications that have come on the market in the last several years, the ante has been raised. Today's potent drugs carry even greater risks. More than ever, people now need access to information on the medicines they take most often. I hope this completely rewritten *The People's Pharmacy* will help people be vigilant so that the cure does not become worse than the disease.

Fortunately, patients have become more sophisticated about their medications and their health. Few consumers these days are willing to swallow pills passively without any knowledge of what drugs are supposed to do. And they want to be informed about how to take their medicine, what the potential side effects may be, and what other medications they need to avoid. Yet many physicians are still reluctant to inform their patients. According to the FDA, "medications are taken improperly up to 50 percent of the time."[1] For example,

**Doctors show concern that patients fail to take their medications properly; 72 percent report that patients frequently fail to take all their medicine as needed.**

**But only 7 percent of the doctors say they tell patients
to finish their prescriptions of the antibiotic tetracycline,
which must be taken in full to be effective.[2]**

Pollster Louis Harris conducted a survey for the FDA and
discovered that "Only about one out of four patients recalls
having been told of side effects by the physician or someone in
his or her office."[3]

But people are wising up. They know that ignorance is *not*
bliss, especially when it comes to drugs. People are taking more
responsibility for finding out what they need to know about
medications. While they may still be intimidated by their doctors
(only 2 percent to 4 percent ask questions in the physician's
office),[4] millions are turning to books and other sources for critical information.

And yet patients are swallowing more pills than ever before,
and at an unprecedented price tag. In 1976, I reported that
Americans were spending about $11 billion on prescribed drugs
and $2.6 billion on over-the-counter medications. Today, hospi-
tal and drugstore sales of prescriptions amounts to over $20
billion.[5, 6] And Americans shell out up to $9 billion on nonpre-
scription drugs "with an estimated 40% of the U.S. population
using an OTC product in any given 48 hours."[7]

Now *that* is one big pile of pills! Keep in mind that most of
these medications can't cure anything. At best they can only
temporarily relieve symptoms. Tranquilizers like **Valium** (diazepam) and **Tranxene** (clorazepate) don't solve the problem of
anxiety. Arthritis meds like **Motrin** (ibuprofen), **Naprosyn** (naproxen), **Clinoril** (sulindac), or **Feldene** (piroxicam) don't really
eliminate the agony of arthritis. And pain relievers such as **Tylenol with Codeine** can soothe pain only temporarily.

And there is almost always a price to be paid for such relief.
The FDA estimates that there are over six million drug-induced
adverse reactions each year in this country.[8]

Simply stated, too many drugs are prescribed in our pill-
popping society. Whether it's **Tagamet** (cimetidine) for ulcers or
**Dalmane** (flurazepam) for insomnia, the evidence is growing that

doctors have been far too casual in the way they hand out such prescriptions and inform patients about proper use.

Drug companies spend over a billion dollars each year promoting drugs to doctors. Their marketing techniques are sophisticated and successful. Doctors often buy the pitch—hook, line, and sinker. The only problem is that *they* don't swallow the drugs: *We* do.

What distinguishes our modern-day practitioners from their predecessors is not so much the greater quantity of new agents at their disposal (though that in itself is a gigantic difference), but rather their heavy reliance on this form of treatment. Today's overworked doctor may have less time to talk with patients and come up with nondrug alternatives. So instead of helping a patient with high blood pressure develop an effective weight-loss program with exercise and nutritional counseling, out comes a prescription for **Dyazide** (triamterene and hydrochlorothiazide) or **Inderal** (propranolol). By the way, these are the two most commonly prescribed brand-name drugs in the United States today.

This book is not meant to replace a trip to the doctor, but rather to explain in everyday English just what those pills your doctor prescribes really do. For far too long, people assumed that they were incapable of understanding "medical language," but all that is changing. The demystification of medicine is a fact. Magazines and books such as *Medical Self-Care* are providing people the tools they need to take better care of themselves.

In the chapters that follow, you will learn about side effects, precautions, and dangerous drug interactions that physicians rarely mention. The unexpected (and usually undesirable) effects of combining more than one drug at a time can be life-threatening.

The frequently prescribed ulcer drug **Tagamet**, for example, may increase blood-alcohol levels when you drink. As a result, a person who normally would not be drunk after only a couple of beers or several glasses of wine may unexpectedly be a menace on the highways, or be arrested for driving while intoxicated.

Drug-to-drug reactivity is an especially acute problem when

you are receiving prescriptions from two or more doctors simultaneously (a very common situation these days). The cardiologist who puts you on **Inderal** for angina and high blood pressure may be unaware that the rheumatologist has you on **Indocin** (indomethacin) for arthritis. The combination could well decrease the ability of **Inderal** to lower blood pressure effectively. The information in this book could be lifesaving when two or more drugs "don't mix."

On a lighter note, you will find some fascinating home remedies—without a doubt my favorite chapter. I included some in the original *People's Pharmacy* almost as a lark. To my surprise, people loved them. So here, completely revised, are some exciting new home remedies for everything from hiccups, heartburn, and motion sickness to poison-ivy itches, removing imbedded ticks, and fighting fingernail fungus. I even offer something for the common cold (besides chicken soup and Vitamin C).

The chapter on over-the-counter (OTC) remedies will bring you up to date on the latest developments coming to pharmacy shelves. Self-treatment is a growing phenomenon, but you can't take good care of yourself unless you're fully informed about nonprescription medications. We will reveal brand-new secrets about OTC sleeping pills and antacids. You will learn why **Tums** or **Alka-2** may be better than **Mylanta** or **Maalox** for some people. You will get specific recommendations for "best buys" so you can spend your health dollars efficiently.

Chances are you've been reading about the aluminum and Alzheimer's disease connection. We'll do our best to bring you up to speed on this controversy. Use an underarm deodorant? Stay tuned for some cool tips. How about dandruff shampoo? With all the brands on the market, it's no wonder you have a hard time picking the right brand. We'll try to help. And we've got good news for athlete's foot sufferers. A new drug called **Micatin** (miconazole) is revolutionizing the treatment of this common problem.

If you or anyone you know suffers from allergies or asthma, you will want to read the latest update on new medications. Drugs like **Beclovent, Nasalide, Nasalcrom,** and **Procardia** are changing the way we treat these ailments. And this revised edition of *The People's Pharmacy* has lots of new information on high-blood-pressure medicines.

If you are using any form of birth control, you will want to read the latest information about the Pill, especially the new "triphasic" tablets that are supposed to mimic Mother Nature. We will also tell you the inside story on **Today**, the new spermicidal sponge that has become so popular. And you will discover the most recent findings on the safety of vasectomy. Any couple contemplating a family had better pay close attention to the new material on pregnancy. And if you already have children, there is lots of crucial information on common childhood problems like diarrhea, ear infections, and bed-wetting.

Anyone who is watching the budget will be delighted to learn about some exciting new tips on how to save money in the drugstore. With some of the most popular prescription products coming off patent (**Aldomet, Ativan, Dalmane, Inderal, Motrin, Valium**, and so many more), there are extraordinary savings to be had if you just do your homework. We'll give you the ammunition to fight back.

Finally, for those of you who want to know more about stocking your medicine chest, we have a completely rewritten chapter about self-treatment (subtitled "Hiking in the Himalayas, or What to Do When the Doctor Won't Come"). Discover the state-of-the-art treatment for traveler's diarrhea, and what to do about urinary-tract infections.

The goal of this book, then, is to provide you with basic information regarding some of today's most commonly used medications. It will give you the power to take a far more active role in your own health care by giving you information on both the benefits and the risks of those medicines the physician prescribes most often.

My hope is to continue enabling people to understand how the medicines they take work in their bodies, and how to approach simple medical problems before, during, and after professional medical intervention. I trust you will get some chuckles out of all this material, along with some practical advice. This totally new and revised *People's Pharmacy* may help save you some money, but more importantly, it may save your life.

## References

1. Miller, Roger W. "Doctors, Patients Don't Communicate." *FDA Consumer* 17(6):6–7, 1983.

2. Ibid.

3. Ibid.

4. Ibid.

5. "Consumer Expenditure Study." *Product Marketing* 13(8):18, 1984.

6. Baum, Carlene, et al. "Drug Use and Expenditures in 1982." *JAMA* 253:382–386, 1985.

7. Boyd, J. R. "Self-Care and OTC Medicines." *Facts and Comparisons Drug Newsletter* 4(2):11, 1985.

8. Harris, Patricia. Statement on Patient Package Inserts. *HHS News,* Sep. 10, 1980, p. 1.

# 2

## What Is a Drug?

When is a drug not a drug? This may sound like a child's riddle, but the question is actually far more serious. Some hucksters have figured out that if they can claim their product is a solvent, an herb, or a food supplement, they may not have to meet federal standards for drugs. Though most people would agree with the Food and Drug Administration (FDA) that anything that acts like a drug is one, that is sometimes hard to prove and harder yet to enforce.

The law says that drugs must be safe and effective in order to be marketed. But the problem is that the legal definition of a drug is somewhat murky. As a result, the FDA has to spend quite a bit of its time arguing about the exact classification of various pills and potions.

Not long ago, for example, several companies excitedly announced that they would soon be offering pills to sober you up after an evening of too much drinking. These "sobriety aids" were to be called things such as **Sober Up Time, Sober-Up**, and **Sober-Aid**. The potential market was huge, as were the potential profits. No wonder the companies were excited.

As it turned out, the first ones to get sobered up were the pill makers. The FDA, in a memo to its field offices, declared the sobriety aids to be "unapproved new drugs when offered for such use." The significance of the memo was hardly lost on the companies. Once classified as a new drug, the sobriety aids would require long clinical trials to produce evidence that they were safe and effective.

"Obviously," said the president of one of the firms, "it would make it a heck of a lot easier if it were classified as a food."[1] That's putting it mildly. Before it's marketed, a new drug requires a New Drug Application to be filed and approved. This legal document, containing all the scientific and clinical studies done to prove that the drug is safe and effective, can run several feet thick and tens of thousands of pages. We're talking big bucks here, so you better be damn sure you've got a winner before you go into the drug-testing biz. But some folks want a shortcut.

Another company's president hurriedly insisted that his sobriety aid contained no drugs, but only ingredients that were "harmless and even beneficial."[2] He'll get a chance to prove it, because the companies' worst fears came true a few months later when the FDA put them on official notice that sobriety aids were drugs. "There is an obvious danger if motorists rely on a product's unsubstantiated claims that it will sober them up," remarked then-Commissioner of the FDA Arthur Hayes.[3] To combat this "threat to the safety of motorists and pedestrians," the agency promised action against any firm trying to market such pills unless it could prove they really could sober up people and that their ingredients wouldn't do harm of their own.

How did the FDA decide that sobriety aids were drugs, not food supplements? When is a food a drug? For that matter, when is a drug a drug, and how can you tell food from drug? As a pharmacologist, I would maintain that any substance that affects the body should be considered a drug. But the FDA has learned the hard way that the lines are not always easily drawn. According to the official definition from the Food and Drug Act, drugs are:

> **Articles intended for use in diagnosis, cure, mitigation, treatment or prevention of disease in man or other animals. Articles intended to affect the structure of or any function of the body of man or other animals.**[4]

That seems clear enough, doesn't it? Rice is a food, **Valium** is a drug, and starch blocker, made from a bean, is a . . . a drug? Welcome to the Alice-in-Wonderland world of drug regulation and marketing.

## Fattening Up on Starch Blockers

Starch blockers were the fat fad of the early 1980s. We seem destined to "discover," every year or so, one thing or another that is the sure cure for that spare tire so many of us carry around our middles. The only thing these products ever permanently lighten is the wallets of those using them, but the cycle never ceases, proving anew each time that P. T. Barnum was right. At any rate, 1982 was the Year of the Starch Blocker. Starch blocker is a substance, derived from a common bean, said to inactivate an enzyme needed to digest starch. You could pop a few pills, gobble several pounds of pasta, cake, or bread, and never gain an ounce—according to the ads.

The response was immediate, immense, and highly profitable for the companies involved. People bought starch blocker pills by the millions. Health food stores were, at first, the only place you could get them, but it wasn't long before they started turning up in the same drugstores that sold prescription drugs and FDA-approved over-the-counter remedies. With most of the country feeling at least a bit overweight, the market was just too large and profitable to ignore, even though the drugstores must have known they were peddling something that was of dubious value.

They were supplied by more than one hundred companies that sprang up within months to produce the pills.

The only fly in the ointment was the FDA. Officials believed that anything that altered the digestive process by manipulating enzymes sounded suspiciously like a drug and might have side effects. But when the feds started making unhappy noises, the companies producing starch blockers assured everyone the pills had to be safe. They were, after all, made from a wholly natural ingredient which was even a food. The problem with this logic is that lethal poisons can be made from all sorts of plants, many of them foods when suitably prepared. Native peoples the world over have been doing it for thousands of years.

When reports of unpleasant adverse reactions began to roll in, the FDA was finally goaded into action. People were showing up in hospital emergency rooms suffering with gas, nausea, vomiting, diarrhea, and stomach pains. And no wonder. Undigested starch is not something the human intestinal system is equipped to handle. Since the starch blocker manufacturers had never submitted any proof that their pills were either safe or effective, the FDA declared them a drug and demanded that sales cease until such proof was produced.

You would think that would be the end of it. But oh nooo! Remember, we're talking about that green folding stuff people love to put in their wallets. The companies had their lawyers appeal this "unjust" ruling. To get the issue resolved, the FDA had to slug it out in court with ten of the diet-pill peddlers.

If it looks like a drug and acts like a drug, gets marketed like a drug, and the FDA says it's a drug, then, the court agreed, it must be a drug. End of starch blockers! By the way, a scientific study completed around the same time showed that the starch blockers didn't even work the way they were supposed to.[5] Worse, there was real doubt that they worked at all. One researcher writing in the *New England Journal of Medicine* put it this way:

> We also recently completed a study in which a starch blocker was proved to be ineffective. In a double-blind

crossover trial in six healthy male subjects, we were unable
to demonstrate any effect on three markers of starch digestion—namely, serum glucose, insulin, and breath hydrogen
. . . the bottom line is that [starch blockers] do not result
in excess calorie loss in the stool . . .[6]

*Your* bottom line should be distrust. When something sounds
too good to be true, ninety times out of a hundred it is! I don't
care whether it's some super-duper arthritis diet, the latest
weight-loss scam, or a wrinkle remover, be skeptical. And if the
label banners the buzzwords *natural* and *organic,* be extra wary.

## Drawing the Line

Though these regulatory shenanigans are of recent vintage,
drugs themselves are nothing new. Probably the oldest "medication," fermented beer, dates back some six thousand years.
Winemaking was well established in the early Stone Age. The
ancient Egyptians were masters of drug therapy—one medical
papyrus lists more than nine hundred prescriptions. In fact, it is
very likely that as long ago as 2000 B.C. Egyptian physicians
treated wounds and infections with a chemical derived from a
fungus that's probably a near relative of penicillin. There's even
a suggestion in some ancient manuscripts that Egyptians might
have had a birth-control pill.

Almost every culture has taken advantage of the chemicals
nature provides in the form of leaves, roots, and bark to fashion
remedies and cures. Before dismissing these as myth and magic,
remember that such staples of modern therapeutics as aspirin,
digitalis, and quinine (first used for fevers, then malaria) are
derived from plants. The white-coated creator of laboratory miracle drugs is a relative newcomer, and even he owes much of his
knowledge and some of his raw materials to substances found in
the wild.

Given the confusion, misinformation, and misapprehension
about drugs in our society, most people don't realize how many

different things the term *drug* can mean. Worse yet, a lot of Americans don't even recognize the drugs they use every day. Just think about the various sorts of drugs, and you'll see what I mean.

First off, there are prescription drugs, also referred to as ethical or pharmaceutical drugs. These are substances which by law are dispensed only by a licensed pharmacist upon order of a properly licensed physician. There is much mysticism and ritual surrounding the writing of a prescription, which still begins with an ancient incantation of Rx and is often drawn up in a strange scrawl and language known only to initiates. Because of this, most folks accept prescription medications as "real" drugs without any argument.

Of course, for a lot of people the word *drug* suggests images of junkies and cocaine snorters. But while drugs of abuse are certainly drugs, with a capital *D*, they're really not the topic of this book.

What about aspirin, cold remedies, laxatives, and deodorants? These over-the-counter (OTC) products can be purchased without a prescription by anyone who can get to a drugstore or supermarket. Because they are both accessible and familiar, people tend to forget that they are still substances capable of exerting a powerful influence on the body, complete with the potential for side effects and interactions.

And that, you may think, covers the subject. But wait—there are still others, which I'm inclined to think of as "hidden" drugs. No, no one's deliberately hiding anything from you. These are substances you might never think of as "drugs," because they're not medications. But alcohol, caffeine, nicotine, sun screen, many food additives, and even oxygen have unquestionable pharmacological effects—a highfalutin way of saying they act like drugs.

Now, sorting out all these chemicals you use isn't going to be easy. After all, even the FDA has had a few problems drawing the fine line between food and drug, as you'll recall. So don't be embarrassed if some of this seems bizarre.

Consider vitamins. Most people would say vitamins aren't

drugs. But what about Vitamin C in the megadoses suggested by Nobel Prize–winner Dr. Linus Pauling to prevent and treat colds? Or Vitamin A prescribed in large amounts to clear up acne? One eighteen-year-old woman found herself in the hospital with severe headache, blurred vision, sleep disturbances, and signs of mental illness. The initial diagnosis was a brain tumor. The right diagnosis turned out to be an excessive dose of Vitamin A. Perhaps we'd better consider vitamins to be drugs more often, especially if they're taken in the humongous doses recommended by health "experts" to help you live forever.

Aspirin is a drug most Americans take without thinking twice. So many billions of pills are swallowed that the mind boggles. It's an over-the-counter drug considered by almost everyone to be completely innocuous. But is it really? Uh-uh. One study showed that every dose of aspirin produces at least some damage to the tender lining of the stomach within twenty-four hours.[7] Those who take large doses of aspirin in order to reduce the inflammation and pain of arthritis often have problems with stomach upset and even ulcers.

That's just the beginning. Aspirin can interact with more than forty other drugs, including Vitamin C. Aspirin has the unfortunate tendency to prevent ascorbic acid from getting into cells, so you don't get the full benefit from this vitamin.[8-12] This is really a case of getting double-teamed. You feel a cold coming on and, heeding both Dr. Pauling and past experience, take a few aspirin and some Vitamin C. But these *drugs* act differently when together in your body than either one would by itself.

Or how about this one. Take more than a couple of aspirins and chances are you will experience an upset stomach. What will you reach for? Probably **Pepto-Bismol**, since it says quite clearly on the label that this medicine is especially good for "upset stomach." No big deal, right? Wrong! The main ingredient in **Pepto-Bismol** is bismuth subsalicylate. Okay, that's a mouthful, but the part to remember is the salicylate part. That sounds vaguely reminiscent of acetyl*salicylic* acid—in other words, aspirin. In fact, if you were to swallow the whole dose of **Pepto-**

**Bismol** recommended on the label, it would be equal to taking eight aspirin tablets. That, added to the aspirin you already took, could add up to an aspirin overdose and that, my friend, can cause problems. You see, it gets *very* complicated. If you want to know more about what happens when drugs get together in your body, make sure you don't skip Chapter 6.

My immediate goal is to demonstrate how tricky and difficult drug awareness can be. As you can see from just the few examples given above, it's not always obvious or easy to determine what a drug is, let alone what some of its effects might be. When you start to combine substances, the problems seem to rise a whole lot faster than the number of drugs you're taking. Potentially, anything can interact with everything else, and the result can be a whole lot of trouble.

Add to that the fact that in many cases doctors don't know everything a patient is taking, either because they haven't asked or because the patient hasn't mentioned something he or she considered unimportant. Lots of times it's just a simple case of a communications gap. The doctor asks if you're taking "any other drugs" and you say no. Would you think to tell the doctor about the megadose of Vitamin C you take daily when he suggests aspirin for your arthritis? Not if you don't think Vitamin C is a drug.

There is a growing movement in this country to reject all forms of drug therapy. The cry "I never take anything" (usually delivered in a tone of moral superiority) can be heard with increasing frequency as people protest the dangers in their chemical environment. With news of toxic spills and toxic pills crowding the nightly news, it's no surprise that many people have retreated to a corner and refuse to take anything.

While resisting unneeded medication is admirable in a culture where we've been taught that there's a chemical answer for everything, taken to extremes this attitude, too, can be unhealthy. It's neither wrong nor immoral to take a drug so long as it is the necessary and appropriate treatment for what ails you.

## If One Is Good, How 'bout a Dozen?

Part of determining what's "necessary and appropriate" involves knowing—or being told—how much of a drug to take, and this is indeed fertile ground in which advertisers have planted plenty of misinformation.

We enter here the mysterious realm of "dose-effect relationships." Simply put, in too weak a concentration, no drug can do its job; but in too high a concentration, it may do you more harm than good. The trick is to find the level which, as Goldilocks put it, is "just right."

Forget pharmacology for a minute and think about baking a cake. What if instead of following directions, you added twice the shortening and sugar called for in the recipe or doubled the amount of frosting? Instead of a sweet treat, you would end up with a gloppy disaster. Not only would you *not* improve your cake with such improvisation, chances are good you would end up with a bellyache.

And yet physicians and patients improvise with drug dosages all the time, often more carelessly than a chef would with the ingredients in his recipes. Taking twice as much of a useful drug may or may not produce twice the level of that drug in your blood or tissue; in most cases, though, it won't improve the drug's ability to do its job, whether that's knocking out pain or fighting infection. And in some cases the extra dose can put you in the trouble zone, where the body has entirely too much of a good thing on its hands . . . and in its kidneys and its liver and other sensitive parts through which drugs pass . . . and no way to cope with the excess.

Here again, what seems to make sense may well not be true, and it's often difficult to know when what you're being told is really nonsense. Consider, for example, the **Anacin** ad that crowed about having "more of the pain reliever doctors recommend most." Their much-touted exotic pain reliever, I'm happy to reveal, is plain old unadulterated aspirin, available in plain, unadvertised bottles at any pharmacy for a fraction of the cost of the same stuff labeled **Anacin**. They also add a little caffeine (32 mg), the benefits of which are controversial.

What's true about the **Anacin** claim is that two of their pills *do* contain 800 milligrams of aspirin, versus 650 milligrams for competing products such as **Alka-Seltzer, Ascriptin, Bayer, Bufferin,** and **Empirin**. It really has more active ingredient (aspirin, remember?) than these products, and the margin over **Excedrin** and **Vanquish** is even greater.

Common sense tells us that more has got to be better. This seems even more obvious when you're sitting there with a splitting headache and would do almost anything for a little relief. If two are good, surely four would be twice as strong or twice as quick to relieve the pain, right? Research says that's nonsense, and so are the ads which imply greater effectiveness.

The Great Aspirin Controversy has been examined scientifically many times, and the results keep coming up the same. Take two aspirin—any two aspirin—and you probably won't have to call anyone in the morning. The aspirin in **Anacin** won't do you any more good than two plain-wrap aspirin. If you really needed more of the painkiller, you could get it by stalking a third aspirin, catching it unaware, and cracking it down the middle with a knife. Hopefully, this will yield several smaller pieces. Swallowing an additional half a tablet would give you about as much aspirin as one of the highly advertised brands (800 mg) and a whole lot more money in your pocket. Maybe now you are getting the idea how silly and misleading these "extra-strength" ads are. The thing that's annoying is that the people who make up such advertising *know* better, and yet they play on your lack of knowledge to turn nonsense into profit. No more, because now you know too.

What you should also know is that aspirin is as good or better than a lot of expensive prescription painkillers and arthritis remedies. If you had a bad sprain or a sore back and went to the doctor asking for something "really strong," the painkiller you have in mind might be something like **Darvon**. Ready for a surprise? A Mayo Clinic study tested **Darvon** and several other prescription products against aspirin on people with pain from inoperable cancer. Neither doctor nor patient knew what was being administered to whom, and it's a good thing—because nobody taking aspirin would have believed they were getting something more effective than **Darvon** for pain. Yet that's just what the results showed.

In the words of the investigators,

**". . . simple aspirin at a dosage of 650 mg was the superior agent for relief of cancer pain among the tested marketed analgesics. Indeed, among all analgesics and narcotics available for oral use, none have been demonstrated to show a consistent advantage over aspirin for the relief of any type of pain."[13]**

Take a close look at that conclusion, folks, because it could be worth a small fortune to you. In dollars-and-cents terms, you're being told by some of the best medical authorities in the country to stop wasting your dollars on fancy pain relievers when it's possible to do the job for pennies.

## Mind over Matter, or Why the Mind Matters

By now, you are probably ready to say that Joe Graedon is full of beans. I can almost hear you protesting, "My brand does *too* work better than plain aspirin." And by golly, would you believe there's a medical study to prove you're right, too? It turns out that the degree of relief you experience from an advertised analgesic is far more complicated than just a matter of chemistry.

In a fascinating study, two British researchers proved that psychological factors contribute enormously to the relief of pain. They found that headache pain was often substantially reduced even when people were given an unimpressive-looking and inactive placebo—the medical word for inert potions and pills. A placebo made to resemble a popular brand-name product was quite a bit more effective, but the clear winner was the active medication in its brand-name guise. According to the investigators, the aspirin in the brand-name pain remedy accounted for about two thirds of the pain relief experienced, but as much as one third of the benefit could be attributed to the brand name on the tablet. As the investigators pointed out, "Patients' expectations that medication will help them increases the likelihood of response. . . . Such expectations and beliefs are influenced by non-active aspects of the medications, such as color, taste, dosage, and size of tablets."[14]

The finding that 40 percent of the people receiving the ordinary-looking tablet with no active ingredients in it felt better is not as amazing as it may seem. Study after study has demonstrated that a very large percentage of the people given placebos get relief from what ails them. Aches and pains, itches and twitches, warts, ulcers, headaches—you name it, placebos cure it.

Are water and sugar pills drugs? By the technical definition, no. Yet they can be incredibly effective, sometimes as good as "the real thing" if the people using them expect them to work. If this sounds as implausible and miraculous as the claims of some faith healers, it may be that indeed they are all working the same way—acting not on the body, but on the mind, which controls to a large extent how we feel. A distinguished dermatologist, A. M. Kligman, once took a group of people who were sensitive to poison ivy and gave them what they thought was an immunizing drug. It was in fact a "remedy" with absolutely no active ingredients, but when these folks were reexposed to the offending plant, lo! A miracle, or something. Some suddenly found themselves immune.[15]

Or consider the case of the disappearing peritendonitis, a painful inflammatory disorder of the shoulder, hip, and Achilles tendon. Patients with peritendonitis often show good recovery when treated with ultrasonic therapy, so researcher H. J. Flax "treated" some people for the problem with an ultrasonic machine that wasn't plugged in. They thought they were being treated, though they were actually being given the business. Not that it mattered, because these patients had a definite decrease in the amount of calcification and pain.

It's only in the last few years that we've discovered that the brain can manufacture its own drugs, the endorphins and enkephalins, for pain control. Most researchers assume this is just the tip of the chemical iceberg. In years to come, science may discover and learn how to duplicate some of the substances the body manufactures to stay healthy, or even heal itself from illness or injury. The hottest drug research going these days revolves around biotechnology and natural substances like interferon, interleukin II, and epidermal growth factor. These are the "drugs" of the future that someday could help us understand how to speed wound healing or cure cancer.

These findings may help us figure out how sugar pills and unplugged machines make us feel better. The power of the placebo is awesome, and though we may never unlock all its secrets, researchers are learning that they may discover a lot more about making drugs by looking inside instead of outside the body. In a society that's been brought up on "better answers through chemistry," it may be time to stop asking "What is a drug?" and instead start asking, "How can we learn how to help the body heal itself?"

## The Myth of Organic Purity

Any mention of natural healing power brings to mind the term *organic.* Everyone, it seems, is looking for safe and simple solutions to what ails them. And nowhere is this more apparent than in the trusty twosome, *natural and organic,* which appears on many a box and label and has become almost an article of faith for some people.

Just what does the word *organic* mean, and what is all the fuss about? The word *organic* has almost come to take on a life of its own, partially in response to legitimate concern about unneeded, unwanted chemicals. Organic, just like drug, has a strict definition and then some common-use definitions. In a strict sense, something is organic if it contains a certain chemical structure involving the element carbon. Since anything that is or has been alive qualifies, all plants and animals are organic.

Then what is organic food, as widely advertised and sold? In that sense, *organic* is a marketing term that has come to mean that the meat or vegetable or whatever is being hawked contains no chemical additives. Organic Vitamin C, for example, is presumably derived from a virginal plant source while other Vitamin C has been synthesized in a lab. The chemical structure is identical. If one wants straight Vitamin C, spending additional money for the organic variety doesn't make sense.

To quote Dr. Linus Pauling: "So-called synthetic ascorbic acid is natural ascorbic acid, identical with Vitamin C in oranges and other foods. There is no advantage whatever to buying 'all natural Vitamin C,' 'Wild Rose Hip Super Vitamin C,' 'Acerola Berries Vitamin C,' or similar preparations."[16]

Nonetheless, when it comes to food, nobody sets out to buy a free load of pesticide, fumigant, preservative, coloring agent, artificial flavor, or emulsifier. Most people suspect, probably quite rightly, that a lot of those chemicals could be bad for human beings as well as bugs, molds, and bacteria. If buying organic food means you're not getting those nasty chemicals, most people would prefer it, all things being equal. But there are two problems: first, the label "organic" doesn't guarantee anything, and second, all things aren't equal—especially when it comes to price.

The health-food market is now a billion-dollar-a-year industry, and a lot of evidence says much of that money is being wasted by people who think they're paying a premium to obtain food that's either purer or more nutritious, shampoo that's better, or vitamins that will make them live longer. In many cases they're not getting what they pay for. There is no evidence that organic foods have a greater variety or higher quantity of nutrients than their ordinary supermarket equivalents.

Of course, organic food is supposed to be raised without nasty additives, thus justifying its inevitably higher price. Yet various consumer agencies have found that as much as 50 percent of the food labeled "organic" is identical in every respect—including the amount of pesticide residue it contains—to the average supermarket stuff. Some rip-off health-food stores simply buy the same food from the same suppliers, mark it 80 percent to 120 percent higher than the local market, label it "organic," and laugh all the way to the bank.[17]

Now don't get me wrong. I enjoy the succulent fruit and delectable vegetables that come from my local "natural food" market as much as anyone I know. When the product is what it claims to be, you're certainly better off from a health point of view buying things that aren't covered, impregnated, or saturated with strong chemicals. The difficulty lies in finding out whether what you're buying is truly worth the price. When possible, grow your own; otherwise find a grocer you can trust. And as far as all those "natural and organic" snack foods, shampoos, and skin creams are concerned, don't pay extra for a slogan that has virtually no meaning.

## How to Be a Wise Drug Consumer

Let's face it, we all take drugs in one guise or another. Some people may use a brand-name product, while others go for a natural and organic herbal tonic. No matter what's on the label, everyone needs an opportunity to make an informed decision about the drugs they purchase and use. The purpose of this book is to provide information that can make a dramatic difference in your consumer role. No longer will you be the passive recipient of a hastily scrawled prescription for something you don't know anything about, may not need, and perhaps don't want.

Most people seem to feel prescription drugs are safe, and they think they're safe just because the doctor prescribed them. In a 1972 study by the Food and Drug Administration, 86 percent of the people rated prescription drugs as "safe," and the most frequently cited reason for feeling that way was "doctor reliability."[18]

The truth is, doctors often don't have the time to keep track of all the reported difficulties with the many drugs they prescribe. Far too often their information comes not from medical journals but from drug company "detail men"—salespeople who visit the office, peddling their wares, and whose presentation of "facts" about their products usually emphasizes the benefits with much less attention paid to risks. Doctors are supposed to read more detailed information about the drug before prescribing, but in many cases they don't. That leaves you with responsibility for your own welfare and suggests that a lot less blind faith might be in order.

After finishing this book you will be, I hope, a more aware partner in the health-care relationship. You should also be less easily manipulated by the annoyingly pervasive and persistent barrage of advertising for over-the-counter remedies whose ingredients range from the inert to the dangerous. In the following chapters we'll be providing the information and tools you need to sort the good from the bad, the helpful from the hurtful, the economical from the economically wasteful.

In many cases we'll be telling you about prescription and nonprescription drugs that either don't do what they oughta, or do their job only at considerable risk to you. We'll suggest some ways to assess the usefulness of various drugs, sort out when you do and don't need some of the riskier ones, and point out the economic considerations that can come into play when considering whether or not a particular drug is the right one for you at a given time.

Many of these risk and economic considerations aren't carefully or fully taken into account by physicians when they blithely write out a prescription for the latest "wonder drug." What they ought to wonder about is whether you can afford it, whether it exposes you to risks too great for the benefits you'll be getting, and whether you wouldn't in fact be better off with something less costly or less potent at least as a first step in assisting your body to use its extraordinary capability to heal itself. Until the day arrives when we can cure ourselves more with our minds than with drug therapy, we must learn how drugs work and how we can protect ourselves from their potential dangers.

# References

1. "FDA Plans Action on 'Sobriety Products.'" *Los Angeles Times,* Jul. 21, 1983, p. 5.

2. "Sobriety Aids Promise FDA Cooperation." *Advertising Age,* Oct. 25, 1982, p. 20.

3. "FDA Moves to Cut Firms Off on Drunkenness Pill." *Washington Drug Letter,* Jul. 25, 1983, p. 5.

4. Food and Drug Act. 21 USC Section 201(g)(1).

5. Carlson, G. L., et. al. "A Bean Alpha-Amylase Inhibitor Formulation (Starch Blocker) Is Ineffective in Man." *Science* (219):393–395, 1983.

6. Li, B., and Ulysses, K. "Starch Blockers." *N. Engl. J. Med.* 308:902, 1983.

7. Graham, David, et al. "Gastric Adaptation Occurs with Aspirin Administration in Man." *Dig. Dis. and Sci.* 28(1):1–6, 1983.

8. Wilson, C. W. M. "Vitamin C: Tissue Saturation, Metabolism and Desaturation." *Practitioner* 212:481, 1974.

9. Sahud, M. A., and Cohen, R. J. "Effect of Aspirin Ingestion on Ascorbic Acid Levels in Rheumatoid Arthritis." *Lancet* 1:937, 1971.

10. Loh, H. S., et al. "The Effects of Aspirin on the Metabolic Availability of Ascorbic Acid in Human Beings." *J. Clin. Pharmacol.* 13:480, 1973.

11. Loh, H. S., and Wilson, C. W. M. "The Interactions of Aspirin and Ascorbic Acid in Normal Men." *J. Clin. Pharmacol.* 15:36, 1973.

12. Russel, R. I., et al. "Ascorbic-Acid Levels in Leucocytes of Patients with Gastrointestinal Haemorrhage." *Lancet* 2:603, 1968.

13. Moertel, C. G., et al. "A Comparative Evaluation of Marketed Analgesic Drugs." *N. Engl. J. Med.* 286:813–815, 1972.

14. Branthwaite, A., and Cooper, P. "Analgesic Effects of Branding in Treatment of Headaches." *Br. Med. J.* 282:1576–1578, 1981.

15. Kligman, A. M. "Hyposensitization against Rhus Dermatitis." *Arch. Derm.* 78:47, 1958.

16. Pauling, Linus. *Vitamin C and the Common Cold.* New York: Bantam Books, 1971, p. 88.

17. Jukes, Thomas H. "The Organic Food Myth." *JAMA* 230(2):-276–277, 1974.

18. Grahn, Joyce L. "Relationship of Consumers' Perceptions of Drugs to Drug Use." *Public Health Reports* 98(1):85–90, 1983.

# 3

# Drug Safety and Effectiveness: There Are No Safe Drugs, Only Safe Patients

*Side-effect horror stories: Selacryn, Oraflex, and Zomax • The weakest link in the chain: postmarketing surveillance • The safety and danger of aspirin • The safety and danger of Indocin • The safety and danger of Inderal • Drug Safety: Protect the bod—it's the only one you've got • Sexual side effects: Doctors' lips are sealed • Buying and storing drugs wisely • Taking your medicine: Harder than you think • DES: A tragedy that never should have happened • Getting rid of ineffective drugs • Are the benefits worth the risks?*

Now that you know what a drug is, you might as well know what it isn't. It isn't necessarily safe for everyone, and it isn't guaranteed completely effective. If you find that a bit surprising, don't feel lonely. Most people think that FDA approval is drugdom's version of the Good Housekeeping Seal of Approval. But it isn't that simple.

Let's suppose, for a moment, that the Consumer Product Safety Commission tested one thousand toasters of a certain manufacturer. While nine hundred of them worked fine, the other one hundred caused a variety of problems ranging from minor cases of burned toast to life-threatening electrical shocks. There would be righteous indignation and no Seal of Approval for such a bread burner. Yet drugs are often approved with a 10 percent incidence of adverse effects, and in some cases the numbers go much higher. Even death (which we can think of as the ultimate adverse effect) is a risk that the FDA considers acceptable for a surprisingly large number of drugs.

Perhaps even more shocking, everybody but the consumer already has this information. The drug manufacturers know that even the best of their medicines always cause problems for at least some people; the FDA knows it; and your doctor knows it. The hitch is, the FDA talks to the drug companies; the drug companies talk to the doctor; and more often than not, the doctor doesn't talk to you. So guess who's left holding the bag full of problems? Take one and pass it on.

How can the FDA go on approving drugs that cause problems or don't work? Elementary, my dear Watson: The feds understand, as you must too, that people are different. What cures Alfred can make Bertha sicker than a dog, and Charlotte may take the same drug and get neither sick nor better. Safety and effectiveness are the two factors being weighed as a drug moves from being a gleam in someone's test tube to being an FDA-approved product. When the scale tips in favor of the patients, the drug does get approved, but it can be a long way from being either perfectly safe or perfectly effective.

I remember writing a newspaper column once about DMSO (dimethyl sulfoxide) and why the FDA had not yet approved this chemical for use in treating arthritis. Within days, my mailbox was stuffed with letters from readers. Some were outraged that the drug wasn't legal and insisted it worked wonders for their aching joints. Others were equally adamant that DMSO was a rip-off and hadn't done a thing for their arthritis. The official jury is still out on DMSO, but this example illustrates just how hard it can be to decide whether something works well enough to merit marketing.

The law says that drugs must be "safe and effective." Nice and simple, right? Wrong! Nothing could be more complex. The Food and Drug Administration has the ultimate responsibility for deciding what those words really mean with respect to the medicines we take, but it's not a precise science. Nowhere does it say that in order to be licensed a drug must do what its manufacturer says it does 100 percent of the time. Even aspirin won't take away everyone's headache all the time. And nowhere does it say a medication can't cause problems for more than 5 percent of the people taking it. There are no numbers, no absolute standards to which any drug must adhere. The FDA has to balance risks and benefits to determine which little druggie goes to market and which little druggie stays home.

It wasn't always that way. Before the turn of the century, just about anybody could sell anything, and just about everybody did. The Federal Pure Food and Drug Act went into effect in 1906, but it didn't say anything about safety or effectiveness. It did, however, require that the ineffective or possibly dangerous drug you were getting was pure. Sometimes progress works in mysterious ways.

It was not until the horrifying revelation of birth defects associated with thalidomide in the early 1960s that the Harris-Kefauver Amendment to the Food and Drug Act finally demanded both safety and effectiveness as prerequisites for marketing. Once that amendment passed, manufacturers were supposed to prove through extensive testing that their new drugs (a) worked, and (b) would not create side effects worse than the original condition. As reassuring as that may sound, believe me when I tell you that the FDA's risk/benefit equation does not shield you completely from danger. It offers some protection, but it's certainly no guarantee.

For one thing, some kinds of side effects, even serious ones, don't always show up while the drug is being tested. Back in 1980, a rather remarkable blood-pressure medication called **Selacryn** (ticrynafen) had to be yanked off the market only seven months after it had been introduced. At first, this drug had seemed to be a godsend for those suffering from both gout and hypertension (high blood pressure). Unlike most hypertension medicines, which raise uric-acid levels and make gout worse, **Selacryn** actually *lowered* uric-acid levels along with the blood pressure. It had only one serious flaw, as it turned out, but that one was horrible indeed. Some people developed liver damage and died while taking this wonderful new drug.

This lethal side effect was pretty rare, affecting about one person in five thousand. None of the four thousand people who had taken **Selacryn** during its testing stages reportedly had come down with liver problems due to the drug. But with a few hundred thousand patients swallowing it, the "rare" reaction became *unacceptably common*.

Unfortunately, this kind of story is becoming far too familiar. Over the past several years, such promising drugs as **Oraflex** (benoxaprofen) for arthritis and **Zomax** (zomepirac) for pain have given some people unexpected and nasty reactions. **Oraflex** was pulled off the market soon after it had been introduced—but not soon enough to prevent scores of deaths. **Zomax** was on the market almost two years before the manufacturer removed it because of severe allergic reactions. You see, despite the rigorous testing new medicines are supposed to undergo before the FDA will give them the green light, almost anyone taking a drug within the first year or two of its introduction is actually serving as an unpaid, often unwitting, guinea pig.

Now please don't get me wrong. The folks at the FDA are not setting you up for a fall. These people are conscientious in their attempts to protect the public, but the drug-approval process does have limitations. When the wizards who work in top-secret drug company labs think they have come up with some exciting new compound, the manufacturer submits to the FDA a proposal setting forth the basis for the claim, what's known about the chemistry of the drug, its relationship to other drugs of

similar chemistry, and the proposed screening process by which
the company will meet its legal obligation to prove that the drug
is "safe and effective."

The FDA then approves a carefully controlled series of tests,
starting with animals, proceeding to small groups of human
volunteers, and then finally using a larger group of patients. The
drug company must document safety and effectiveness at each
step before being allowed to proceed to the next one.

But even when the whole process is finished, the drug will have
been taken by a relative handful of people—anywhere from a few
hundred to a couple of thousand. Such a small sample cannot
possibly reflect accurately the population that will eventually be
using the medicine. In fact, the way the process is currently set
up, the drug probably won't be tested at all on people who are
very young, very old, or who have underlying ailments. In other
words, experimental subjects are usually the least likely to have
drug reactions of any kind.

As a result, when a drug is first released, it is essentially still
being tested for safety and effectiveness! Think about the consequences of taking a medication when it first comes on the market. If you're over sixty, suffer from chronic illnesses, or take
other medications, it's entirely possible that nobody like you has
ever swallowed the drug before! In effect, you're taking part in
an uncompleted experiment.

Sometimes the experiment doesn't turn out well. That was
what happened with **Selacryn, Oraflex,** and **Zomax.** In the testing phase, these drugs breezed through with relatively minor side
effects. It took more than fifteen million people before anyone
realized **Zomax** was causing cases of severe allergic reactions.
The problems with **Oraflex** and **Selacryn** appeared more
quickly. Within months of being marketed, the cases began to
pile up. Cases of liver failure due to **Selacryn**; cases of liver and
kidney problems associated with **Oraflex**; cases with death cer-
tificates attached for all three.

Substantial numbers of patients had taken each of these medicines before the sheer weight of statistical probability brought
the difficulties to light. So you can see there's a lot riding on the

system by which drugs are tracked *after* approval. Let's take a look and see how that's done.

## The Weakest Link in the Chain

Once a drug makes it over the FDA hurdle, is approved, and is being taken by hundreds of thousands (if not millions) of people, it enters the murky world of "postmarketing surveillance." That means everyone is supposed to be keeping an eagle eye out for unexpected or unusually severe reactions. Drug companies are required to report any such problems to the FDA; doctors and consumers are also encouraged to do so.

That's the way it's supposed to work, but far too often the system breaks down. Take **Oraflex**, for example. Company officials knew that twenty-nine people had died while taking this arthritis medicine in Europe before it was even marketed in the United States. They failed to report these deaths to the FDA, on the grounds that they were an "expected reaction to a drug of that kind."[1]

If pharmaceutical companies have a hard time deciding what is and what isn't an expected side effect, think how hard it must be for doctors and patients. Theoretically, the doctor prescribing the drug is supposed to pore over all the labeling information cleared by the FDA and supplied by the drug company, and then relay the pertinent parts to the ailing patient.

But in the real world quite the opposite often takes place. Doctors usually try to put the drugs they prescribe in the best possible light. They may feel that most of the side effects are relatively infrequent and that telling you about them will just tend to plant a seed of suggestion that could sprout into an annoying phone call in the middle of the night asking if you're throwing up from the drug rather than the two anchovy pizzas you had for dinner.

Then again, the doctor may not know what all the side effects and interactions are. Think about this. When was the last time you saw a doctor look in a book to check on the adverse reactions

and interactions while prescribing a drug? You've probably
never seen it happen, any more than you've seen the pilot of a
747 reading the operating handbook right before takeoff.

The 747 pilot, however, *does* use a checklist during every
phase of the flight, to make certain that no routine-but-critical
step has been omitted. Your doctor, on the other hand, probably
attempts the impossible feat of remembering everything there is
to know about dozens or even hundreds of drugs he prescribes
regularly. Even if the busy doctor did once take the time to
carefully and critically read the detailed labeling with all the
warnings on interactions and side effects, is it reasonable to
expect him to remember *everything* weeks or months later?

But perhaps you are fortunate enough to have a fantastic
physician. She reads the official package insert carefully, keeps
up with the latest medical literature, and communicates *all* the
important drug information you need to know in language that
is easy to understand. Great, but even in this best of all possible
worlds, will she report an adverse reaction to the FDA that is
unusual or unexpected? Maybe, but the chances are slim to nil.
Without that critical information, postmarketing surveillance is
a joke.

As you may suspect by now, adverse reactions aren't particularly unusual. As many as six million people suffer adverse drug
reactions (ADRs) every year.[2] And one authority says, "We can
conjecture the range of 60,000 to 140,000 ADR deaths to be
probably extremely conservative."[3] Now, an ADR can be nothing more than a slight rash or an upset tummy, but look at those
numbers again. You can die from the medicine that was supposed to make you better, and every year thousands of people do
just that.

If that's just a bit frightening, maybe it will jolt you into taking
your medicine—and the way it's prescribed—a bit more seriously. I repeat: **THERE ARE NO ABSOLUTELY SAFE
DRUGS!** There can only be safe patients: those who are concerned and informed enough to ask the right questions about
what they're being given, why they're taking it, and what the
known adverse effects are.

## The Safety and Danger of Aspirin

It's important not to take *any* drug for granted. Even one that seems completely safe can sometimes be dangerous, the more so because you don't expect any trouble. That's certainly the case with plain old aspirin. The adage about familiarity breeding contempt often applies to aspirin (acetylsalicylic acid). Many people don't even consider the lowly aspirin tablet a drug. But it is one, perhaps even the closest thing to a true wonder drug that we have. Aspirin is consumed in enormous quantities that may range as high as twenty thousand tons per year in the United States alone.[4] A lot of people think that because aspirin is available without a prescription, it must not be very strong, and that it's therefore totally safe. They're wrong on both counts.

Aspirin is useful for a lot of what ails you. Most of life's pains are relatively minor, and aspirin has the ability to soothe a lot of them, from minor aches to fever and the inflammation of arthritis. Aspirin is now being used experimentally as a "blood thinner" to try to prevent strokes and heart attacks. There is even hope it may be useful in slowing or halting the progression of cataracts.

Aspirin is the reference standard against which newer painkillers and anti-inflammatory drugs are tested, because it reduces pain as well as any nonnarcotic drug and helps arthritis as much as most prescription medications do. Even things many of us tend to think are much stronger, such as **Darvon** (propoxyphene) or **Motrin** (ibuprofen), for example, don't really work any better than plain aspirin.

Because it has been around so long, aspirin has been thoroughly studied. We know a lot about how, why, and where it works in the body, although until fairly recently the mechanism by which aspirin relieved pain was a mystery. There has never been any doubt that it works. But like other drugs, it also has its share of side effects.

So far I've used the term "adverse drug reaction" to mean the side effects from a normal dose of a drug. Now it's time to look at another "downside": toxicity. Toxic effects are those resulting from an overdose of a drug, whether accidental or otherwise. What had been intended as a cure becomes a poison, with results that range from mildly uncomfortable to life-threatening.

Aspirin's toxic effects are well known, though little publicized. The **Anacin** and **Bufferin** ads don't mention the more than ten thousand cases of serious aspirin overdose occurring in this country every year, nor do they point out that many of the victims will be children.[5] As little as 10 grams (about twenty "extra-strength" tablets, or about thirty regular aspirin) have been fatal in adults, and it takes far less in a child. At least for children, childproof caps help decrease the chances of an accidental poisoning.

Taking too much aspirin over a longer period of time can lead to a more chronic condition known as salicylism. This is characterized by ringing in the ears (tinnitus), headache, dizziness, vision and hearing problems, and mental confusion. Aspirin is definitely a dangerous drug when overused.

Even when taken in normal doses, aspirin can have many adverse effects. By now almost everyone has heard that "the pain reliever most recommended by doctors" can produce stomach upset that ranges from simple heartburn all the way up to nausea and vomiting. These symptoms occur in about 5 percent of all people taking regular doses of aspirin.

Less well known is the fact that everyone who swallows regular aspirin suffers some bleeding. Between 40 percent and 70 percent of those taking a dose of aspirin will lose as much as a teaspoonful of blood a day. This is usually no big deal, but if it continues over a long period of time, iron-deficiency anemia may result.

People really get into trouble when they have a few drinks and then pop some aspirin with the idea of heading off a hangover. NO GOOD! Alcohol makes the stomach incredibly sensitive to aspirin, and the combination will make the stomach bleed and bleed and bleed. ALWAYS take aspirin with a full glass of water or milk, or with some food. Do NOT take aspirin if you have any sort of ulcer, or have had ulcers in the past.

Aspirin decreases your blood's ability to clot normally. This isn't a problem with a small cut, but it can be dangerous in other circumstances. Women who have taken aspirin during the last few weeks of a pregnancy may bleed more when giving birth, and their babies may also be at risk. If you go in for surgery, you will probably be advised not to take any aspirin for at least a week prior to the operation.

While relatively rare, severe bleeding is possible after taking aspirin; it's estimated that fifteen out of every one hundred thousand hospital admissions are due to aspirin-induced hemorrhage. People who are taking anticoagulants ("blood thinners") are at much higher risk of having a serious hemorrhage, as are hemophiliacs. A black, tarry stool is a serious sign of such hemorrhaging and requires immediate medical attention.

If you have gout, small doses of aspirin can make your problem worse. Uric acid, which is the culprit for gout patients, normally exits via the hardworking kidneys. Aspirin, however, can interfere with this elimination and thus precipitate a gout attack. (Paradoxically, large doses of aspirin may do just the opposite.)

And then there's aspirin allergy. Very few people have ever heard of this problem, but for those who are susceptible it can be serious indeed. Asthmatics and people who suffer from hives are at special risk; 20 percent are likely to be allergic to aspirin. Symptoms can range from an itchy skin rash to shortness of breath, severe asthma, or life-threatening shock. What is especially insidious about this reaction is that it can be delayed several hours. This often makes it hard for an asthmatic to know if an attack just occurred out of the blue or was a drug side effect.

Aspirin-sensitive people are at increased risk of being allergic to certain other drugs such as **Butazolidin** (phenylbutazone), **Clinoril** (sulindac), **Feldene** (piroxicam), **Indocin** (indomethacin), **Motrin** (ibuprofen), **Nalfon** (fenoprofen), **Naprosyn** (naproxen), or **Tolectin** (tolmetin). They are also often sensitive to a yellow food dye called tartrazine, known as FD&C Yellow #5, which is used in many types of foods and even some drugs.

Since many prescription and over-the-counter products contain aspirin or related compounds (salicylates), people with aspirin sensitivity must read labels carefully and be constantly vigilant. This is especially true, since manufacturers rarely mention in their ads what their wonderful extra-strength pain reliever really is. Salicylates crop up in drugs you might never think of, such as indigestion aids, cold remedies, and menstrual medications. Here is just a partial list: **Alka-Seltzer, Anacin, Arthritis Pain Formula, Ascriptin, Aspergum, BC Powder, Bufferin, Cama, Congesprin, Cope, Coricidin, Doan's Pills, Duradyne, Empirin, Excedrin, Goody's Headache Powder, Midol, Pepto-Bismol, Sine-Off, Triaminicin,** and **Vanquish.**

By now you might be getting the mistaken impression that I am down on aspirin. No way. I *still* believe that aspirin is about as close to a wonder drug as anything we have. Not only is it an excellent pain reliever, but as we've mentioned, it seems to be extraordinarily effective for preventing heart attacks and strokes. The point is that we must all be aware that every drug, even good old over-the-counter aspirin, can be dangerous for some people.

## The Safety and Danger of Indocin

If you didn't know it before, you should now be convinced that almost any medication that can help also has the potential for doing some harm. But even that awareness wouldn't have helped in the "good old days" (only a few decades ago) when drug information was not entrusted to consumers. Finding out about side effects was almost impossible. Over-the-counter drugs didn't even list their ingredients (trade secret, don't you know?), and prescription medicines were obtained only after the patient carried a mysterious piece of paper bearing an illegibly written message in a Latin code from the doctor to the pharmacist.

All that has changed. Today all nonprescription drugs must list ingredients and most come equipped with labeled warnings, precautions, and drug-interaction information. In fact, it is often easier for a concerned consumer to find out about the side effects of over-the-counter medications than of the pills the doctor prescribes.

Now you would think it would be just the other way around. After all, prescription drugs are theoretically more potent and hazardous than the OTC drugs you can buy right off the shelf. What's more, to get a prescription medication, the consumer has to go through two health professionals, the doctor and the pharmacist. Shouldn't that mean information about side effects and other problems will be dispensed along with the drug?

It should, of course, since that is part of the rationale for restricting some drugs to prescription-only status. Unfortunately, the system breaks down far more often than the pros like to admit. There are still many physicians who don't take the time to communicate with their patients, and pharmacists are often too busy counting, pouring, licking, and sticking to take time to talk. But these professionals do have the information you need, because the FDA tells manufacturers what information must go into the Physician Package Insert. This official labeling language must accompany all ads in medical journals, and it also comes to the pharmacist with every bottle of medication.

Now, this label is not one you're likely to see. It's almost always removed before the drug is dispensed to the consumer. Besides, it's written in medical jargon that is not easy for most of us to understand. It is, however, one of the ways manufacturers talk to doctors. Another way is through the *Physicians' Desk Reference,* or *PDR.* This prescriber's "bible" is essentially a collection of these inserts, written by the drug manufacturers and their lawyers, and approved by the FDA. In a sense it is paid advertising; drug companies must spend a lot of cold hard cash to get their drugs into the *PDR,* which is then given away free to doctors.

Let's see what it says about **Indocin** (indomethacin), a drug that is very widely prescribed for relieving the pain and inflammation of some kinds of arthritis. Here's what Merck Sharp & Dohme, the manufacturer, tells physicians about **Indocin** in the *PDR:*

**INDOCIN cannot be considered a simple analgesic and should not be used in conditions other than those recom-**

mended . . . INDOCIN has been shown to be an effective
anti-inflammatory agent, appropriate for long-term use in
rheumatoid arthritis, ankylosing spondylitis, and osteoar-
thritis. INDOCIN affords relief of symptoms; it does not
alter the progressive course of the underlying disease.

This means that Indocin does not cure or reverse the damage
caused by the arthritis, but only provides relief from the pain and
swelling. Still, if you or someone in your family suffers from
rheumatoid arthritis, you know that relief from the symptoms is
most welcome! Don't stop there, though; keep reading over the
doctor's shoulder:

Because of the variability of the potential of INDOCIN to
cause adverse reactions in the individual patient, the following are strongly recommended:

1. The lowest possible effective dose for the individual patient should be prescribed. Increased dosage tends to increase adverse effects . . . without corresponding increase
in clinical benefits.

2. . . . As advancing years appear to increase the possibility
of adverse reactions, INDOCIN should be used with
greater care in the aged.

The *PDR* continues in the same vein:

If minor adverse effects develop as the dose is increased,
reduce the dosage rapidly to a tolerated dose and OB-
SERVE THE PATIENT CLOSELY. If serious adverse
reactions occur, STOP THE DRUG. After the acute phase
of the disease is under control, an attempt to reduce the
daily dose should be made repeatedly until the patient is
receiving the smallest effective dose or the drug is discontinued. Careful instruction to, and observation of, the individual patient are essential to the prevention of serious,
irreversible, including fatal adverse reactions.

Okay, now that is just the introduction. Next come the special warnings, precautions, and adverse reactions. (The comments in brackets are the author's):

**ADVERSE REACTIONS:**

[These adverse reactions occur in about 3 percent to 9 percent of patients]: nausea (with or without vomiting), dyspepsia (including indigestion, heartburn, and epigastric pain), headache [occurs in over 10 percent of patients taking this drug], and dizziness.

[Reactions occurring in over 1 percent are]: diarrhea, abdominal distress or pain, constipation, vertigo [a whirling sensation], somnolence [sleepiness], depression and fatigue, and tinnitus [a ringing in the ears].

**WARNINGS:**

Single or multiple ulcerations, including perforation and hemorrhage of the esophagus, stomach, duodenum or small intestine, have been reported to occur with INDOCIN. Fatalities have been reported in some instances . . .

Ocular [eye] Effects: corneal deposits and retinal disturbances . . . have been observed in some patients who had received prolonged treatment with INDOCIN. It is advisable to discontinue therapy if such changes are observed. Blurred vision may be a significant symptom . . . Since these changes may be asymptomatic [you might not notice them], ophthalmologic examination at periodic intervals is desirable in patients where therapy is prolonged.

Central Nervous System Effects: INDOCIN may aggravate psychiatric disturbances, epilepsy, and parkinsonism . . . INDOCIN may cause drowsiness; therefore, patients should be cautioned about engaging in activities requiring mental alertness and motor coordination, such as driving a car. INDOCIN may also cause headache. Headache which persists despite dosage reduction requires cessation of therapy with INDOCIN.

    **Gastrointestinal Side Effects: Because of the occur-
rence, and at times severity of gastrointestinal reactions
to INDOCIN, the prescribing physician must be continuously alert for any sign or symptom signalling a possible
gastrointestinal reaction.**

    That's some list! And I didn't even mention the sixty-odd
other side effects that occur in fewer than one patient out of a
hundred. Your doctor won't tell you about those either, you may
bet, since the chances are about 99 to 1 you won't have to worry
about them.

    I don't mean to imply with all this that **Indocin** is a "bad"
drug. It is a potent drug that can be very effective against crip-
pling arthritis. But it *is* a medicine with many other effects,
including some potentially very dangerous ones, and a lot of the
people taking **Indocin**—perhaps as many as half—will have serious problems with it.[6]

    If you take **Indocin**, did your physician warn you to stop
taking it immediately if a headache persists? Did he emphasize
that it must be taken with food, milk, or an antacid to minimize
the stomach upset so often encountered? Did he suggest that you
start with a low dose and gradually increase it until you reach
the recommended level?

    Did your doctor recommend occasional blood tests to discover
anemia, if it develops, in its earliest stages? Did she stress that
you should not drive when you take **Indocin**, because your mental alertness and motor coordination may not be up to par? And
did she urge you to try to get off the drug as soon as the acute
flare-up of your arthritic condition is under control?

    If your doctor left out more than a few of these warnings, he
or she is not following the guidelines set down by the manufacturer and the FDA. It's easy to see how a harried doctor could
be the weak link in the crucial chain of communication about
adverse drug reactions.

    Your doctor also may not have kept up with the medical
literature and consequently might not *know* all the latest adverse-reaction information. The rather frightening truth is that

far too much of what doctors know about the new drugs they prescribe comes from two sources: ads in medical journals, and drug company sales representatives ("detail men"), traveling minstrels who whisk in and out of doctors' offices with their spiels and free samples in hand. Since the sales rep has only moments to pitch his company's line, you can bet he doesn't spend a whole lot of time telling the doctor the real "details" about what Drug X, Y, or Z can do to a patient besides cure him of some disease.

## The Safety and Danger of Inderal

Before we go on to consider physician-patient communication in greater depth, I want to take a detailed look at one more drug so you will realize how much *can* happen, and how little the average patient is usually told.

**Inderal** (propranolol) is one of the most widely prescribed drugs in the world. It is used to treat heart problems, high blood pressure, and even migraines. As you read these words, millions of people will be faithfully following doctors' orders and swallowing their hexagonally shaped pills. Most will have been assured it's just what they need to fix them up. That's what the doctor says to the patient. Wouldn't you like to see what the company making **Inderal** says to the doctor?

Turning again to the *Physicians' Desk Reference,* we'll just peek at some of the things Ayerst Laboratories (and the FDA) thinks your doctor should consider before giving you **Inderal**:

> **Because of the potential for adverse results, treatment should be carefully monitored. The patient should also be reevaluated periodically since the dosage requirement and the need to continue INDERAL may be altered by clinical exacerbations or remissions.**
>
> **There is no simple correlation between dose or plasma level and therapeutic effect, and the dose-sensitivity range as observed in clinical practice is wide.**

Translation: This drug may take a lot of "fiddling" to get the dose right. It's not the sort of medicine a physician can prescribe and walk away from. Do not wait until the next annual checkup to evaluate the dose.

There's more:

**IN PATIENTS WITHOUT A HISTORY OF CARDIAC FAILURE, continued depression of the myocardium [heart muscle] over a period of time can, in some cases, lead to cardiac failure. In rare instances, this has been observed during INDERAL therapy.**

**Inderal** is *not* unusual, nor is it particularly dangerous—at least no more so than the majority of drugs in common use. The kinds of statements reprinted above are, in fact, typical of those accompanying most modern medications. If they sound a bit more ominous than the vague murmurs of assurance the doctor offered with *your* last prescription, then keep reading. We're about to take a look at the warnings on adverse reactions:

**Cardiovascular: bradycardia [slow heartbeat], congestive heart failure; . . . hypotension [low blood pressure]; . . . arterial insufficiency . . .**

  **Central Nervous System: lightheadedness; mental depression manifested by insomnia, lassitude, weakness, fatigue; reversible mental depression progressing to catatonia; visual disturbances; hallucinations; an acute reversible syndrome characterized by disorientation for time and place, short-term memory loss . . .**

  **Gastrointestinal: nausea, vomiting . . . abdominal cramping, diarrhea, constipation . . .**

  **Respiratory: bronchospasm [asthma]**

  **Miscellaneous: reversible alopecia [hair loss] . . .**

That's just a selection from a much longer list—and as I said before, **Inderal** isn't unique in either number or severity of adverse reactions it can create. Perhaps by now you're getting the feeling there's something the doctor didn't tell you about your last prescription? Or perhaps that there's a LOT he or she didn't tell you?

## Drug Safety: Protect the Bod—It's the Only One You've Got

By now we know that there is no such thing as a drug that is perfectly safe, never has any side effects, and always works for everyone. So who's going to make certain that what you get is safe? Ultimately, *you*.

And you'd better be prepared to do your job almost every time you go to the doctor, because a recent study conducted by the National Center for Health Statistics found that drugs were prescribed or dispensed at 62 percent of the office visits.[7] That means almost two times out of every three you visit the doctor, the solution to your problem will involve drugs. Learning to be an aware drug consumer isn't just desirable—it's a matter of life and death.

Drug safety depends on communication; yet in two surveys conducted by the FDA, 70 percent of the people said their doctors don't inform them of precautions for and possible side effects of drugs, and only 2 percent to 4 percent of the people took the initiative and asked questions about their prescriptions.[8]

What are the other 98 percent doing? They're meekly accepting prescriptions that could bring on all kinds of problems, instead of asking fundamental questions like "How do I take this medicine?" or "What are its side effects?" You're going to have to take the responsibility for insisting on getting good information. Only by becoming an impatient patient will you become the safest possible drug consumer.

Few things are as critical in health care as good communication. The working partnership that you should have with your doctor and the rest of the health-care team is as important as all the medications and fancy high-tech equipment they can throw at you, perhaps even more so. In a 1982 commencement address for medical students at George Washington University, Norman Cousins pointed out:

> **Words used by the physician can be gate openers or gate slammers. They can open the way to recovery, or they can make the patient dependent, tremulous, fearful or resistant.**
> **The right words can potentiate a patient, mobilize the will to live, and set the stage for heroic response. The wrong words can produce despair and defeat or impair the usefulness of whatever treatment is prescribed.[9]**

Besides those hard-to-measure benefits that a positive attitude has on the healing process, there are other, more tangible rewards for good communication. If you know what drug you're taking, why you're taking it, and the risks and potential benefits of taking it, you will be more likely to take your medicine when and how you should. Or, in the paternalistic jargon of the medical profession, you will be more "compliant" with your medication program.

(By the way, being noncompliant—not taking your medicine —can put you in the hospital. One study done in Israel showed that almost 3 percent of hospital admissions to a major medical center were due to noncompliance.[10] The authors urged doctors to educate patients better so as to "increase patient participation in the therapeutic process.")

It is your doctor's responsibility to communicate with you about the medicines he or she prescribes. It is absolutely essential that you as the patient and consumer understand the nature of your illness and the consequences of treatment. Dr. Barry Blackwell, writing in the *New England Journal of Medicine*, puts it eloquently:

> **Prescriptions written in illegible Latin abbreviations may serve as a secret shared with the pharmacist but are a poor start to communication with the patient. As has been pointed out, they often do neither and tend instead to cause confu-**

sion and inaccuracies. It is better to write the prescription in plain English and to explain what it means, encouraging the patient to ask questions and make comments on whether the regimen matches his daily activities.[11]

Remember, your physician is providing you with a service. If the doctor treats you with less than total openness and candor, then it's time for a change, even if he or she is the "greatest" doctor in town.

Your pharmacist, too, shares in the responsibility for informing you about medications. A pharmacist should do something for you besides count tablets and type labels. Providing those stickers that read, "Take with Food or Milk" or "Do Not Drink Alcohol While Taking this Medication" is not enough.

The results of a 1979 Schering Drug Company study show that while 74 percent of pharmacists said that they were available to counsel patients on their medications, only 34 percent of their customers said that the pharmacists were easy to approach for information.[12] Only 52 percent of the pharmacists stated that they were available to explain prescriptions. Only 2 percent of pharmacy customers realized the extent of a pharmacist's drug-related training (at least five to six years of college work and up to four years of postgraduate study). Yet even given these dismal statistics, nine out of ten customers said that they respected the judgment of their pharmacist.

You should choose your pharmacist with as much care as you would your physician. He or she should be available to talk with you about any aspect of your medications, help protect you from drug interactions, and help you save money. But no pharmacist I know can read minds. If you have questions, *you* have to ask them.

## Sexual Side Effects: Doctors' Lips Are Sealed

There's one other reason the doctor (or the pharmacist, for that matter) may not give you the straight poop about side effects:

embarrassment. You see, one not-infrequent side effect of many drugs has to do with sexual performance, and many doctors still are as uncomfortable talking about sex as the rest of us.

Here's the story: There are a number of drugs that reduce sexual performance or desire. Both men and women can be affected, although more research attention has been focused on the sexual side effects on men. For men, drug-related problems fall pretty much into three categories: less interest in sex (decreased libido), difficulties in gaining and sustaining an erection (impotence), and inability to ejaculate normally. Women may also suffer from decreased libido and have trouble achieving orgasm.[13, 14]

Sexual function is highly complex and poorly understood, and it is readily affected by expectations, stress, illness, and hormonal imbalance, as well as by drugs. But only in the last several years have researchers begun to appreciate fully the extent to which drugs can contribute to sexual problems. In a study of more than a thousand middle-aged men which found 34 percent of them to be impotent,[15] the most common cause of impotence was the medication these men were taking.

The authors write, ". . . the medications most often implicated were diuretics, antihypertensives, and vasodilators . . . In many instances the patients stopped taking the medications but were hesitant to tell their physician why." These drugs are used to treat high blood pressure or heart problems, and they can be real lifesavers when taken properly. But what man wants a chemical castration?

Sex *is* a sensitive subject, for doctors and patients alike. That's no excuse, however, for everyone to avoid it, especially since the consequences are potentially quite harmful. Problems, like drugs, interact. When a patient, without expecting to, suddenly suffers impotence, the psychological burden can be enormous. It can even lead to chronic depression or marital problems, and all because nobody would talk about sex.

If you're going to be taking a medication that might interfere with your sex life, you DO want to know about it. First, you're entitled to know what to expect, so that the physical problem doesn't become a psychological one. Second, you and your doctor may want to evaluate the need for a particular medication in light of the possible side effects. And third, you should be given the opportunity to discuss the possibilities of alternate medications that might be equal or nearly equal in effectiveness, in case the prescribed medication turns out to have sexual side effects for you.

There are a whole lot of factors that can contribute to sexual problems, and sorting them out isn't easy. For example, many men with untreated hypertension are impotent, but medications for high blood pressure can cause identical problems. Mental depression can be an important source of sexual difficulty, yet antidepressant medication that may banish the depression can inhibit orgasm. It's a vicious cycle that you'll want to keep yourself out of if at all possible, and one way to do that is by being aware of some of the specific offenders so you can raise the subject if the doctor doesn't.

One of the drugs with the worst reputation for affecting sexual performance is guanethidine, prescribed under the brand name **Ismelin**. It's estimated to cause sexual side effects in from 20 percent to 30 percent of the men taking it.[16] It is a very potent and effective drug for people with hard-to-manage high blood pressure. Unfortunately, many men who discover for themselves that their pill prevents ejaculation just stop taking it. This could produce potentially disastrous long-term results. A physician should determine whether or not his patient would tolerate such a side effect should it occur, or whether another drug might be more appropriate. An article in the *British Medical Journal* suggests, "High risk drugs . . . are probably best avoided in younger men . . ."[17] That advice applies equally to sexually active men and women of all ages.

Other antihypertensive medications that can interfere with sexual performance in some people are **Aldomet** (methyldopa), **Serpasil** (reserpine), **Catapres** (clonidine), **Eutonyl** (pargyline), and in higher doses, **Apresoline** (hydralazine). **Inderal** (propranolol) belongs in this list too. It may cause impotence or loss of libido in both sexes.

Diuretics, or "water pills," are also frequently used for high blood pressure. These drugs have a lower, but still real, incidence of adverse sexual side effects. Included among these drugs are: **Hygroton** (chlorthalidone), **HydroDIURIL** (hydrochlorothiazide, or HCTZ), and in higher doses, **Aldactone** (spironolactone).

Drugs affecting the mind rarely do so without affecting the body, and several such products have a well-known tendency to act on sexual function. The common antianxiety drugs ("minor tranquilizers") such as **Valium** (diazepam), **Librium** (chlordiazepoxide), and **Serax** (oxazepam), among others, may cause changes in libido. Common sleep medications may also be added to the list.

**Mellaril** (thioridazine), a "major tranquilizer" or antipsychotic medication, is often blamed for causing ejaculatory problems. Three drugs used to treat psychological depression, known to doctors as "MAO inhibitors," are reported to cause impotence. They are **Nardil** (phenelzine), **Marplan** (isocarboxazid), and **Parnate** (tranylcypromine).

Some antiparkinsonism drugs such as **Cogentin** (benztropine) and **Artane** (trihexyphenidyl) affect male sexuality fairly commonly. However, there are scattered reports that one antiparkinsonism drug, **Larodopa** (levodopa or L-dopa), might actually increase male libido. Researchers are still arguing over whether this is due to the psychological benefit of symptomatic relief or to some physiological aphrodisiac effect.

**Tagamet** (cimetidine), a very popular ulcer medication, is associated with adverse sexual side effects, including impotence and enlarged breasts in men, when it is taken in very high doses. Even birth-control pills may have a dampening effect on female libido. And, of course, drugs of abuse, including alcohol, can interfere with sexual performance.

This is far from being a complete list of drugs with sexual side effects. In fact, a complete list would probably include almost every drug at one time or another. Keep in mind that people are highly variable in their responses to drugs. While one drug that frequently causes sexual problems might cause you no anguish, another one *not* commonly thought of as having sexual consequences could give you trouble.

## Buying and Storing Drugs Wisely

The person who fills your prescription will be a licensed pharmacist—someone with years of training devoted entirely to drugs. Your pharmacist has a certain accountability when it comes to filling the prescription. Taking pills out of a big bottle and putting them into a little one isn't enough, nor does the responsibility end with typing your name and address on the label. It's part of the pharmacist's job to see that you know what you're taking, how and when it should be taken, and what it does and doesn't mix with.

Let's start with the name of the medication. The pharmacist should put this on the container. There is no circumstance under which you shouldn't be told what you're getting, and there are a lot of reasons why you ought to know. This information could become a matter of life and death.

Another important bit of data that should be on the label is the medicine's expiration date. When your pharmacist receives a shipment of drugs, it always has an expiration date stamped on it. When you buy most nonprescription drugs off the shelf, they too have the expiration date on the package. This is because of a federal Food and Drug Administration ruling in 1971, which said that all drugs subject to deterioration had to meet appropriate standards and "at the time of use, the label of all such drugs shall have suitable expiration dates which relate to stability tests performed on the product."

What does this date mean? Well, most drugs are chemically complex substances that can deteriorate over time. When factors such as light, heat, and humidity all gang up, they speed the downhill slide in the usefulness of a drug's active ingredient or ingredients. Manufacturers are required by law to test their drugs under various storage conditions and to determine how long they will last. The expiration date, therefore, is pretty much the manufacturer's guarantee of potency. Of course, the drug doesn't just magically disintegrate on the appointed date. On the other hand, after that time nobody, especially not the manufacturer, is making any promises that you'll be getting what you should out of the pills you're taking.

Speaking of magic, here's some you can do. Want to make a drug disappear? Just store it improperly. The ability of the drug to do its job properly can disappear just as thoroughly as if someone had made the package vanish.

Everyone has read the instructions to "Store in a cool, dry place," just as everyone has ignored those instructions. If you don't believe me, go look in your bathroom cabinet. If you have medicine in there, think about what it's like inside that cabinet each morning as you take your shower and the mirror fogs with steam. A "cool, dry place"? Not exactly.

Most drugs will do just fine if kept in a secure, dark place where the temperature isn't too extreme. But a few need special handling. Insulin, for instance, is best stored in the refrigerator. Suppositories with a cocoa-butter base are designed to melt at body temperature and will also need to sit in the cooler if you live in a hot climate.

Light is detrimental to many drugs or vitamins (especially riboflavin). Some major tranquilizers (**Thorazine, Mellaril,** and the like), certain high-blood-pressure medications (**Hydropres, Rauzide,** reserpine, **Salutensin, Ser-Ap-Es, Serpasil**), and various antibiotics may also be affected. A well-sealed dark-colored or opaque container helps. Since no drugs really benefit from exposure to light, you can play it safe by storing everything where direct sunlight can't wreak havoc.

Doctors have long noted, with some wonder, the highly variable response of patients to nitroglycerin. This drug is used by people whose heart arteries bog down during exertion, bringing on the chest pain known as angina. The mystery was solved with a study[18] showing that the packaging and storage of nitroglycerin were the most important factors in the uneven response. One three-month-old bottle had lost 84 percent of its original oomph. The label, stuffed inside the bottle, had absorbed most of the drug the patient was supposed to get!

The plastic vial in which the tablets were stored also absorbed some of the drug, and the cotton filler plug got a phenomenal one-third of the active ingredient . . . in just one week of storage!

Reformulation of most nitroglycerin tablets has improved the situation, but nitroglycerin still requires careful handling. It should be dispensed in the manufacturer's original glass container and should be kept tightly sealed and in a dry location. NEVER store nitroglycerin in a plastic pill box.

Before leaving the pharmacy, ask if there are any special storage requirements for your prescription. And then take a close look at the directions. If it says, for example, "Take three times daily," are you certain you know what that means?

## Taking Your Medicine: Harder than You Think

You got your medicine safely home—you *didn't* leave it in a hot car all day, did you?—and you're ready to start taking it as prescribed. Those instructions seem so simple: "Take three times daily."

But it's not nearly as easy or as obvious as it appears, and making the wrong choices can muck up either the safety or the effectiveness of the medication. And if you're taking more than one medication, the situation can get *really* complicated.

Just think for a moment about the seemingly simple direction to take some antibiotic on an empty stomach. This means at least one hour before or two hours after eating; otherwise it won't be effective. But often it's easier to give such instructions than to follow them. What about the commuter who has barely enough time to grab a bite of breakfast in the morning before dashing to catch the train to the city? Or the accountant who may have to stay late to catch up on work? Trying to fit in four doses a day, on an empty stomach, can be tough in our on-the-go, eat-and-run lives.

And that's not all. A patient faced with two medicines labeled "take four times daily" would probably gulp them together at six-hour intervals, or as close to that as possible without getting up in the middle of the night. Of course, if the two drugs cancel each other out when consumed at the same time, that could lead to big trouble. But imagine the alternative: How would you take two drugs, four times a day, at evenly spaced intervals on an empty stomach, but not within two hours of each other? This sounds like the sort of problem you'd need a computer to unscramble, and it may grow more difficult with each additional medication. If you ever do get a logical schedule worked out, you might have to change your life-style to fit it.

All this effort is necessary because some medicines interact with food. Tetracycline is a classic example. It's an antibiotic that goes by the brand names **Achromycin V, Panmycin, Sumycin, Tetracyn, Tetrex,** and many others. Just about everybody, at some time or another, gets a prescription for tetracycline. If you are one of the millions who have received this drug, did your doctor *emphasize, stress,* or almost scream that you must NEVER take this drug with milk or any other dairy product, including cheese, yogurt, ice cream, or cream in your coffee? The calcium in milk grabs onto the tetracycline in the stomach and prevents it from ever getting into the bloodstream.

That also goes for magnesium, iron, aluminum, bismuth, and zinc, all commonly found in antacids, vitamin combinations, and other products. You may be sorely tempted to wash your tetracycline down with some **Pepto-Bismol** or **Maalox**, or to take it with a **Tums**, since this antibiotic can upset the stomach. But if you do, your high-priced prescription will be rendered useless. Resist temptation, and take it with nothing but a full glass of plain water.

Actually, a tall glass of water isn't a bad idea for almost all pills, regardless of when you must take them. Many folks try to be stoic, or macho, or something, gulping tablets and capsules down dry or with just a sip of water. There are no awards for this sort of bravery, and no rewards either, since the pill that is not washed down well could become stuck in the esophagus and damage tissue there. Doctors have found this is far more common than was once thought, especially in patients who take their medicines while lying in bed.[19]

One reader wrote to tell us that he couldn't see why anyone would make a fuss about swallowing pills. When he has to take a pill, he pours himself a glass of bourbon and branch, and the pill goes down painlessly! But this novel approach also has its dangers, you may be sure. Any kind of alcohol in combination with aspirin, as we've said, can really mess up the lining of your stomach. Don't do it. And when you are taking certain kinds of medication, especially those in time-release capsules, you should stay away from booze altogether.

Many drugs can make you drowsy, and adding alcohol can multiply this effect dangerously. NEVER drink alcohol if you are using sleeping pills such as **Dalmane** (flurazepam), **Seconal** (secobarbital), **Benadryl** (diphenhydramine, or DPH), and others.

You'd be wise to turn teetotaler, too, when taking antihistamines. Combination cold/allergy products like **Contac, Sudafed Plus, Actifed, Coricidin**, and oodles of others contain antihistamines that can make you quite drowsy, especially if you're elderly or very young. In fact, **Benadryl**, listed above as a sleeping pill, is really an antihistamine, but it made people so sleepy that the companies decided to put this side effect to good use. DPH is now the prime ingredient in the recently reformulated nonprescription sleeping pills like **Nytol with DPH, Sominex Formula 2, Compoz**, and **Sleep-Eze 3**. It's a pretty good sleeping preparation if used wisely—but remember, NO ALCOHOL!

Other medications that can make you drowsy include antidepressants, tranquilizers, some painkillers, and many, many more. These drugs all by themselves may impair your motor coordination and attentiveness, so use extra caution when driving your car or performing any potentially dangerous task. Better yet, find someone else to do it for you, and stay off the sauce.

There are plenty of horror stories about people taking their medicines incorrectly. Each pharmacist has a favorite. For instance, one child came in to the doctor to have an antibiotic capsule, meant only for oral use, removed from his ear. His mom thought that since he had an ear infection, that's where the capsule belonged.

Another gentleman returned to the pharmacist, complaining that his rectal suppositories were causing him pain. It turned out, after careful questioning, that he wasn't removing the sharp foil wrappers. Still another man was heard to comment on how good his medicine tasted—but his prescription was prepared in cocoa-butter suppositories intended for rectal use. These anecdotes may sound amusing, but the consequences are not. Moral: Be ABSOLUTELY sure that you know the correct way to take your medicine. In other words, ASK.

## Effectiveness: A Bitter Pill?

Now you know how to be a careful, cautious, and intelligent patient. If only you could just sit back and trust that the medication you are being so good about taking would really do its job.

Sadly, though, there's disturbing evidence that some doctors prescribe medication based more on their responses to advertising, salesmen, personal experience, and anecdotal tales rather than on a dispassionate reading of the scientific literature. Far too many doctors fail to keep up. They may continue prescribing a certain drug long after it has been found to be harmful or worthless.

Sometimes, after a drug has been available for a long time, it's found to be hazardous, yet prescriptions for it continue rolling in. The results can be most unfortunate, as they were for many diabetics taking certain oral medications.

People who contracted diabetes as adults used to be placed immediately on oral drug therapy. In 1970, a long-term study involving more than eight hundred diabetics shook the medical profession to its foundation. The study demonstrated that two of the most commonly used diabetes drugs, **Orinase** (tolbutamide) and **DBI** (phenformin), put people at increased risk for heart attacks and other problems.[20]

In fact, the results of the study were so dramatic that investigators removed patients from the **Orinase** therapy before the experiment had even run its course. They were unable to justify continuing exposure to a drug which carried twice the risk associated with either insulin or dietary therapy. Many diabetologists have critized this study, and there were flaws in its design. Nevertheless, **DBI, Meltrol**, and all other phenformin-containing diabetes drugs were eventually banned on July 25, 1977, but not before hundreds of people were made seriously ill. Many died needlessly because physicians failed to heed the warning flags in the medical literature. Why? Apparently, because habit and advertising can speak louder than science.

## DES: A Tragedy That Never Should Have Happened

Another drug that didn't do what it was supposed to do was diethylstilbestrol (**DES**). Unfortunately, it *did* cause one of the biggest tragedies in recent medical history.

**DES** was first developed in 1937 as a potent synthetic estrogen, a mimic of one of the body's important female hormones. It was approved by the FDA in 1947 for use in pregnant women, but had been used for research purposes since about 1940 on the theory that miscarriages were often the result of a maternal lack of estrogen. **DES** was given to women considered at "high risk" of miscarriage: those who had had previous miscarriages, difficulty in conceiving, diabetes, or vaginal bleeding.

Sometimes, though, it was prescribed for women in their first pregnancies with no particular risk factors, and later **DES** was given to all sorts of women "just to be on the safe side." The drug was prescribed with the best of intentions, but not with the best of results. This first became evident as early as 1953, when it was reported that **DES** did *not* improve a woman's chances of bearing a healthy child. In spite of that, the drug continued to be widely prescribed.

Between 1966 and 1969, Dr. Arthur L. Herbst at the Massachusetts General Hospital noted eight cases of an extremely rare form of vaginal cancer in young women between the ages of fifteen and twenty-two.[21] The mothers of seven of the eight had received DES; the eighth had received a similar drug. A search of the medical literature revealed only three other cases ever reported in women under thirty-five years of age. DES, a drug that didn't do its job, was doing something else—causing cancer in the offspring of those who took it.

Since that discovery, more than 425 cases of this rare and potentially fatal cancer have been reported. No one now disputes that DES taken by a pregnant woman can have disastrous effects on the unborn child. However, it wasn't until 1971 that the FDA officially warned physicians of the dangers of DES, including a wide variety of problems in both female and male children exposed in their mothers' wombs. One author estimates that 69 percent of all DES daughters have some anatomic deformity.[22]

In addition, the mothers who took DES while they were pregnant are now experiencing a higher rate of breast cancer than would be expected.[23] This has led Health Research Group Director Dr. Sidney Wolfe to state, "DES thus becomes the major environmentally identified cause of breast cancer, and this epidemic of breast cancer will increase as years go by."

Dr. Wolfe estimates that such exposure may increase the risk of breast cancer by 41 percent, perhaps leading to as many as twenty-five thousand additional cases among these women. The risk increases sharply about twenty-two years following the pregnancy during which they took DES.

This should not lead to panic. In both mothers and daughters, cancer is still quite uncommon. Nevertheless, women who were exposed to DES either while they were pregnant or before birth should have screening tests at least once a year and should do self-examination of the breasts every month.

Another legacy of DES is, ironically, an increased risk of miscarriage and problem pregnancies among DES-exposed daughters. So we see this drug actually causes in the daughters the very problems it was meant to prevent in their mothers.

DES is a painful reminder of the fact that there is ALWAYS a risk in taking anything, and that benefits must be clear-cut and demonstrable in order to justify the risk. In the case of **DES**, an estimated two to three million women and their children were exposed to a drug that wasn't effective—and many of those women were exposed long after serious doubts were raised about its efficacy. The price for that error is being paid by people who did not even take the drug themselves.

## Getting Rid of Ineffective Drugs

There ought to be a law. Actually, there is a law. It's just working slowly. As I said back at the beginning of the chapter, the law now requires drugs, prescription and over-the-counter (OTC) alike, to be both safe and effective. But the responsibility for getting unsafe or ineffective products off the market lies with the FDA, and the agency has been slow to fulfill its mission.

In 1966, the FDA began analyzing both prescription and OTC drugs to see if they were "safe and effective." They found that of 512 common ingredients in nonprescription drugs, only 25 percent were both safe and effective for their stated purpose.[24] On the basis of this evidence, the FDA decided it better take a closer look at all OTC drug products.

The OTC Drug Review, begun in 1972, has been a monumental undertaking. Somewhere between two hundred thousand and three hundred thousand OTC medications are available in the country. And that means gobs of green—as much as $9 billion in annual sales. Unfortunately, what the FDA discovered was that much of what is shelled out on nonprescription medicines is wasted. After spending over ten years analyzing more than seven hundred active ingredients in thousands of OTC products, the experts concluded that only about one third were safe and effective for their intended uses. What that means is that millions of Americans swallow nonprescription pills every day that expose them to some risk without offering any potential benefit. And it will be years before the FDA gets all the worthless products off pharmacy shelves.

Some drugs have already been removed from the market as a result of the drug review. Methapyrilene, an ingredient once used in **Nytol, Sleep-Eze, Sominex,** and other OTC sleep aids, was voluntarily recalled in 1979 after scientists found it might cause cancer. Hexachlorophene was removed from nonprescription soaps and baby powders in 1972 after it was associated with brain damage in infants.

All right already. So what if a bunch of over-the-counter drugs won't live up to their claims. Surely the medicines that "really" count—prescription drugs—are doing the job. Not so fast, my friend. This may come as a bit of a shock, but there are hundreds of products prescribed on a daily basis to millions of people that have never been proven effective. While it's true that all medicines marketed since 1962 must pass rigorous tests, there are a whole slew of compounds dating back to the 1940s and 1950s that never received close FDA scrutiny. Many are of dubious value but still get prescribed in humongous quantities.

For a list of these drugs, I refer you to the book *Pills That Don't Work,* by Dr. Sidney Wolfe and the Health Research Group founded by Ralph Nader. While I don't agree with Dr. Wolfe about all the medications included in his book (some definitely *do* work, even though they have not yet received official approval), this is one publication you should add to your library.

## Are the Benefits Worth the Risks?

By now I'm sure you'll agree that taking medication is, or should be, a carefully considered balancing act. Everyone—physician, pharmacist, nurse, and patient—must weigh risks and benefits. Every drug, prescription and OTC, has risks, but so does being sick. Every drug has (or is supposed to have) benefits. When the benefits outweigh the risks, you've got something worth taking. But remember, since you will be the person swallowing that pill or potion, YOU should make the final decision. To make that decision wisely you will need information from your physician and your pharmacist.

According to the American Medical Association, "A physician must obtain the consent of his patient before he can render any form of treatment."[25] Consent in this context means IN-FORMED consent. Now that you know the inside story on "safe and effective," you'll be a more informed consumer of medication. And that should mean a consumer with a *lot* of questions to ask next time the doctor starts to reach for a prescription pad, or the next time you start to reach for a remedy on the shelf of the local pharmacy. Never forget that there is no such thing as a 100-percent-safe drug.

# References

1. Mintz, Morton. "Lilly Official Knew of Deaths before U.S. Approved Drug." *Washington Post,* Jul. 22, 1983, p. A8.

2. "Statement by Patricia Roberts Harris," press release, Dept. of Health and Human Services, Sep. 10, 1980.

3. Tally, Robert B., and Laventurier, Marc F. "Drug-induced Illness." *JAMA* 229:1043, 1974.

4. Flower, R. J.; Moncada, S.; and Vane, J. R.; "Analgesic-Antipyretics and Anti-Inflammatory Agents; Drugs Employed in the Treatment of Gout." In Gilman, A. G.; Goodman, L.S.; and Gilman, A., eds. *The Pharmacological Basis of Therapeutics,* 6th ed. New York: Macmillan Publishing Co., 1980, p. 688.

5. Ibid, p. 695.

6. Davies, D. M. "Epidemiology—Incidence of Adverse Drug Reactions." In Davies, D. M., ed. *Textbook of Adverse Drug Reactions.* Oxford: Oxford University Press, 1977, pp. 3–9.

7. "Psychotropic Drug Study Notes Prescribing Habits." *Medical World News,* Sep. 12, 1983, p. 139.

8. "The Doctor Isn't Talking; the Patient Isn't Asking." *Medical World News,* Sep. 12, 1983, p. 47.

9. Cousins, N. "The Physician as Communicator. *JAMA* 248:587–589, 1982.

10. Levy, M.; Mermelstein, L.; and Hemo, D. "Medical Admissions Due to Noncompliance with Drug Therapy." *Int. J. Clin. Pharm. Ther. Toxicology* 20:600–604, 1982.

11. Blackwell, B. "Drug Therapy Patient Compliance." *N. Engl. J. Med.* 289:249–252, 1973.

12. "Pharmacy/Consumer Prescriptions on Pharmacy Services." *F-D-C Reports* 49 (44):T&G 12–13, 1979.

13. *The Medical Letter on Drugs and Therapeutics.* 25:73–76, 1983.

14. Marks, R. G.; Fuentes, R. J.; and Rosenberg, J. M. "Sexual Side Effects—What to Tell Your Patients, What Not to Say." *RN,* Feb. 1983, pp. 35–41.

15. Slag, M. F., et. al. "Impotence in Medical Clinic Outpatients." *JAMA* 249:1736–1740, 1983.

16. Wartman, Steven A. "Sexual Side Effects of Antihypertensive Drugs." *Postgrad. Med.* 73(2):133–138, 1983.

17. Editorial. "Drugs and Male Sexual Function." *Brit. Med. J.* 6195:883–884, 1969.

18. Shangraw, R. E. "Unstable Nitroglycerin Tablets." *N. Engl. J. Med.* 286:950–951, 1972.

19. Evans, K. T., and Roberts, G. M. "Where Do All the Tablets Go?" *Lancet* 2:1237–1238, 1976.

20. University Group Diabetes Program "A Study of the Effects of Hypoglycemic Agents on Vascular Complications in Patients with Adult-onset Diabetes II. Mortality Results." *Diabetes* 19 (Suppl.):789, 1970.

21. Herbst, A. L.; Ulfelder, H.; and Poskanzer, D. C. "Adenocarcinoma of the Vagina: Association of Maternal Stilbestrol Therapy with Tumor Appearance in Young Women." *N. Engl. J. Med.* 284:878, 1971.

22. Kaufman, R. H., et. al. "Upper Genital Tract Changes Associated with Exposure *in utero* to Diethylstilbestrol." *Am. J. Obstet. Gyn.* 128:51, 1977.

23. Greenberg, E. R., et al. "Breast Cancer in Mothers Given Diethylstilbestrol in Pregnancy." *N. Engl. J. Med.* 311:1393–1398, 1984.

24. Gilbertson, W. E. "The FDA's OTC Drug Review." In *Handbook of Nonprescription Drugs,* 7th ed. Washington, D.C.: American Pharmaceutical Association, 1982, pp. 1–7.

25. Simonaitis, Joseph E. "Photographs of Patients." *JAMA* 229:844, 1974.

# 4

---

# Sexy Trade Secrets
# and Home Remedies

---

*Home remedies: Chicken soup—good
for what ails you • Hiccups • Help for
heartburn • Preventing Chinese-Restaurant Syndrome • Curing Cecil the
Seasick Sea Serpent • Hot Cha-Cha:
Spices to clear your lungs • Running
cold on hot: First aid for burns • The
Sting: Meat tenderizer to the rescue •
Things that go bite in the night • Poison-ivy protection • Beating back the
bugs: DEET comes in many guises •
The tick trick: Nail polish and Vaseline
• A rose is a rose is a primrose: Routing
rashes with flower power • Breaking the
cycle of brittle nails • Fighting fingernail fungus • Fire-Feet for icy toes • A
cure for the common cold? • The dangers of home remedies.*

---

Once upon a time there was something called a family
doctor. He [there were relatively few female physicians in
those days] was often known as a GP [general practitioner],
and more likely than not he was a family friend and confi-
dant. Besides administering an occasional medication

(which he might have made up himself), he was very big on common sense and practical advice.

Unfortunately, the old family doc has been replaced by a new species known as a specialist, who is long on up-to-date modern scientific techniques but a bit short on patience and friendly suggestions. Let us see if we can bring back some of those old-fashioned home remedies and perhaps add some new ones.[1]

Since I wrote those words almost a decade ago in the first edition of *The People's Pharmacy,* there has been an explosion in self-care. People are more interested than ever in taking good care of themselves, but they are increasingly reluctant to rely on doctors or drugs to solve simple health problems. There has been a growing interest in how-to books for everything from allergies and backaches to hemorrhoids and headaches. Publications like *Our Bodies, Ourselves* and *How to Be Your Own Doctor, Sometimes* have been enormously popular.

Americans have become disenchanted with a medical system that seems preoccupied with treating disease rather than preventing illness. More and more people are interested in striving for optimal health rather than settling for some doctor-defined "norm." We have become a nation of health nuts, and it's about time! Nutrition and exercise have almost become national obsessions. Nondrug alternatives are growing in acceptability.

People are using audio relaxation tapes for stress management instead of popping **Valium, Librium**, and **Dalmane**. They are turning to vitamin and mineral supplements, herbal remedies, acupuncture, and massage. As folks watch the cost of doctor-dispensed health care skyrocket, many have rediscovered a host of simple treatments that go back to Grandma's time and beyond.

A recent survey provides some fascinating statistics.[2] When confronted by simple problems like insomnia, minor anxiety, cuts and scratches, indigestion, or diarrhea, over one third of the people questioned did not treat the symptoms. Instead, they applied a wonderful remedy called "Tincture of Time." About a third used an over-the-counter medication and 14 percent tried a home remedy. Only 9 percent called or went to the doctor. Over 80 percent said "they prefer to fight symptoms without taking medication," and 96 percent said "they know that medication should only be taken when absolutely necessary."[3]

Now that's progress! Let's hear it for good old-fashioned common sense. In this chapter we are celebrating a return to home remedies. We will examine some things you can do without a doctor to relieve a wide range of minor problems. Some of these ideas have been tested and reported in such prestigious publications as the *New England Journal of Medicine,* while others are just passing notes whose appearance is justified simply because they seem to make sense. And if you have a handy-dandy home remedy you'd like to pass along, please send it to us for inclusion in the next edition of this book.

## Home, Home on the Range

Home remedies are folk medicine. If that conjures up visions of backward people in backward places, think again. We know quite a few octogenarians who grew up with the pioneering attitude that they'd rather do for themselves. Faced with everyday ailments, they came up with their own treatments to relieve pain, reduce swelling, or cure infections. Some of the folks who've gotten by on home remedies without seeing a doctor for fifty years are better off than they would be if they had received a fancy prescription for every complaint.

Of course, much of what they thought worked did nothing. Some of it, we later learned, actually did harm. But through it all, a few things persisted and were later incorporated into "orthodox" medicine.

Some home remedies have been passed from generation to generation by word of mouth. Others have come to the attention of medical people, who either laugh at them or adopt them, depending on how a particular remedy seems to fit into scientific knowledge of that time.

The doctor may have the corner on high-tech medicine, but

he doesn't have a monopoly on everything that works. The home remedies we're about to discuss are available without a prescription, and are easy to use.

Take, for example, chicken soup. In fact, taking chicken soup is just what the *Mayo Clinic Health Letter* recently said you should do for a cold![4] There has actually been some research on the uses of Grandma's favorite "antibiotic," and there's evidence the stuff really does the job better than other hot liquids.

"Chicken soup," says the distinguished clinic's health letter, "particularly the homemade variety with chicken parts, vegetables, herbs, spices, and noodles, is a safe, effective treatment for many 'self-limiting' illnesses (those not requiring professional attention). It is inexpensive and widely available. Side effects are few, with the notable exception of weight gain if it is used excessively.

"Next time you come down with a head cold," the letter concludes, "try hot homemade chicken soup before heading for the pharmacy. We believe chicken soup can be an excellent treatment for uncomplicated head colds and other viral respiratory infections for which antibiotics ordinarily are not helpful."

So there you have it, straight from one of the most respected sources in American medicine. A home remedy works. It works well. It works better than anything modern medical science has to offer and, like most home remedies, it does the job cheaper than anything you can buy to treat the problem.

There's no doubt about it, home remedies can be great. But that doesn't make *all* home remedies great, or useful, or even safe. Like all medication, home remedies have to be used carefully. By that I mean not so much *how* they're applied, as *when*.

The trick to doctoring yourself is knowing when not to do it. Most of the conditions we'll discuss in this chapter are benign ones. They can be uncomfortable, irritating, sometimes even maddening. But hopefully few will be life-threatening, and it's unlikely anyone would be much the worse for wear if another day or two passes without medical attention while a home remedy gets its chance at bat.

In fact, the Secret Factor in a lot of that fancy, expensive, doctor-dispensed medicine is that many minor illnesses are *self-limiting*. That's fancy doctor talk for saying it will go away by itself in seven days if you take medicine, or in a week if you leave it alone. That will be thirty-five dollars, please.

With the national medical tab running close to a cool billion bucks a day, I think there's a strong argument to be made for each of us doing what we can to take care of ourselves in situations where such an attempt doesn't run any serious risk of doing damage. With that in mind, we present *The People's Pharmacy* guide to doing it yourself. Here are the sexy trade secrets and home remedies that just might help.

## Hiccups

We'll start with this one because it's common, because it's a favorite topic of doctors, and because the remedies really do work. Curing hiccups has almost become the physician's answer to Trivial Pursuit, with lots of letters-to-the-editor in prestigious medical journals, describing a new cure.

First, let's take a stab at understanding hiccups. The diaphragm, a muscle between your chest and abdomen, supplies the power behind every breath. When the phrenic nerve, which stimulates this muscle, becomes irritated, it can produce a spasmodic contraction of the diaphragm. This in turn causes the voice box to close suddenly, which is what makes the distinctive hiccup sound.

Now let's cure it. Get a cotton swab. Have the hiccupping victim open his or her mouth. Place the swab on the roof of the mouth, right where the surface changes from hard (in front) to soft (towards the rear). Rub gently for a minute or so, and begone, damn hiccups. This one was first suggested in a letter to the *New England Journal of Medicine* and republished in the Mayo Clinic's health newsletter, so it's nothing to sneeze—or hiccup—at.[5]

But why does it work? Probably the same reason many of the traditional hiccup remedies have worked. It irritates the phrenic

nerve someplace other than where it's already irritable, and the
two irritations cancel each other out, or so overload the system
that it just shuts down.

Among the other remedies also reputed to do some good are
eating crushed ice, placing sugar at the back of the throat, and
pulling the tongue. Each of these stimulates the rear of the
throat, and that may well be the key.

The sugar cure also appeared in the *New England Journal of
Medicine*. Dr. Edgar Engelman reported that "one teaspoonful
of ordinary white granulated sugar swallowed dry resulted in
immediate cessation of hiccups in 19 of 20 patients."[6] Twelve of
these poor souls had their hiccups longer than six hours, and
eight of them had endured anywhere from a full day to six weeks
of hiccup suffering.

I've found brown sugar a bit more palatable, but the white
may do the job more consistently because of its texture. It has
been suggested that for younger patients a few drops of water
with the sugar will also help it go down.[7]

In case the Q-Tip or sugar cures don't do the job, here are
several other tips from the pages of the *New England Journal of
Medicine*. Dr. Jay Howard Herman offered the following suggestion titled "A Bitter Cure."

Hiccups (singultus) have plagued humanity for ages, often
at awkward times. Therapy is tedious, with frequent fail-
ures. Granulated sugar taken orally has been previously
reported as highly effective; it probably activates a local
pharyngeal reflex. Hiccups are commonly associated with
ethanol [alcohol] ingestion. We wish to report our success
with an alternative remedy that is well known to bartenders,
but that we cannot find in the medical literature.
All subjects had ethanol-induced hiccups that were unre-
sponsive to traditional treatment. . . . Treatment consisted
of oral administration of a lemon wedge of the size served
in bars; the wedge was saturated with Angostura bitters and
rapidly consumed (except for the rind). Small amounts of
granulated sugar were occasionally used to enhance palata-

bility, but they did not increase efficacy. Response was defined as at least a two-hour cessation of hiccups within one minute of treatment. The total response rate was 88 percent (14 of 16 cases), including two cases of initial treatment failure that was overcome after a second treatment within five minutes.[8]

Dr. Herman's home hiccup remedy spurred another note to the *Journal.* "No doubt the remedy of Herman . . . is good, but one does not always have a lemon in the house. I am 81 years old, and I have always found the following to cure hiccups.

"Fill a glass to the top with water, then bend over as far as you can from the waist, and drink all you can from the far side of the glass. You will find that the hiccups disappear."[9]

I told you that doctors love hiccup remedies. But here's one I've never seen in any medical journal. A friend swears he has seen a woman cured by having someone hold a twenty-dollar bill just above her extended thumb and first finger. The person promises her she can have the bill if she'll just catch it as it slips between her fingers. By talking constantly and releasing the bill at unexpected times, it has invariably fluttered untouched to the ground, and the hiccups have consistently disappeared after just a few rounds. Don't blame me if you lose money trying this.

A final word to the wise: If you know someone suffering from prolonged, incurable hiccups, take note. They could be a sign of something serious, including diseases of the liver, pancreas, esophagus, or bladder. Even some drugs (Decadron, Hexadol) can cause hiccups.[10] So if none of our handy-dandy home remedies does the trick and those hiccups persist, hie thee to a doctor for a complete physical examination.

## Help for Heartburn

Ask most people what you should do for heartburn and they will undoubtedly suggest an antacid. (See Chapter 5.) But I've got a better idea. If you liked my spoonful of sugar for hiccups, you should love the candy-and-chewing-gum home remedy for heartburn.

Okay, I admit that candy and chewing gum sound like the last thing you would want if you suffer from "gastroesophageal reflux," otherwise known as heartburn. But once again, the *New England Journal of Medicine* offers us a simple and elegant home remedy for one of mankind's most common plagues.

When stomach acid splashes back up into the esophagus (sometimes referred to as the gullet), it causes irritation and pain. After all, we're talking about hydrochloric acid here—nasty stuff. The body's natural response to this assault is to swallow, which gets most of the acid back into the stomach, where it belongs. But that may not be enough. To help nature along, sucking on a piece of hard candy or chewing gum can stimulate saliva production. This helps in two ways. First, it washes the acid down by promoting swallowing; and second, it serves to neutralize any residual acid left in the esophagus.[11]

Though doctors once thought that it would take too much saliva to be able to neutralize the acid that sloshes up and causes heartburn, this research by doctors at the Medical College of Wisconsin shows sucking on candy can increase saliva production by eight or nine times, so that the acid is easily neutralized for most people.

Drugs such as **Pro-Banthine** (propantheline), which dry out the mouth and suppress the swallowing reflex, would probably be counterproductive. Nevertheless, such medications are commonly prescribed for people with "acid" problems. So here's a case where the home remedy could be better than the expensive prescription approach.

## Simple Prevention for Chinese-Restaurant Syndrome

Have you ever gone out to eat Chinese food and afterwards suffered from heartburn, flushing, headache, chest tightness, lightheadedness, tingling, or even asthma? For reasons that are still mostly a mystery, some people react strongly to monosodium glutamate (MSG), frequently used in Chinese, Japanese, or Southeast Asian foods.

Up until recently, this has meant that sufferers had to forego these delectable cuisines. But now, there may be an antidote. Researchers have found that Vitamin $B_6$ (pyridoxine) seems to be involved. Students who reacted to MSG took 50 mg of $B_6$ a day for twelve weeks. When they were then dosed with MSG again, they no longer reacted to it.[12]

Now I can't guarantee this home remedy. Although it did appear in a respectable publication called *Nutrition & the M.D.*, that doesn't mean it will work for everyone. If you're supersensitive to MSG, I wouldn't recommend that you gobble some Vitamin $B_6$ and then pig out on Chinese food. Test the waters gently. Gradually increase pyridoxine intake for a couple of months and perhaps then you could sample the egg rolls or wonton soup. If you have no reaction, the next time out you could be a little more adventuresome.

## Curing Cecil the Seasick Sea Serpent

One of the most popular phrases of the last decade has been, "If we can put a man on the moon, why can't we . . . ?" You get to fill in the blank with whatever it seems should be cured with a dose of high technology.

Now NASA is joining in the game, asking why, if they can put a man on the moon, they can't keep him from throwing up en route. It turns out that even experienced fliers who have spent thousands of hours in the air lose their lunch when they get into outer space. Almost half the space shuttle pilots have had to cling to airsick bags like nervous passengers on a bumpy flight.

I can sympathize. As the parent of a susceptible five-year-old, I think twice before setting out on any trip likely to last longer than twenty minutes. "Daddy, I feel sick" has become an all too familiar refrain.

Motion sickness can strike sensitive people almost anywhere

—in a car, bus, plane, or train. And let's not forget boats. Anyone who has really been seasick knows that death can seem like a reasonable alternative.

So what causes motion sickness in the first place? Why is it that some poor souls suffer when the car hits a few bumps, while others can ride a roller coaster with glee? The problem is thought to arise when the brain receives confusing signals from the inner ear. It is the inner ear, after all, that is responsible for our sense of which end is up in the world. When the messages that are relayed to the brain from the ear conflict with what makes sense, bad things happen to good people, or at least some of them.

There are lots and lots of motion sickness remedies around, and just about everyone who's ever been seasick has tried at least one of these, such as **Dramamine** (dimenhydrinate), **Bonine** (meclizine), or **Marezine** (cyclizine). The results are usually mixed, at best, with some getting some relief and others still left hanging over the railing. And of those who do get relief, some of them pay for it with side effects such as extreme sedation, which hardly adds to the enjoyment of a day of sailing.

If you visit the doctor for some powerful prescription medicine, chances are he will prescribe scopolamine. This is no space-age miracle medicine, however. The belladonna plant it is derived from was used by physicians before the Roman Empire to cure a multitude of sins. The latest version of this ancient remedy is **Transderm-Scop**. Instead of swallowing a pill, you apply a coated adhesive patch (about the size of a nickel) behind your ear. Gradual absorption of the drug through the skin is supposed to provide sustained relief from nausea and vomiting. While reasonably effective, **Transderm-Scop** can cause dryness of the mouth, drowsiness, difficult urination, disorientation, memory disturbances, and blurred vision.

If you're motion sickness–prone and facing an irresistible invitation to go sailing, there's still hope. Recent research says that you just might get good relief by bypassing the expensive over-the-counter and prescription remedies in favor of a couple capsules of ground ginger.

That's right, ginger, the spice. In a test of ginger's ability to control motion sickness, two researchers subjected thirty-six people who were highly susceptible to motion sickness to a motor-driven revolving chair. This is the sort of device which brings out—and up—the worst in those whose systems are motion sickness–prone.

About twenty minutes before being blindfolded and entering the torture device, the people were dosed with either **Dramamine**, two capsules (a total dose of 940 milligrams) of powdered ginger, or an inert placebo. When the world began to whirl, each person was asked to rate his or her feelings of stomach upset.

When the results were tallied, the winner in suppressing motion sickness was ginger, which was almost twice as effective as **Dramamine**.[13] None of the people who received a placebo or **Dramamine** was able to stay in the chair for the full six minutes. But surprisingly, over half the subjects who received powdered ginger made it all the way through the experiment.

"We don't recommend that people just take a spoonful of ginger, because it's rather caustic," says one of the researchers on the project. "But a small bit of ginger root ground up and put in a gelatin capsule just might be effective for people who have tried everything else with no effect."

Now you probably won't be able to find ground-up ginger in your pharmacy, but the local health-food store may have ginger capsules available. And of course the kitchen spice shelf should already be well stocked. You might want to whip up a batch of extragingery gingerbread before heading off on your next wild adventure. The kids should love it. Happy sailing!

## Hot Cha-Cha

As long as we're speaking of spices, here's a quick and easy remedy. If you have one of those miserable winter colds where the gunk in your chest is thick and hard to get up and out, go out to dinner!

But not just any dinner. A hot, spicy Chinese or Mexican meal is what we have in mind. Dr. Irwin Ziment, chief of medicine at Los Angeles County-Olive View Medical Center, says the spicy stuff gets the respiratory tract to pouring out secretions, making it easier to cough up the mucky mucous.[14]

If going out is more than you're up to, he says you can accomplish the same thing at home with a gargle of about twenty drops of **Tabasco** sauce in eight ounces of water.

By the way, be aware that there's almost no remedy short of sedation for the terrible burn resulting from handling hot jalapeno or red peppers. This type of injury typically strikes people not raised in the Southwest, who decide for the first time in their life to make a "real" Mexican (or Chinese) meal.

Unaware of the burning power built into one of these chilies, our poor intrepid chef washes, seeds, and slices the chilies by hand, instead of wearing rubber or plastic gloves. Within an hour, the poor soul will be uselessly plunging his or her hands into ice water, seeking to put out the fire.

The fire, though, is caused by an oily, alkaline resin called *capsaicin*. It's insoluble in water, so all the soaking in the world won't help. You have, for all intents and purposes, plunged your hand into a barrel of lye.

If you get Hunan Hand, or Chili Fingers, or whatever you choose to call it, the only things that can help are (a) the passage of time . . . you will, believe us, live; though this may not seem a preferable alternative for a while, (b) mild pain relievers such as aspirin, and (c) possibly a prolonged soak in vinegar. The acid will eventually neutralize the highly alkaline capsaicin.

## Running Cold on Hot

If the burning feeling on your hand is caused by grabbing a hot pan instead of hot chilies, the remedy is very different. Most burn injuries happen at home, and this is an instance where a home remedy is not only possible, but actually very important. Action taken in the first few seconds can have a strong effect on how serious the burn injury will be.

For many years, medical people were ready to argue at the

drop of a match over what was appropriate first aid for burns. For a while, there almost seemed to be a "burn treatment of the year" club. Among the heralded treatments were butter, baking soda, and nothing.

But at long last, there's an unequivocal answer about what to do with a burn. The application of cold water or a cold, wet compress is the treatment of choice.[15] This treatment, applied for twenty minutes, "has been shown to reduce the depth of the injury."[16]

Another researcher reported a reduction of up to two thirds in total treatment time and burn severity when immediate cold water immersion was employed on one hundred fifty patients suffering a variety of chemical, heat, and electrical burns, some quite severe.[17] All infections were prevented.

This is an instance where too much of a good thing could be bad. Do not rush in with ice. Used directly it's just too cold, and you can wind up causing tissue damage from the cold on top of the tissue damage already present from the burn. A few ice cubes added to a pan of water, however, is okay.

Once a person is burned, get moving with that cold water or cold compress! Seconds count, and it doesn't take long to make the difference between a nasty blister and no obvious skin reaction.

For reasons that elude us, there's been a trend toward burn ointments and sprays. This can be dangerous. Most of these preparations contain a local anesthetic (benzocaine is one of the most common ingredients). It can cause a reaction, especially when applied to skin where the first layer or two may already be missing.

Sometimes this skin reaction can actually be worse than the original burn! Where there's a deep burn, you can get in double trouble due to greater absorption of the ointments into the body. Remember, they've been tested and found safe as *topical* ointments, not as drugs to be taken internally.

The cold-water treatment is safe and proper first aid for any burn, but anything greater than a first-degree burn confined to a small area should be seen by a doctor. A first-degree burn is one where there's slight reddening, comparable to sunburn. It's perhaps the most uncomfortable kind of burn, since the tissue is all very much alive and hurting.

Anything beyond a first-degree burn represents a substantial medical threat from infection, lost fluids, and many other complications. Don't play doctor with one of these burns, and don't make later medical help more difficult by gooping up the scene with butter, oil, ointments, or anything else. Get cold water on it, then get the person to a doctor or emergency room.

## The Sting

What's the first thing you do after being stung by a bee or insect? Most people probably scream a little, make futile efforts to remove the stinger, or perhaps make a compress of mud or baking soda. (One old remedy calls for rubbing fresh horse manure on the sting, but this cure is definitely horses--t.)

What does work is meat tenderizer. That's right, meat tenderizer, the stuff sitting right there on the spice shelf dressed up as **Adolph's** or one of a dozen other brands. About a quarter teaspoonful dissolved in a couple teaspoons of water (enough to make a paste) should stop pain pronto, according to Dr. Harry L. Arnold of the Health Insurance Institute.[18] A little dab will do ya.

How does meat tenderizer get the job done? It turns out that the stuff contains *papain,* an enzyme extracted from the fruit of the tropical papaya tree. In addition to breaking down muscle tissue and thus tenderizing meat, papain also does a job on the proteins that make up bee-sting and other insect venom. When it is rubbed into the skin immediately after a sting, the toxic chemicals are broken down before they do damage.

If you want something fancier (though not necessarily better) than off-the-shelf meat tenderizer, you can go to your friendly neighborhood pharmacist or health-food store and ask for a "digestive aid" containing papain. Mail-order vitamin companies will often offer natural papaya enzyme in tablet form. The

Parke-Davis drug company even manufactures such a product under the brand name **Papase**. All you have to do is smash up the tablet and make a paste.

An even better method is to have the stuff ready to go, in ointment form. This is the Cadillac of sting treatment, and you can buy it in the form of **Panafil Ointment** (Rystan Company, P.O. Box 214, Little Falls, NJ 07424). This ointment also contains urea, and is intended for munching up dead tissue around injuries, so it will require a prescription. You'll need the cooperation of a friendly physician if you want a "scrip" for **Panafil**, but it might be worth the effort. Of course, you can always fall back on meat tenderizer in a pinch.

A final tip on using anything containing papain. Do NOT cleanse the wound first with hydrogen peroxide. The hydrogen peroxide inactivates any papain you apply. Just remove the stinger (without squeezing or pushing on it, which will release more venom) and slap the tenderizer on there ASAP (as soon as possible).

And if you have any reason to believe that you, or anyone who has been stung, is truly allergic to bee or insect stings, then get them to an emergency room instantly. People who suffer severe reactions to insect venom can have a life-threatening reaction within minutes.

## Things That Go Bite in the Night

Mosquito and flea bites aren't so dangerous, but the itching can drive you crazy. What happens when a dive-bombing mosquito selects your juicy bodily fluids to extract? What do you do if your dog's fleas decide that they would like some variety in their lives and want to try you on for size? How do you respond to the plague of poison ivy?

If you're like most people, you swear a little and then smear, spread, or spray some over-the-counter anti-itch gunk on your sad skin. Some of these products work, some don't, but fortunately, there's an incredibly simple and effective home remedy.

It's available everywhere and is as cheap as anything could ever be. What is this wondrous stuff? Nothing more exotic than water. Hot water, to be precise.

According to some dermatologists, applications of hot water for a brief period of time can provide almost instantaneous relief of itching. And the effects last up to three hours.[19]

I know it sounds crazy, but it really works. The water should be hot enough to be slightly uncomfortable but not so hot as to burn—about 120 to 130 degrees Fahrenheit. If it's not warm enough, the itching can be made worse.

You can either stick the affected spot under the running water for a second or two, or you can use a washcloth. Several applications should do the trick for a few hours.

Obviously, an extensive skin involvement should not be treated in this manner, nor should poison ivy that has blistered. Keep in mind that prolonged heat may be dangerous in certain kinds of skin problems, so make the applications short and sweet.

How does this one work its magic? Interestingly enough, much the same way as the hiccup cure—that is, by overloading a nerve network, in this case the fine nerves in the upper layer of your skin. By short-circuiting the itching reflex, your urge to scratch is reduced or eliminated.

Of course the most desirable approach in dealing with pruritis (a doctor word for itching) is to remove the underlying cause. But when the problem is a mosquito or flea bite, mild poison ivy, or atopic dermatitis (a chronic condition with no known cause or cure) hot-water therapy can be a cheap and fast temporary treatment. And it certainly is readily available.

## Poison-Ivy Protection?

Wait. What's that I hear? A roaring sound. Must be the faithful standing up to be counted on behalf of their **Caladryl, Ivy Dry, Ivy-Chex, Ivy-Rid, Poison Ivy Cream,** or other preventives or remedies for poison ivy.

Well, I hate to disappoint you, but there isn't a whole lot

you can do about poison ivy once it's on your skin more than a few minutes. A few helpful treatments can be applied right at home without the dubious aid of expensive store-bought remedies. And some pharmacy products can actually do more harm than good.

A common ingredient in many anti-itch products is diphenhydramine (**Benadryl Antihistamine Cream, Caladryl, Didelamine, Surfadil, Ziradryl**). Yet dermatologists have known for years that this drug itself can produce "contact dermatitis," that is to say a nasty red, itchy rash in some people.[20-23]

Imagine the poor soul with poison ivy. He goes to the drugstore for relief and buys an over-the-counter poison-ivy product containing diphenhydramine. On it goes over the red, itchy skin. But instead of getting relief, he may soon discover the rash has spread. Thinking the poison ivy is getting worse, he applies more medicine, which may in turn make the itching and redness worse.

What's going on here, of course, is the nastiest of catch-22s. The poison-ivy remedy can end up causing the very symptoms it is supposed to be curing.

So what should you do if you discover that the weeds you have been busily pulling up in the backyard are really poison ivy? The first line of defense is soap and water. You've got ten minutes or less after exposure before the active ingredient in the poison ivy enters the skin and sets off an allergic red alert. Some people claim that rubbing alcohol solubilizes the poison ivy or poison oak resin and is also helpful in getting the gunk off the skin. And there's a report that alcohol towelettes will also work to cut the poison oak oil.[24]

By the way, just because you wash your hands or other affected areas doesn't guarantee you will be safe. The resin can easily get on clothing, gloves, tools, and on animals. When your skin comes into contact with these things, even days later, you can get zapped.

Once the process is in motion, about all that can be done for anyone is to lessen the discomfort a bit. Here's another home remedy from the pages of the *New England Journal of Medicine:*

The itching associated with poison-ivy dermatitis can be mitigated or stopped when the crushed leaves of the common plantain . . . are rubbed on the affected areas of the skin. We used narrow-leaf plantain. Plantain can grow profusely on any lawn in the United States . . .

A group of 10 people—family and friends, all sensitive to poison ivy—were treated with plantain last summer. The cessation of itching in all cases was rapid . . . This treatment is a blessing for those who must have a constant supply of calamine lotion or cortisone during the warm months . . .

Bibliographical research reveals that the therapeutic effects of plantain have been known at least since the 16th century.[25]

That folk wisdom comes courtesy of Serge Duckett, M.D., Ph.D., of Jefferson Medical College. If you want to bolster this home remedy with some drugstore soaks, you can try a dilute solution (1:20) of aluminum acetate, which the pharmacist may sell you as "Burow's solution." Cold compresses for about half an hour, four to six times a day can be excellent. Pure calamine lotion is also a safe bet and you may find that hydrocortisone ointments and creams (**Cortaid, Cortil, Dermolate, Hytone, Lanacort, Resicort, Rhulicort, Wellcortin**) provide significant relief.

If the skin reaction is very extensive, it's time to call the dermatologist. Poison-ivy reactions can be severe, and may call for treatment with powerful steroids or antihistamines. Do *not* play doctor for any serious skin irritations.


## Beating Back the Bugs


The best cure for itching from things that go bite in the night is to keep them from biting. Now, there are about as many home remedies for scaring off biting critters as there are fishermen, hunters, and lumberjacks who've crawled around on the ground. Through the millennia, humans have rubbed themselves with a veritable cornucopia of disgusting things in the hopes that mosquitoes, black flies, gnats, biting fleas, and chiggers would also be disgusted and move on to a more palatable meal.

Rancid bear grease was a favorite home remedy with American Indians. And according to one authority, when Henry David Thoreau got fed up with mosquitoes around Walden Pond he "concocted a mess of turpentine, oil of spearmint and camphor that he finally decided was itself more unpleasant than the insect bites."[26] The original **Old Time Woodsman's Liquid Fly Dope** contained pine tar, camphor, and citronella, and many lumberjacks in northern New England swore by the stuff. But it's possible that friends and lovers also did a lot of swearing when they got close enough to smell anyone so coated.

Well, what should you use if you decide to head for the hills? The truth is, one thing has been proven superior to the competition at keeping skeeters and such at bay. That stuff is a chemical called N,N-diethyl-meta-toluamide which for obvious reasons is usually called DEET.

DEET got its seal of approval from no less than the U.S. Army. Those folks have tested everything anyone could ever dream up (and a few you'd hope nobody would dream up) for keeping bugs away from our service-men and -women. After sifting through more than nine thousand things, the Army pronounced DEET the chemical of choice.

For a while about the only way you could lay your hands on this bug repellent was to join up, but in 1956 a dilute version became available under the brand name **Off!** It worked, but for heavy-duty campers and sportsmen it wasn't quite strong enough, since they had to keep applying the stuff every couple of hours to keep bugs away.

**Enter Charles Coll, a Truro, Nova Scotia, paint chemist and outdoorsman. He read of Deet in 1959, ordered some from a chemical company and put it in little bottles. Mr. Coll called his product Muskol and sold it himself. Because it was 100% Deet, undiluted by alcohol, Muskol would keep bugs from biting most of the day. Mr. Coll wasn't much of**

a marketer, but over the course of 20 years, word-of-mouth advertising finally made Muskol popular enough in Canada to attract competitors. About five years ago, Muskol entered the U.S. market.[27]

The success of **Muskol** is now apparent, as it was recently bought up by Schering-Plough, Inc., a pharmaceutical giant better known for **Coricidin** and **Chlor-Trimeton** cold tablets, **Coppertone** lotions, **Maybelline** cosmetics, and **Dr. Scholl's** foot gear.

So off you go to the pharmacy to look for an insect repellent. And there you find a bewildering array of brand names. How to choose the best? Easy. Turn the bottle over and see what percentage of DEET (also listed as diethyl toluamide) it contains. The winner is the one with the biggest number. Notice I said "the bottle." Avoid spray-on preparations in aerosol cans. They usually cost more and are less efficient.

The consumer is in luck because there is now an amazing collection of high-potency DEET-containing products available on pharmacy shelves. The battle for your bucks is heating up. After all, Americans are now spending almost $75 million each year to keep bugs at bay, and competitors are scrambling to produce the most concentrated concoctions.

Among the brands with virtually 100-percent pure DEET are **Muskol, Ben's 100, Jungle Plus, Maximum Strength Deep Woods Off!, Jungle Juice 100,** and **Repel 100**. But for some folks, these high-potency products may be overkill. If you are not particularly tempting to mosquitoes and other sucking insects, you can probably get by with less concentrated protection. Other brands with a reasonable percentage of DEET include **Skram Insect Repellant** (74.5 percent), **Space-Shield II Insect Repellant** (75 percent), **Sportsmate II Premium Insect Repellent Cream** (55 percent), and **Cutter Cream Formula** (30 percent).

Nothing works if you don't put it on. Repellents are repelling to people, there's no doubt about it. They aren't exactly French perfume, they usually leave you feeling like a greased pig, and there's the sense that you've just dosed yourself with some kind of poison that is seeping into your interior. In fact, DEET is absorbed into the body and can occasionally cause toxic reaction, especially in babies and children. A few youngsters have experienced convulsions or encephalopathy. Skin rashes in adults as well as children are not uncommon. But if you insist on exposing your flesh to biting insects, you will either put on a dose of DEET or be eaten alive.

There's another option besides the smear-and-smell one. Among the insect repellent remedies that people have both sworn by and sworn at is Vitamin $B_1$ (thiamine). As long ago as 1943 there were published studies saying the vitamin, taken orally, could repel insects, particularly mosquitoes.[28] Mexican dermatologists later reported that thiamine was effective in reducing insect bites and diminishing itching when administered in doses of 200 milligrams daily to adults and 100 milligrams to children.[29]

Another study, reported by Dr. H. L. Meuller, concluded that

**Thiamine hydrochloride taken internally has been reported to be a repellent for mosquitoes and fleas. In our experience, over 70 percent of 100 insect-sensitive patients given doses of 75 to 150 milligrams of thiamine hydrochloride daily reported that insects bothered them little or not at all while taking it, but the effect wore off rapidly if the thiamine was omitted.[30]**

Thiamine is a plain old everyday vitamin, though the recommended dose for chasing bugs is certainly far larger than the Recommended Daily Allowance. One of the reports cited above, however, found no evidence of adverse reactions even in doses of more than 300 milligrams.

Unfortunately, none of the studies on Vitamin $B_1$ has been very scientific, and there are newer reports in the literature disputing the efficacy of thiamine as an insect repellent.[31] Without a carefully designed experiment, it's hard to engage in unrestrained cheering. Nevertheless, I have received enough letters from faithful readers praising this vitamin as an insect repellent that you might consider giving it a whirl if you're the sort who's popular mosquito meat.

## Getting Ticked Off

While we're on the subject of things that bug us, consider the tick. There you are, merrily hiking away on a lovely day in the beautiful countryside. Pausing for a drink at a mountainside stream, you look at your leg and see . . . a tick. Yecch! There goes the fun.

I'll never forget the panic in my son's voice when he discovered that a tick had lodged in his scalp. As my wife, Terry, held him, I tried to remove the critter as calmly as possible. It wasn't easy and as a result of my bumbling he still has a fear of anything remotely resembling a tick.

While tick bites are not terribly painful, they can be pretty hazardous. Ticks are *vectors*—carriers, that is—of several serious diseases, most notably Rocky Mountain spotted fever.

Once one of these little fellow travelers leaps aboard, he sets up housekeeping by planting his paired pincers into your skin for a blood sundae. In the course of doing that, all manner of nasty things go from tick to Rick . . . or Sally, or Sam, as the case might be.

Over the years all sorts of ways have been suggested for getting ticks to let go of their hold on people. The first temptation, of course, is to grab the little bugger by the butt and yank him out. After all, there sits the tick, head buried in your arm or leg, tail end waving in the breeze.

The problem with that approach, however, is that such violence tends to cause the tick to lose his head, which will remain buried in your skin, where it can get infected and may continue transmitting whatever disease it might have had to offer.

The tick trick is to get the thing to back out, on its own accord. You're then welcome to carefully burn it to a crisp or set it free, depending on how great a nature lover you are.

How to do it? The old macho wild west approach used to be

to light up a cigarette, take a few deep drags to get the tip red hot, and then touch the cigarette to the tick's hind end. I've also heard tell that some folks used to pour a little lighter fluid on the tick and light it! That was back when men were men, when John Wayne was still around, and when most people carried Zippo lighters. It also didn't work very well. Both techniques have been known to produce some rather bad burns, and to just kill the tick in place.

More modern cures are available. Three of the best we've seen appeared recently in medical journals. If you insist on using a heat technique, you could follow Dr. Joseph Benforado's suggestion as published in the *Journal of the American Medical Association:*

**The materials needed are a pocket knife (or similar blade), large nail (eight- to ten-penny size), and matches.**

**The procedure is as follows.**
   **1. Warm the tip of the nail in a match flame.**
   **2. Slide the flat of the knife blade under the tick's abdomen.**
   **3. Place the heated nail tip on the tick's dorsal surface [back] so that the beastie is sandwiched between the knife blade and the nail.**
   **4. When the tick's legs begin to wiggle (a response to the heat), turn the knife blade 90 degrees so that the tick, now at right angles to the skin, is "standing on its head."**

**Keeping the tick sandwiched, raise the blade and the nail slowly away from the skin. The live tick, having released its mouthparts, comes away easily and is then appropriately disposed of. If the legs do not wiggle, the nail is not warm enough and a reattempt is needed. However, the object is to "annoy" the tick rather than to roast it.[32]**

As a camp physician, Dr. Benforado apparently had ample opportunity to try out this approach on an almost daily basis. He claims it has never failed him.

If, however, the nail-and-knife technique sounds a tad complicated, not to mention a little dangerous, you could try the fingernail-polish trick. This one comes from Dr. Warren Sherman, who generously credits it to the real discoverer—his fifteen-year-old daughter:

**I would like to report a simple and successful method of removing an embedded tick from the skin. This method was suggested to me by my daughter, a 10th-grade student. It was applied successfully on two occasions involving other members of my family, during a recent visit to Cape Cod, Massachusetts.**

**Approximately two drops of clear fingernail polish are allowed to fall from the brush and completely cover the tick. Within seconds the tick will release its bite and back out of the wound. The tick can then be easily wiped from the skin and properly disposed of.[33]**

A California physician reports in the *Western Journal of Medicine* that a little petroleum jelly will also do the trick quite nicely:

**A simple and safe method of tick removal is to coat the tick with petroleum jelly (such as Vaseline), wait ten minutes and then gently remove the tick with forceps, grasping it very close to the skin of patient or pet. The tick can be removed intact without problems associated with application of strong chemicals or burning. In addition, petroleumjelly-based ointments are readily available in most homes.[34]**

One theory to explain the petroleum-jelly tick trick is that the goo so completely covers the tick that it can't breathe. Ticks do breathe, by the way. Faced with suffocation, it begins to let go and back out. I have tried this technique and can vouch for its success, though patience is required. Waiting ten minutes can seem like an eternity when you have one of those beasties embedded in your skin.

Of course prevention is still the best approach of all. By checking frequently for ticks while hiking, it should be possible to spot them soon after they've come aboard, which often means before they've even had time to head in for dinner. If they've already become attached to you, do not panic. Reach for the clear nail polish or the petroleum jelly.

## A Rose Is a Rose Is a Primrose

Quick and easy cures for long and difficult ailments are, of course, much appreciated by long-suffering patients. If, that is, the cures really work. The problem is that sometimes a drug that shows even the slightest sign of helping with any one problem suddenly gets elevated to cure-all status. This is especially true of items available without a prescription for do-it-yourself dosing.

A case in point is something called evening primrose oil. This oil, made from the flower of that name, is enjoying a run of popularity among the natural-food set. Proponents claim it's good for hangovers, alcoholism, overweight, diabetes, high blood pressure, heart disease, premenstrual syndrome, schizophrenia, brittle nails, asthma, arthritis, and almost everything else for which we have few or no medical answers.

What evening primrose oil seems to do is affect the production of prostaglandins in the body. Prostaglandins have been one of medicine's most fertile research fields in the last few years. We know that these substances are produced by the body and control a wide range of physiological processes, including pain, inflammation, respiration, reproduction, and the contraction of certain types of muscle tissue.

Too much or too little of one or another prostaglandin (there are many different types) may be a factor in pain, arthritis, ulcers, psoriasis, eczema, and menstrual cramps. And we now know that many painkillers, including aspirin, get at least part of their effectiveness from an ability to temporarily slow or still the body's production of prostaglandins.

Enter evening primrose oil. It's a substantial source of a substance called gamma linoleic acid (GLA), from which the body produces a prostaglandin called PGE1. Supporters claim that raising the body's level of PGE1 can relieve or cure a number of human afflictions. Among the claims are that it can help lower blood pressure and cholesterol, reduce the risk of blood clots, stimulate the immune system, prevent hangovers, control overweight, improve eczema, and relieve menstrual cramps. Whew.

There is scientific evidence, from a good study, that evening primrose oil can be effective in relieving the symptoms of atopic eczema.[35] Patients with long-lasting severe itchy, red skin rashes (allergic in origin) were entered into the research program. Two to six capsules of **Efamol** (one brand of evening primrose oil) were taken daily for twelve weeks. At the end of the test the improvement ranged from 30 percent to 43 percent, depending upon the dose of **Efamol** employed. The larger the dose, the better the response.

That's good news, especially since the eczema had been hard to treat previously. But lest you get too excited with this news, researchers have found it ineffective for weight control, mental illness, and rheumatoid arthritis. The jury is still out on whether or not evening primrose oil offers any benefits in treating alcoholism.

For the moment we'd have to classify evening primrose oil as a home remedy with promise, most of it unsubstantiated. We can't help but note that the substance gets its name because the plant produces a flower that grows, blossoms, and dies all in a single evening. Let's hope this self-help remedy doesn't do the same. If it eventually proves to do even a quarter of what its proponents claim, that would be substantial progress for home remedies.

## Breaking the Cycle of Brittle Nails

Okay, it's nail inspection time. Get 'em out there, let's have a look. You there, with the dry, chipped nails. What are you doing to improve the situation? Gelatin? Baloney. The "evidence" to support the use of gelatin to strengthen nails is thin.

If you're a woman, maybe you get your nails treated with a "nail wrap" consisting of nylon, acrylic, or some other nail-hardening agent. That may give the temporary appearance of improvement, but it may actually make the situation worse, since the treatment tends to make hard, brittle nails even harder and more brittle.

Ready to give up? Well, we just might have a simple solution for you. Dr. Lawrence Norton, an expert on nail disorders, reported to a meeting of medical writers conducted by the American Academy of Dermatology that people should soak their fingers in water fifteen minutes a day, three to five times a week. After soaking, the moisture is sealed in with a phospholipid-containing hand cream such as **Complex 15.**

"The fluid content of nails determines to a large extent their pliability and capacity to withstand breakage," reported Dr. Norton. "The relative lack of water in nails is a primary reason for their hardness."[36]

The trick is in getting the nail to absorb some water and then hold onto it. The prolonged soak is needed because the dense protein tissue of the nail is reluctant to suck up water at first. Once you get it in there, applying a cream or lotion should help keep the moisture in. Dr. Norton advises against overuse of nail-polish remover or excess exposure to soap or detergent. These chemicals tend to dry the nails out and make them more brittle.

## Fighting Fingernail Fungus

While we've got your nails out there for a look-see, it's apparent that some of you are suffering fungal infections that make the nail look munched upon, ragged, and generally yucky. The fungus can thicken and discolor the nail to a sickly yellow-brown hue.

You've undoubtedly been told by a dermatologist that fungal infections in the nail are notoriously difficult to eradicate, and that about the only way to do it is through yanking the nail off. Faced with what sounds like medieval torture, many people choose to simply suffer their infections quietly and keep their hands in their pockets.

If you're one of those people, here's a chance to get your hands out of those pockets and into the light. It's a trade secret that even many dermatologists may not have heard of, so you might have to help your doctor out by providing the literature reference.

The secret potion is a mixture of urea, white petroleum jelly, lanolin, and beeswax. The chairman of the Department of Dermatology at Stanford University, Dr. Eugene M. Farber, discovered the urea ointment treatment while traveling in the Soviet Union. He learned that Russian doctors have apparently been using urea plasters "for many years to remove fungus-diseased nails."[37]

After protecting the skin around the infected nail, the goop is applied and covered with a piece of plastic wrap. "Booties" or plastic gloves can also be used to keep the nail completely dry. After seven to ten days, you return to the doctor and the nail is removed with no strain or pain.

One of the amazing things about this treatment is that normal nail is not affected. The only thing that comes off is diseased nail. "The procedure," say Dr. Farber and his collaborator, Dr. David South,

**has several distinct advantages. It is a nonsurgical method, and therefore intrinsically inexpensive for the patient. Multiple abnormal nails can be treated in one session. The procedure is essentially painless, and apparently without risk of infection or hemorrhage, making it ideal for treating patients with diabetes and others with vascular insufficiency [circulatory problems].[38]**

Once the diseased nail has been removed, it is possible to attack the underlying infection with a topical antifungal ointment. **Tinactin** (tolnaftate), **Micatin** (miconazole), and **Loprox** (ciclopirox) may be effective. Japanese researchers have reported impressive results using a 2 percent tolnaftate ointment along with a 20 percent urea ointment.[39]

There is one problem, however. Your physician and local pharmacist probably do not have a urea paste available. Until fairly recently, this ointment had to be specifically compounded by a pharmacist for each patient according to Dr. Farber's formula[40] (*Cutis,* volume 25, June 1980, p. 609). There was no commercial source, perhaps because once again there's no way to win an exclusive patent and thus no way to make a huge profit. Now, however, there is a company making the urea ointment for physicians. Your doctor can obtain it from Dermatological Laboratory & Supply Co., 201 Ridge Street, Council Bluffs, IA 51501. If your doctor wishes to call, the company's toll-free number is (800) 831-6273.

## Fire-Feet for Icy Toes

How many times have you climbed into a cold bed with freezing feet that made it hard to fall asleep? Or perhaps it's your spouse who suffers with frigid tootsies and warms them on your vulnerable body. Maybe you'd like to try the "home remedy" Minnesota Vikings kicker Benny Ricardo uses to keep his feet warm during a long football game.

"We stand around a lot," Mr. Ricardo says, "and when you go to hit the ball, it feels like a brick."

Another fan is Frederick Caito, trainer for the Chicago Bears. Some of the staff members used WarmFeet during the team's last home game, when the temperature with the wind-chill factor was minus 38. "We were a little hesitant about using it on the players because we didn't want to get everyone taped and dressed and then find out their feet were burning," he says. "Now that we know it doesn't cause any side effects, we'll probably use it for the players next year."[41]

So what is in this strange remedy variously called **WarmFeet** or **Fire-Feet**? It is a concoction of powdered herbs containing ground capsicum, zingiber, and brassica—roughly the same as hot pepper (cayenne), ginger, and mustard. Anyone who has ever chewed on a hot pepper knows it can produce a distinct feeling of warmth. It is supposed to do much the same thing for your feet.

Samantha Stevens tried about fifty different combinations of herbs before settling on these three. She was trying to come up with something to keep her tootsies warm while skiing. She was so successful that various national retailers are now selling her product.

Miss Stevens recommends that "users sprinkle the powdered concoction in their socks, massage their feet and wait at least twenty minutes before going out in the cold."[42] Theoretically, the herbs in **WarmFeet** dilate blood vessels and counteract the usual effect of cold weather.

Now I can't make any guarantees about the effectiveness of this product. All I'm going on is the testimonial reports of some frozen football players. It's unlikely the Food and Drug Administration will ever require safety or effectiveness tests since it's not technically a medication. And there are some cautions:

> **Bob Reese, head trainer for the New York Jets, says his players liked it, "but a couple of the linemen said it made their feet itch."**
>
> **Even Mr. Ricardo of the Vikings has a word of warning: "You have to wash your feet off with cold water. If you wash off with hot water, your feet will stay warm for two or three days."[42]**

Dermatologists advise that diabetics should stay away from a potential irritant like this, as should anyone with sensitive skin. If you decide to give **WarmFeet** or **Fire-Feet** a whirl before hiking or skiing, start cautiously with just one foot and a tiny spritz. If it works you can become bolder.

Where can you get this product? It is distributed nationally by

Divajex Inc., 1551 Redhill Avenue, Tustin, CA 92680. You may also see it advertised in catalogues like "Early Winters" or "Eddie Bauer."

## A Cure for the Common Cold?

Speaking of cold weather, what do you do for those sniffles and sneezes so common in winter? If you're like most people you moan and groan and head for the nearest pharmacy. The American public throws away $1.6 billion on over-the-counter cough and cold remedies.[44] I say "throws away" because so many of these products contain a sinkload of ingredients—antihistamines, decongestants, cough suppressants, expectorants, pain relievers, not to mention alcohol and caffeine.

Sometimes these ingredients work at cross purposes. For example, the expectorant is designed to loosen mucous and help you cough it up. But when combined with a cough suppressant that keeps you from coughing, there is no way for the expectorant to work. There may also be a decongestant like ephedrine, which can be stimulating to the nervous system, combined with an antihistamine designed to put you to sleep. And of course there will likely be aspirin. Believe it or not, there is some evidence that aspirin, the pain reliever found in so many cold remedies, can actually increase the multiplication and shedding of cold viruses. This may make you sicker longer, or at the very least a source of contamination for friends and loved ones.[45]

So what should you do? We discussed the benefits of chicken soup earlier in this chapter, but that is more for the symptoms of a cold than for its cure. What about Vitamin C? Well, I do confess to being a bit of a vitamin nut myself. I do take ascorbic acid (Vitamin C) regularly, and when I come down with the sniffles I increase my intake accordingly.

But the research results on this vitamin are controversial and equivocal. Depending upon your point of view you can find a number of studies to bolster your position. Some investigators have found that Vitamin C does not prevent the common cold, nor does it seem to speed recovery. Others offer data that suggests it will indeed decrease your days sick once you come down with a respiratory infection.

But there are a couple of other alternatives. Scientists at the University of Texas in Austin have found that zinc seems to help cold sufferers get well faster. They started the zinc study after they discovered that

> **a leukemic child refused to swallow a 50-mg zinc gluconate tablet and dissolved it slowly in her mouth instead. When her accompanying cold symptoms disappeared within hours, the investigators looked into the ability of zinc ions to halt replication of diverse viruses . . .**[46]

The Texas researchers took sixty-five people with fresh cold symptoms and gave half of them zinc gluconate lozenges (23 mg) every two hours during the day for a week. The remainder got placebo lozenges.

The results were impressive. More than four fifths of the people getting zinc got over their colds in less than a week, while more than half of those taking the placebo were still suffering after seven days.[47] A number of those in the zinc treatment group got rid of their cold symptoms almost immediately: 11 percent reported cold symptoms gone within twelve hours, while 22 percent said their colds disappeared in less than a day.

There were only two drawbacks. Zinc lozenges can be nasty tasting and irritating to the mouth, and they can cause nausea on an empty stomach. It is not clear whether you have to suck on zinc lozenges or whether you would get the same benefits by swallowing zinc tablets. So there is still a lot of research to be done before we can give zinc the brass ring award for curing the common cold. But initial results are tantalizing.

One final bizarre home remedy for curing the common cold comes from the Nuremberg International Inventors Fair in West Germany. An enterprising inventor claims that a nose clip "will cure a cold in 24 hours. The trick is to press the nose wings together to dry out the mucous membranes."[48] His invention looks something like a clothespin for the nose, though I rather imagine you could achieve much the same "benefit" by using the kind of noseclip swimmers use to keep water out.

Again we make no guarantees, but there is another possible explanation for how such an invention might work. Pinching the nostrils together may raise the temperature within the nose, which in turn might make it harder for viruses to survive and multiply. Of course any theoretical benefit from such a technique could be offset by the silly way you will look walking around with a clothespin or a noseclip stuck on your nose, breathing through your mouth.

Will we ever have a truly effective cure for the common cold? Investigators think so. Research is now proceeding on many fronts, and we may one day have an interferon nasal spray that really works. Until then, however, we recommend good old chicken soup. It is still the safest, tastiest, and cheapest treatment we know of.

Well, there you have it. Home remedies for everything that ails you from the nose to the toes. But before we take leave of this chapter, there is an important warning.

## Danger: Home Remedy Ahead

Up until now, I've told you about a wide variety of helpful home hints, each of which has a fair amount of evidence supporting its safety and efficacy.

I'd be remiss not to remind you, however, that home remedies have their dark side. Many home remedies don't do anything. There's probably little danger in that except for prolonging your discomfort a bit. However, there are many cures which can be far, far worse than the problems they're supposed to treat.

Take, for example, something so simple and obvious as putting baking soda on an infant's diaper rash. This remedy is based on the logic that (1) the problem is an acidic environment caused by the baby's urine, which should be offset by the alkaline baking soda, and (2) baking soda soaks are often recommended as first aid for adult rashes, bites, and other skin irritations.

The problem, according to an article in the medical journal *Pediatrics,* is that baking soda applied to an infant's rash may be absorbed much more readily than it would be in an adult. The infant, with an immature kidney function, has a limited capacity for clearing the bicarbonate, and the result can be a serious disruption in the acid–base balance of the body.[49]

When it comes to home remedies, none are more touted and more exploited than herbs. We tend to think of gentle herbs as things with almost magical powers to not only enhance the taste of food but also to do good somehow when rubbed, swallowed, or otherwise applied to the body.

And there are indeed roots and herbs with almost miraculous curative powers. After all, many of our modern medicines are derivatives of herbs. The important heart drug digitalis is from the foxglove plant, and the recently approved treatment for a ruptured spinal disk, chymopapain, comes from the papaya tree.

So what's the problem? Well, there are several. First of all, herbs can be strong medicine, both good and bad. Socrates died drinking an herbal tea, as you may recall.

Because herbs are not well regulated, the potency of herbal remedies varies enormously, particularly since there are so many methods of preparing them. Since systematic clinical testing is rarely done, we know little about the indications and effectiveness of herbal medicines. Worse yet, we may not have good information on adverse reactions, and so we're forced to rely on anecdotes that show that herbs can sometimes cause harm.

One story concerns the eighty-year-old relative of a physician who had suffered diarrhea for two months and had lost considerable weight. The old woman was, needless to say, greatly depleted, and the doctors were about to put her through a grueling series of tests when her relative found a bottle of "dark brown liquid" on the kitchen table.

"She told me," reports the doctor, "that this was an alcoholic extract of herbs, which she had prepared herself according to a recipe she had read in a popular phytotherapeutic magazine . . . [T]he [old Swedish] recipe included laxative herbs such as aloe, senna, rhubarb, and jalap, and diuretic herbs such as juniper berry and radix ononidis (restharrow root) in high doses."[50] Placed on a diet of fruits and vegetables, the woman promptly overcame her diarrhea and regained her former vigor.

Four patients taking Chinese herbal medicines for arthritis or back pain suffered even more serious consequences when they came down with the blood disease agranulocytosis and accompanying life-threatening infections. One of the four died.[51]

The herbal concoctions they had been taking turned out to contain both aminopyrine and phenylbutazone as undeclared ingredients. Aminopyrine was once available as an over-the-counter product, but was removed from sale in 1938 because of its known propensity for causing agranulocytosis. Phenylbutazone is used by physicians to treat inflammation, but is used with great care because it too is known to cause blood abnormalities. Yet the herbal remedy was available without a prescription.

This incident and another in which a woman developed severe lead poisoning from another Chinese herbal cure illustrate the problem: It is impossible to know everything that's in an herbal tea or preparation, since the material isn't subject to consistent quality control or testing. And it's also impossible to know what the dose limits might be, since rarely, if ever, are there any clinical studies that would help establish the boundary between rational and dangerous use of herbal medicines.

Some home remedies now known to be dangerous ought to be avoided. One is the notion that you should rub snow on frostbitten tissue. It makes things worse by further chilling the skin and constricting blood vessels.

Camphor (camphorated oil—a mixture of camphor and linseed oil) is extremely toxic when taken orally and has accounted for far too many poisonings in the past, especially when parents mistook it for castor oil.

Even something as simple as licorice root or sassafras could be dangerous. Licorice can deplete the body of potassium and cause fluid retention, serious consequences for anyone with high blood pressure. Sassafras root bark contains sassafras oil, which has been shown to be a cancer causing chemical in animals.

Many home remedies are helpful and inexpensive. But we need to be careful to keep familiarity from breeding carelessness. Like any medications, home remedies need to be used with caution, moderation, and common sense. Symptoms which persist deserve medical attention.

We hope you enjoyed the home remedies we've discussed. Since most of them came from the pages of the *New England Journal of Medicine* or other respectable medical sources, it's clear that doctors like home remedies, too. While we can't guarantee that ginger will cure your motion sickness, that Vitamin $B_6$ will solve the problem of Chinese-restaurant syndrome, or that zinc will chase away your cold symptoms, we believe they may be worth a try. Please let us know if they work.

# References

1. Graedon, Joe. *The People's Pharmacy.* New York: St. Martin's Press, 1976, P. 53.

2. Highlights of a Consumer Survey of Self-medication. *Health Care Practices and Perceptions,* Proprietary Association: Washington, D.C., Mar. 1984, pp. 14–22.

3. Ibid.

4. "Chicken Soup and the Common Cold." *Mayo Clinic Health Letter* Oct. 1984, p. 5.

5. "Why Hiccups Start and How You Can Stop Them." *Mayo Clinic Health Letter* Sep. 1984, p. 3.

6. Edgar, G., et. al. "Granulated Sugar as Treatment for Hiccups in Conscious Patients." *N. Engl. J. Med.* 285:1489, 1971.

7. Margolis, George. "Hiccup Remedies." *N. Engl. J. Med.* 286:323, 1972.

8. Herman, Jay Howard, and Nolan, David S. "A Bitter Cure." *N. Engl. J. Med.* 305:1054, 1981.

9. Brenn, Ethel. "Sequel on Singultus." *N. Engl. J. Med.* 306:1115, 1982.

10. LeWitt, P., et al. "Hiccup with Dexamethasone Therapy." *Ann. Neurol.* 12:405–406, 1982.

11. Helm, James F., et al. "Effect of Esophageal Emptying and Saliva on Clearance of Acid from the Esophagus." *N. Engl. J. Med.* 310:-284–288, 1984.

12. "Chinese-Restaurant Syndrome." *Nutrition and the M.D.* 8(12):1, 1982.

13. Mowrey, Daniel B., and Clayson, Dennis E. "Motion Sickness, Ginger and Psychophysics." *Lancet* 1:655–657, 1982.

14. "Cold Medicines." *Glamour,* May 1984, p. 345.

15. "Heat and Cold as Analgesics." *Medical Letter* 12:3–4, 1970.

16. Chatten, Milton J. "Disorders Due to Physical Agents." In Krup, Marcus and Chatten, Milton, *Current Medical Diagnosis and Treatment, 1983.* Los Altos: Lange Medical Publications, 1983, p. 963.

17. Shulman, A. G. "Ice Water as Primary Treatment of Burns." *JAMA* 173:1916–1919, 1960.

18. Arnold, Harry L. "Immediate Treatment of Insect Stings." *JAMA* 220:585, 1972.

19. Sulzberger, M. B., et. al. *Dermatology: Diagnosis and Treatment.* Chicago, Yearbook, 1961, p. 94.

20. Cronin, E. *Contact Dermatitis.* Edinburgh: Churchill Livingstone, 1980, pp. 236, 439.

21. Calnan, C. D. "Contact Dermatitis from Drugs." *Proc. R. Soc. Med.* 44:39–42, 1962.

22. Vickers, C. F. H. "Dermatitis Medicamentosa." *Br. Med. J.* 1:-1366–1367, 1961.

23. Coskey, Ralph J. "Contact Dermatitis Caused by Diphenhydramine Hydrochloride." *J. Am. Acad. Dermatol.* 8:204–206, 1983.

24. "The Evil Weed." *San Francisco Examiner,* Sep. 5, 1982.

25. Duckett, Serge. "Plantain Leaf for Poison Ivy." *N. Engl. J. Med.* 303:583, 1980.

26. Bulkeley, William M. " 'Deet,' by Any Name, Doesn't Smell Sweet to a Pesky Mosquito." *Wall Street Journal,* May 26, 1983, p. 1.

27. Ibid.

28. Shannon, W. R. "Thiamine Chloride—An Aid in the Solution of the Mosquito Problem." *Minn. Med.* 26:799–802, 1943.

29. Ruiz-Maldonado, Ramon, and Tamayo, Lourdes. "Treatment of 100 Children with Papular Urticaria with Thiamine Chloride." *Int. J. Derm.* 12:258–260, 1973.

30. Meuller, H. L., and Samter, M. *Immunological Diseases.* Boston: Little, Brown, 1965, p. 683.

31. Smith, C. N. "Repellants for Anopheline Mosquitoes." *Miscellaneous Public. Entomol. Soc. America* 7:99–117, 1970.

32. Benforado, Joseph M. "Removal of Ticks." *JAMA* 252:3368, 1984.

33. Sherman, Warren T. "Polishing Off Ticks." *N. Engl. J. Med.* 309:992, 1983.

34. Shakman, Robert. "Tick Removal." *Western J. Med.* 140(1):99, 1984.

35. Wright, S., and Burton, J. L. "Oral Evening-Primrose-Seed Oil Improves Atopic Eczema." *Lancet* 2:1120–1122, 1982.

36. "New Formula Offers Hope for Chronically Brittle Nails. News Release, Mar. 22, 1984, American Academy of Dermatology.

37. "Diseased Nails Are Easily Shed with Urea Treatment." *Medical World News* Feb. 5, 1979, p. 88.

38. Farber, Eugene, and South, David. "Urea Ointment in the Nonsurgical Avulsion of Nail Dystrophies." *Cutis* 22:689–692, 1978.

39. Ishii, Masamitsu, et al. "Treatment of Onychomycosis by ODT Therapy with 20% Urea Ointment and 2% Tolnaftate Ointment." *Dermatologica* 167:273–279, 1983.

40. South, David A., and Farber, Eugene M. "Urea Ointment in the Nonsurgical Avulsion of Nail Dystrophies—A Reappraisal." *Cutis* 25:609–612, 1980.

41. Hall, Trish. "These Herbs Give Football Players a Warm Sensation—in Their Feet." *Wall Street Journal* Jan. 13, 1984, p. 25.

42. Ibid.

43. Ibid.

44. "Consumer Expenditure Study." *Product Marketing* 13(8):22, 1984.

45. Stanley, Edith D. "Increased Virus Shedding with Aspirin Treatment of Rhinovirus Infection." *JAMA* 231:1248–1251, 1975.

46. "Sniffles and Sneezes? 'Take Two Zincs . . .' " *Medical World News* Feb. 13, 1984, p. 41.

47. News Front. "Zinc: Speeding Recovery from the Common Cold." *Modern Medicine* Jul. 1984, p. 43.

48. AP Laserphoto. "Cure for Cold?" *Durham Sun,* Nov. 14, 1983, p. 3-B.

49. Gonzalez, M. D., and Hogg, R. J. "Metabolic Alkalosis Secondary to Baking Soda Treatment of a Diaper Rash." *Pediatrics* 67:820–822, 1981.

50. Eichler, Ingeborg. "Cryptic Illness from Self-medication with Herbal Remedy." *Lancet* Feb. 12, 1983, p. 356.

51. Ries, Curt A., and Sahud, Mervyn A. "Agranulocytosis Caused by Chinese Herbal Medicines." *JAMA* 231:352–355, 1975.

# 5

# Over-the-Counter Drugs: Snake Oil or Self-Care?

How would you like relief from those television ads for hemorrhoidal remedies, laxatives, antacids, and medicines for gas? An alien scientist from outer space, tuning in on our nightly news, would conclude either that earthlings are plagued and preoccupied with digestive-tract problems, or that we have a love affair with laxatives.

Most people are reluctant to discuss their bad breath, body odor, dandruff, or gas in polite company, but the characters on the tube seem eager to share their most personal problems with millions of viewers. When the authoritative announcer holds up his hands for the umpteenth time to demonstrate how his preparation shrinks swelling of humongous hemorrhoids, aren't you just a little grossed out, or have you developed an immunity to over-the-counter (OTC) drug ads?

You'd think it would be easy to ignore those silly commercials that warn you of the dangers of dandruff, a dreadful disease which is likely to turn you into a social outcast unless you use the company's super shampoo. But most of us do worry, just a little, that we too might offend.

Drug manufacturers are masters at manipulating our insecurities. When they portray some poor nebbish with bad breath or, worse yet, body odor, we all cringe at the thought that if we're not careful it could happen to us. There—but for the grace of **Listerine, Scope, Dial,** and **Ban**—go we.

Hogwash. Now I don't have objections to people using soap or underarm deodorant. But it's high time we stopped falling for the ad man's high-pressure pitch. Americans spend over seven and a half billion dollars annually on nonprescription drugs.[1] And that doesn't even include the three billion we shell out on soaps, shampoos, and deodorants.

Care to know how it all breaks down? First, half a billion gets flushed on laxatives—I told you Americans are ridiculous about regularity. Find that hard to believe? Well, guess what the number-one over-the-counter drug is these days. Bet you'd never think of **Fleets Enema**. But each year it outsells such giants as **Maalox, Nyquil, Mylanta,** and even **Bayer.**[2]

We spend another $1.6 billion stifling sneezes and sniffles, and suppressing coughs. Vitamins and tonics take $1.3 billion, while diet aids, artificial sweeteners, and "natural" food supplements soak up $850 million.

Then there's pain. Americans must be hurting pretty bad, because we fork over $1.6 billion on OTC painkillers. And that doesn't even include the millions spent on arthritis rubs, salves, and ointments. Given our tendency to eat on the run, it's hardly surprising to learn that we burp up $600 million for antacids and other indigestion products. If you throw in the hundreds of millions more we spend on motion-sickness medicine, wart removers, wrinkle creams, hemorrhoidal suppositories, sleep aids, diarrhea drugs, jock-itch products, ear-wax removers, and goodness knows what else, you begin to get the idea that we are a nation of sickies.

When it comes to over-the-counter pills and potions, we are our own worst enemies. Here is one place where we cannot blame anyone else for our stupidity and bad reactions. Sure the drug companies' ads are tempting, but no one stands in the drugstore with a gun at our heads forcing us to buy **Anacin, Contac,** or **Rolaids.** This is where we all get to play doctor—for, by, and on ourselves. It's an interesting game filled with lots of opportunities, both good and bad.

There's the opportunity to save money by skipping a trip to the doctor. Then again, there's the opportunity to waste money on an OTC remedy containing worthless ingredients. You have a crack at relieving the symptoms of something far faster than you can get a doctor's appointment, but also a chance at completely misdiagnosing a condition that may need stronger medicine.

If you're going to play this game, the first thing to know is the rules. The first one is that the companies selling OTC remedies are more interested in marketing than medicine. There are two very good reasons for that.

First, most OTC concoctions differ little if at all from their competitors, so it is marketing, not effectiveness, that establishes a winner in the marketplace. Just walk into your local drugstore and mosey over to the cough and cold section. You will find dozens of products with exactly the same ingredients—antihistamines, decongestants, and painkillers—neatly lined up on the shelf. I don't care whether you pick **Allerest Sinus Pain Formula** over **Coricidin Sinus Headache Tablets**, or **Sinarest Extra Strength Tablets** over **Sine-Off Extra Strength**. They all contain chlorpheniramine, phenylpropanolamine (PPA), and acetaminophen.

Second, many of the OTC preparations just haven't been proven to do anything useful, so getting you to continue buying them is a classic exercise in selling the sizzle rather than the steak.

When the first edition of *The People's Pharmacy* was written, I thought many OTC drugs were at best a waste of money and at worst a definite danger. One report published in the *Journal of the American Medical Association* titled "Drug-induced Illness Leading to Hospitalization" implicated over-the-counter drugs in 18.1 percent of the hospital admissions.[3]

I warned that nonprescription drugs could be just as hazardous as those our physician prescribes. They may aggravate an already existing condition or, worse, mask the symptoms of an underlying disease until it is so bad corrective procedures may not be able to reverse the harm done.

But most folks believe OTCs are simple and safe. After all, you can buy them in supermarkets, convenience stores, even gas stations. With familiarity breeding contempt, many people don't bother to read the warnings on OTC drug containers. The New York Pharmaceutical Society demonstrated that of ten thousand people studied, 85 percent either did not follow the advice written on the container or did not comprehend its significance.

Even when people do take the time to read the label, it may not be very helpful. The print can be so small that you need a magnifying glass to read it. But even if it's legible, that doesn't mean it will be understandable. Often the information is written in gobbledygook that seems designed to confuse rather than to inform.

Next time you go to the drugstore, check out the drug interaction precaution on the back of a bottle of **Nyquil: "Do not take this product if you are presently taking a prescription antihypertensive or antidepressant drug containing MAO inhibitor except under the advice and supervision of a physician."**

What's that again? An MAO inhibitor? Give me a break, already. I find it inconceivable that a drug company would seriously expect a patient to know whether he is taking a blood pressure drug containing an MAO (monoamine oxidase) inhibitor. And how many people will really seek the "advice and supervision of a physician" when they take an over-the-counter drug like **Nyquil**? The answer is damn few!

Warnings and cautions aside, you'd think that by now the FDA would be able to guarantee that all drugs sold on pharmacy shelves would be safe and effective. That doesn't seem too much to ask of the guardian of our health. But so far, about all the agency has done is confirm the worst of my fears.

After reviewing almost all OTC ingredients, the feds discovered that for generations American consumers often had their pockets rather than their sinuses drained. In too many cases they've been relieved of their money, not their symptoms. All this time they've spent billions of dollars on hundreds of thousands of products, many of which have never been proven to do *anything,* let alone what they claimed they would do.

## The Overdue Over-the-Counter Review

How can I assert with such certainty that Americans have been ripped off on so many nonprescription medications? Well, it's all because of a little law Congress passed in 1962. At that time our legislators made a small change in the Federal Food, Drug, and Cosmetic (FDC) Act. Up until then, drugs were required to be proved *safe*—that's all, just safe—before getting put on the shelf. Anything that didn't cause toenails to crumble, hair to fall out, or people to keel over could be marketed to the public.

Given those standards, all sorts of things crawled into bottles, tubes, tubs, and vials. And as far as the manufacturers were concerned, anyone who could be convinced to pay for the privilege to swallow, sip, or smear their concoctions was fair game. And that included some of the biggest and most reputable drug companies in America.

In 1962 the FDC Act was amended to say OTC drugs had to be both safe *and effective*. That may not seem like it's asking very much of companies that are making billions of dollars a year with these products, but you should have heard the howling. A whole lot of manufacturers were not eager to step forward and prove that their products really did something. Maybe they feared it would be an exercise in futility.

At first the FDA didn't appear much more anxious to know the truth than the drug makers were to tell it. It took our faithful watchdog agency four years just to round up a panel of experts from the National Academy of Sciences (NAS) to check out a sample of OTC drugs. Three years later, in 1969, the FDA received a bombshell in its in-box. The NAS experts had found that only about 25 percent of the ingredients people were paying hard-earned money for could actually be shown to live up to their claims. There was no scientific proof of effectiveness for the rest.

You can probably imagine the FDA's reaction to that. Here folks were plunking down billions every year on popular brand-name concoctions monitored by the agency. Then along comes a superprestigious panel saying that three fourths of the ingredients might not live up to expectations. This definitely called for a closer look, and that's what it got . . . eventually.

## Slower than a Sleepy Snail

If you expected the FDA to spring into action, you've forgotten how slowly the wheels of bureaucracy can sometimes turn. After three years of futzing around, the agency began its official Over-the-Counter Drug Review in 1972. For the first time in history the feds hoped to find out which drugs actually worked and which didn't.

Seventeen expert panels were recruited to examine in detail seven hundred or so ingredients found in hundreds of thousands of products. The experts studied vaginal sprays and athlete's foot remedies, cough medicine and dandruff shampoos. They even looked into aphrodisiacs.

It's a big job, the FDA told the public, so please be patient. It will take us three to five years. We should have been so lucky. Eleven years later, in late 1983, the tale was ready to be told. The panels had found only one third of the ingredients to be both safe and effective! That's a little better than the results of the original NAS study, but still not much to be proud of.

In a public statement the FDA hastened to point out that the results didn't mean that only one third of all OTC products were safe and effective. It didn't? No, the FDA told us, because "Most popular products have safe and effective ingredients even if they sometimes contain other ingredients that are ineffective or have not yet been shown to be effective."[4] See, if you put one good thing in with three useless things and claim the whole mess works, that's not really so bad, is it? This is called "FDA math."

Besides, hope springs eternal. The panels classified ingredients into three categories. Category I contained compounds for which there was valid scientific evidence of safety and effectiveness. These things do what they say they do. Good guys, worth paying for if you need them.

Category II was for things that were either unsafe or ineffective. In spite of searching high and low, the panels couldn't find any evidence to justify this junk.

Then there's Category III, for which "available data are insufficient." This might be thought of as the dog-pound category, where hot potatoes, controversial cases, pet projects, and other such things got deposited in the hope they'd be picked up before someone got around to putting them to sleep. In a word, Category III became a wastebasket for drugs that lacked decent data. Rather than throw them out altogether, they passed into regulatory limbo to wait for new research to be completed.

This administrative dodge didn't go unchallenged. The Health Research Group (a Ralph Nader affiliate) sued the FDA. They pointed out that the 1962 law didn't say anything about "maybe" safe and effective. It said either a drug *was* safe and effective, or it *wasn't* to be on the market. Period, end of discussion. The federal judge—Judge John Sirica, of Watergate fame—apparently agreed and ordered the FDA to banish Category III.

The agency acted with its usual dispatch—it took two years to get the regulations in line with the law. Even then they fudged, since the rule allows the companies to keep these questionable substances on your drugstore shelf while testing continues. This gives the manufacturer further opportunity to come up with supporting data, and the American consumer further opportunity to come up with money for a drug that could eventually be yanked off the market when all the administrative games have been played out.

It's a long-running road show. Although all the panels have reported in, the game is far from over. You see, the FDA now publishes a "Proposed Monograph" for each and every one of the categories of product reviewed. It then ponders the comments elicited by these tomes, which you can bet are "bestsellers" to the industry.

This accumulated and digested wisdom merits yet another document, the "Tentative Final Monograph." More comments, more pondering. And finally, we're promised, a "Final Monograph," which will have the force of regulation. By the way, the FDA now estimates that the job will be done around the year 2000. Stay tuned, but please don't hold your breath. It wouldn't be the first time the agency was late.

## What's Really Going On

It's important for you to understand what's happening here, dear reader, because it affects both your pocketbook and your health. Needless to say, the time consumed in accomplishing the whole OTC review is an insult. The FDA has managed to drag the task out for more than *two decades,* and the end is nowhere in sight. All this time we are wasting money on thousands of drugs that probably will never be proven to do what they should.

We're talking big money. The marketers of OTC drugs are some of the biggest, most politically powerful groups in the country. They hire expensive lobbyists, funnel money to elected officials via political action committees, and do everything necessary to get their way. I'll bet you never thought of those as activities that had anything to do with your good health, did you? What's perhaps most amazing is that the 1962 FDC law revision ever got through in the first place.

Think of it as war and you'll have a much more accurate view of the matter than if you consider it a question solely of people who are interested in your health. The fight is for your dollars. The weapons are advertising, marketing know-how, political clout, and money. Especially money. These people would sell you snake oil if they could. In fact, a close look at some of the Review Panel results pretty much says that they *are* selling us the media-massaged, updated, new-and-improved, 1980s version of the very same stuff once peddled from the backs of wagons. If you don't believe that, let's take a look at some favorite American remedies.

## Sleep, Perchance to Dream

Have you ever had trouble sleeping? Most people have, at least once in a while. But while some people shrug off their insomnia, for others it may become an enormous problem. Having worked in a sleep laboratory I can vouch for the fact that many confirmed insomniacs who "never sleep a wink" actually get a far better night's sleep than they think. Subjects who were hooked up to electronic equipment (an electroencephalogram) that monitors brain activity repeatedly slept many hours each night, then claimed in the morning that they had had a horrible night.

Such people were obviously prime candidates for a little OTC magic. And drug companies have been only too happy to reinforce the idea that we all need a full eight hours of sleep every night. The ads imply that their spectacular sleeping pills will bring slumber swiftly and certainly. American consumers have been sold on the notion of sleeping pills to the point where they swallow millions of them every night just in case they might have a little trouble dozing off.[5]

**After aspirin, sleeping pills are the most widely used drugs in the United States. At a cost of more than $175 million, over 1 billion sleeping pills are swallowed every year, enough theoretically to put every man, woman and child in the nation to sleep for 200 hours.**[6]

With so much being spent on sleeping pills you would think Americans would be enjoying sweet dreams. But what the FDA review panel reported in 1978 was that *none* of the ingredients then being used in OTC sleep aids were effective.[7]

That was bad enough, but in 1979 a nightmare came true. A National Cancer Institute report revealed that methapyrilene, then a common ingredient in nonprescription sleeping pills, daytime sedatives, and allergy remedies, caused cancer. Dr. William Lijinsky, an internationally renowned cancer researcher, discovered that when he fed this drug to rats, virtually every animal developed liver tumors.[8] Such a high incidence of cancer is extraordinary and indicated that methapyrilene was an extremely potent carcinogen.

Amazing! Here was an over-the-counter compound used by millions of people to relieve insomnia, relax jittery nerves, and reduce allergic symptoms. It was found in hundreds of products, including **Allerest Time Release Capsules, Alva-Tranquil, Compoz, Cope, Dormin, Excedrin P.M., Nervine, Nite Rest, Nytol, Relax-U-Caps, Seedate, Sleepinal,** and **Sominex.**

What is so damn exasperating is that had anyone bothered to look, they would have known as far back as 1971 that methapyrilene didn't help put people to sleep. That was when two of the leading sleep researchers in this country, Drs. Joyce and Anthony Kales, published results of their tests on **Sominex:**

**The results of our sleep laboratory study of Sominex indicate that such sleep medications at the recommended dosage (2 tablets) are ineffective in relieving moderate to severe insomnia. . . . Results showed that Sominex in its recommended dose did not produce any favorable effects in terms of inducing sleep.**[9]

Now you can't get a whole lot plainer than that. By the way, what held true for **Sominex** should also have applied to drugs like **Compoz, Nite Rest, Nytol, Sleep-Eze,** and **Sure-Sleep**, since they all contained the same ingredient. But the FDA wasn't paying attention. So for years, insomniacs continued to pay for sleeping pills that not only didn't work, but probably increased their risk of cancer. Americans were unwitting guinea pigs while safety tests were conducted *after* products were already on pharmacy shelves.

In 1979, faced with growing evidence that methapyrilene posed a hazard and offered no benefit either as a sleeping pill or as a daytime sedative, the feds finally got around to banning this drug. Not surprisingly, the drug companies put up a howl, claiming that their products were "safe at recommended doses." But the handwriting was on the wall, and additional research proved beyond a shadow of a doubt that methapyrilene was indeed a powerful cancer-causing substance.[10-14]

You might think the manufacturers of OTC sleeping pills would have folded up their tents and disappeared into the night after all this bad news. But never underestimate drug companies. Remember, we're talking big bucks here. These folks were loathe to lose their lucrative market. Showing absolutely no chagrin over having marketed useless and dangerous sleeping pills for decades, they simply turned around and brewed up a new batch.

At first they tried a related compound called pyrilamine, but there wasn't any evidence it worked better than its discredited predecessor. So, they looked around to see which allergy pills made people the dopiest and settled on a drug called diphenydramine (**Benadryl**). Before you could say "**Nytol**," the most popular brand-name sleeping pills contained this antihistamine. That, friends, is why **Nytol** became **Nytol with DPH.**

Now DPH (short for diphenhydramine) is one of the most sedating of all antihistamines. Anyone who has ever had hay fever or hives and received a prescription for **Benadryl** can testify to the fact that the drug will knock you for a loop. I can only describe the reaction as a feeling of walking underwater.

In what should qualify for the chutzpah award, drug companies had turned to marketing a nostrum whose main effect is a side effect! In other words, the drowsiness associated with a prescription allergy medicine was being exploited as an OTC sleeping pill. So besides **Nytol with DPH**, there is now **Sominex 2, Sleepinal Maximum Strength Capsules, Compoz Nighttime Sleep Aid**, and **Sleep-Eze 3 Tablets.** All contain diphenhydramine. In fact, if you have hay fever or hives and have used **Benadryl** in the past, you could probably avoid a trip to the doctor and save money by buying some **Sleep-Eze** or **Sominex 2.** In its infinite wisdom the FDA made diphenhydramine available over-the-counter for sleep in 1982, but for allergies, you still needed a doctor's prescription until 1985. Crazy? You bet!

Well, what can you do for insomnia short of relying on heavy-duty prescription sleeping pills like **Dalmane?** A number of sleep experts suggest that you might be better off trying tryptophan. This is an amino acid, one of the substances from which the body builds proteins. In the body, tryptophan is converted into serotonin, a substance used by the brain to send chemical signals, including the sleep signal. A fair amount of evidence has accumulated over the years saying tryptophan can help a lot of people get to sleep easily, gently, and pleasantly.[15-17] No drug hangover, no hassles.

Where to get tryptophan? It's available at health-food stores, but another source may be even closer at hand—the refrigerator. A good source of tryptophan is milk. This may explain why Grandma's recommendation that you drink a warm glass of milk before bedtime had some validity. Tryptophan is also found in turkey, which could explain why most folks feel so sleepy after a big Thanksgiving dinner.

Here's a tip on how to maximize the tryptophan. Add some carbohydrate, such as a slice of toast, a cookie, or a cracker. It seems the amino acid is carried into the brain with greater ease if you combine it with carbos. A great-grandmother wrote to me with the following home remedy for insomnia—"a drink of warm milk made with instant breakfast and malt." Right on, Grandma! Common sense and practical experience can be worth a lot.

In pill form it may be necessary to take one to four grams of tryptophan to achieve the maximum benefit. The advantage of this therapy, notes an editorial in *JAMA*, is that it gets you to sleep "while producing remarkably little effect on sleep stages and the architecture of sleep."[18] The problem with most drugs given as sleeping pills is that they alter the normal pattern of sleep. It's not just a simple question of eight hours of sleep; you need a certain amount of what's known as "rapid eye movement" (REM) sleep in order to awaken feeling refreshed.

Writes one sleep researcher, "Any drug which further suppresses the slow-wave sleep and/or tampers with the adjustment of REM that appears to have taken place . . . actually exacerbates the insomniac's basic sleep problem, while giving the appearance of helping."[19]

What this means is that once people become regular sleeping-pill junkies (lots of folks take these drugs every night "just in case"), they may discover they now have more problems than they bargained for. What was only an occasional bout of insomnia may turn into a chronic sleep disorder. Even worse, daytime functioning may be affected as a result of REM-sleep deprivation, perhaps coupled with an antihistamine hangover.

Try the glass of milk first. Other possibilities that may make falling asleep easier include vigorous exercise during the day, a nice hot bath before bedtime, and satisfying sex. Then there is progressive muscle relaxation. Dr. Richard Surwitt, a professor at the Behavioral Physiology Lab of Duke University, has prepared a "Progressive Relaxation" tape and workbook that can help you learn how to relax tight muscles. You can buy his materials by making a check out to Duke University Medical Center for $9.95 and sending it to Dr. Surwitt at Box 3926, Duke Medical Center, Durham, NC 27710.

Dr. Surwitt's tape is good, but the Cadillac of relaxation tapes comes from Dr. Emmett Miller. If you want to treat your body and mind to an incredibly peaceful journey you *must* consider "Easing into Sleep" for $10.95. He has also prepared a tape called "The Healing Journey" and "Letting Go of Stress." Each tape is $10.95 and they can be purchased by calling (800) 227-

1617 or in California (800) 772-3545. Ask for extension 514. The address is: P.O. Box W, Stanford, CA 94305.

Believe me, I have no vested interest in Dr. Miller's tapes. If you aren't satisfied, you can return them for a full refund within two weeks of receipt. But I honestly believe this may be the cheapest and most effective way to learn how to relax, and that is a big part of the problem of insomnia.

If all else fails, you should probably seek help from a specialist. And I don't mean a family physician or even a psychiatrist. You may need to visit a sleep disorder center. There are now dozens of such centers around the country where specially trained clinicians can provide a full assessment of your sleep situation. They should be able to decide whether the restlessness is a result of stress, depression, or other causes that need to be dealt with by something besides a pill.

To find the closest center in your area you can write to the Association of Sleep Disorders Centers, P.O. Box 2604, Del Mar, CA 92014. And never forget the most important lesson of all: At their very best, sleeping pills cover up a sleep problem. They can never really resolve it.

## How Do You Spell Relief?

Drug companies have a vested interest in bellyaches. They love to see us bringing on billions of burgers, putting away pizza, pickles, and potato chips by the ton, and slurping soft drinks and coffee on the run. Each belch and bellyache represents another potential customer for all those OTC drugs designed to soothe the savage beast rumbling in our guts.

More than half a billion dollars a year is spent on antacid products alone.[20] **Maalox, Mylanta, Rolaids, Pepto-Bismol,** and **Alka-Seltzer** lead the list of nonprescription nostrums for tummy troubles. Unfortunately, although an incredible amount of money is spent on advertising such products, most consumers are never quite sure whether they should spell relief **R-O-L-A-I-D-S** or **T-U-M-S**.

Anyone with a television set has watched OTC products by the score go plop-plop, fizz-fizz. We have seen desperate souls rummaging in their medicine cabinets for relief from their indigestion and hangovers. TV announcers have soaked up gallons of acid with sponges and shaken flasks filled with gas bubbles. What they haven't told us is that many nonprescription stomach medicines may be dangerous for large segments of the population, and that choosing the right antacid can be a very difficult task.

Take, for example, **Alka-Seltzer Effervescent Pain Reliever and Antacid**. (Though you may be better off if you don't take it.) This one is a classic, achieving its phenomenal success in the marketplace largely by virtue of an extraordinary amount of money spent on advertising over the years. In 1983, for example, the company spent approximately $13 million trying to get us to *plop* and *fizz.* [21]

**Alka-Seltzer** is promoted for "fast relief of UPSET STOMACH with HEADACHE from overindulgence in food and drink." The medicine is supposed to neutralize acid, relieve heartburn, indigestion, and "sour stomach" (whatever that is), not to mention make you feel better after a hard night on the town. How well does it satisfy its claims?

All things considered, **Alka-Seltzer** probably can relieve acid indigestion. After all, it contains a tried and true antacid—baking soda (sodium bicarbonate). **Alka-Seltzer** will also take away your headache, not to mention your other aches and pains, since it relies on good old plain-Jane aspirin.

But the price you pay for this combination is absolutely incredible. A package of twelve foil-wrapped tablets can cost over two dollars. That amounts to only six doses (since the recommended dose is two tablets). For that amount of money you could buy over one hundred aspirin tablets and enough baking soda for hundreds of upset stomachs. Now that combination might not fizz for you, but I am not convinced all those little bubbles are worth the extra money you pay for **Alka-Seltzer**.

Price aside, there are other reasons to be wary. The combination of a painkiller with an antacid is of very dubious medical value. For just a garden-variety headache, you do not need an antacid. If you have indigestion or an upset stomach, the last thing you want is aspirin. That is a little like trying to put out a fire with gasoline. Even though dropping the tablets into a glass of water converts the aspirin to a much less irritating formulation called sodium acetylsalicylate, it offers no benefit for heartburn.

More important, anyone who has had any alcohol in his system shouldn't consume aspirin. In a person who is drinking, the stomach lining loses its protective coating and becomes exceedingly sensitive to the hemorrhage-potentiating effects of aspirin. Of course many people have come to believe that **Alka-Seltzer** is the best hangover remedy money can buy because this is one of the many "overindulgences" for which the drug has been hyped. And while I don't doubt that dissolved aspirin is far easier on the tum than a solid tablet, you'd be better off waiting till the morning after before glugging any potential cures for hangover headaches.

There's one unexpected ingredient in **Alka-Seltzer**, and in a lot of the other OTC antacids, that millions of people should avoid, and that's sodium. For those on any sort of salt-restricted diet, a dose of **Alka-Seltzer** could be the equivalent of falling completely off the wagon. Why? Let's see. There are 551 mg of sodium in an **Alka-Seltzer** tablet. That makes 1,102 mg for the average two-tablet dose. Two doses and anyone trying to keep their sodium to 2 grams or less a day (equal to about one teaspoon of salt) has already blown the show.

Another hidden ingredient in many antacids (fortunately not in **Alka-Seltzer**) is sugar. Take pity on the poor folks who are diabetic, or on a diet, or in any other way facing a restriction on their sugar intake. Should they decide to suck or slurp one of many of the popular antacids on the market, chances are they will get a whopping dose of sugar.

A mere 15 milliliters (about a tablespoon) of liquid, or one tablet, will dose people with the following amounts of sugar:[22]

**Mylanta-II** liquid, 2,000 mg
**Gaviscon-2** tablets, 2,400 mg
**AlternaGel** liquid, 2,000 mg
**Gaviscon** tablets, 1,200 mg
**Gaviscon** liquid, 1,500 mg
**Mylanta-II** tablets, 918 mg
**Maalox Plus** tablets, 575 mg

When we're looking at up to 4,800 mg of sugar for two pills or tablespoonsful, the intake of sugar is far from trivial. For some, it could even be dangerous.

This illustrates a problem that we see time after time with OTC drugs. Instead of selling one effective ingredient to deal with one problem, the companies engage in a veritable orgy of chemical mixing. Like some alchemist gone wild, they toss in all sorts of ingredients, for all sorts of reasons. And many of those reasons have a lot more to do with marketing than they do with medicine.

Perhaps you've heard of simethicone? If you have, it's probably because of the television ads promising that one or another antacid with the added wonder ingredient simethicone would gobble up all that nasty gas that is presumably torturing you.

Actually, the gas problem would be considerably relieved if all the hot air in these commercials were to be released. All simethicone does is make big bubbles out of little ones. When you suffer a bloated, distended feeling after eating, it's usually because you ate too much. It has little if anything to do with "gas," and all the simethicone in Siberia will not do anything to relieve that problem. The solution to our after-eating stuffiness is to lighten up at the table.

That's not to say it's impossible to have gas. Everyone does. It comes either from swallowing air while eating, or as a by-product of the digestion of food in the intestine. Gas is produced from the fermentation of undigested sugars, and some people have a harder time digesting certain foods, particularly beans, broccoli, onions, and cabbage. Now hear this: Nothing—no

OTC remedy—will alter the amount of gas your body produces. Gross though it may be, the only cure is to pass the gas.

## So What's Good for Indigestion?

Well, gee, what about **Tums** and **Rolaids** and all their friends? Aren't antacids good for anything? Sure. Antacids are good for exactly what their name says: for neutralizing acid. At one time or another, most of us will experience indigestion. But what does that mean?

Indigestion is one of those terms that are supposed to cover a multitude of sins. Doctors have taken to prescribing **Tagamet** (cimetidine) or **Zantac** (ranitidine) whenever a patient burps or complains of amorphous stomach pain, but these drugs are expensive and there are some downsides to their use.

Most people reach for an OTC product before they head off to the doctor's office. Ask the average person why he is gorping down **Bromo-Seltzer, Di-Gel,** or **Maalox** and he is likely to complain of belching, heartburn, or "sour stomach." Indigestion is a garbage term that can include everything from stomachache and nausea to gas pains and overstuffing.

Some people even consider their chest pains to be indigestion. This is extremely dangerous, since heart trouble often manifests itself with symptoms many people mistakenly attribute to "indigestion." We now know that up to 25 percent of all heart attacks may go unrecognized.[23] Many of these so-called "silent" heart attacks produce few if any symptoms and "indigestion"-like discomfort may be the only tip-off that something bad is happening to the heart.

It is clear then that people may be treating a multitude of different and complex problems under a single heading—indigestion. In many cases, an ulcer is responsible for the misdiagnosed generalization of heartburn. Unsupervised use of antacids may merely mask a serious situation temporarily, without allowing the ulcer to heal. A physician may recommend antacid therapy, but he will likely prescribe the antacids in a form and dose that will actually do some good.

A few guidelines may serve to help you decide when it is important to see a doctor and when to treat yourself. Certainly an occasional attack of stomach upset is no big deal, especially if you know that it was caused by combining pickles, pizza, and hot peppers. When the attacks start occurring more than once every few weeks over a period of months, however, then it is time to hightail it to a doctor. Equally, *any* severe attack that is associated with difficulty in getting your breath or vomiting is worth a trip to the medic. And if pain starts moving down your arm or up to your jaw, head for the emergency room. You might be having a not-so-silent heart attack.

For the moment, let's assume your occasional heartburn is simply a result of an argument with the boss or a minor dietary indiscretion. What is going on, and what can you do about it? There is a sphincter, or ring of muscle, at the bottom of the esophagus that is supposed to keep acid out. When that ring of muscle doesn't quite do its job and acid from the stomach creeps up and irritates the esophagus, you've got heartburn.

Here are some tips to try before running to the medicine chest. First, please try to give up cigarettes. Stopping smoking is probably the best thing you could possibly do for your digestive tract. Losing weight can also be a big help, and if you can give up alcohol and aspirin, you would also be heading in the right direction. Fatty food, chocolate, coffee, orange juice, and spicy tomato drinks may also be adding to your woe.

After that, give gravity a boost. Sit upright or stand for a while after eating. If you can stand it, try sleeping with the head of the bed elevated eight to ten inches. Also try lying on your left side. That will go a long way toward keeping acid from oozing back up into your esophagus.

In addition to all this, you will undoubtedly find that an antacid can provide gratifying relief, especially for garden-variety indigestion. Before rushing out to buy one, however, take a look in the cupboard. It's very likely you already have on hand one of the best, cheapest, and most effective antacids—plain old baking soda (sodium bicarbonate). If the image of someone drinking baking soda in water seems less macho than the idea of a high-powered executive munching **Maalox** or **Mylanta** (containing aluminum and magnesium), so be it. But baking soda is a reasonable home remedy for indigestion.

Now if you want to go out and spend a lot of money buying virtually the same active ingredient with a brand name and some flavorings, rush for the drugstore and grab **Bell/ans** or **Soda Mint**. **Alka-Seltzer Effervescent Antacid** also contains sodium bicarbonate (as well as citric acid and potassium bicarbonate). Just remember, you will be paying mostly for fancy packaging and advertising.

A word of caution about sodium bicarbonate is in order. Even though a half-teaspoon of baking soda in eight ounces of water will do the trick for indigestion just about as well as many OTC antacids, you should be aware that its sodium content is quite high. It should be avoided by those on salt-restricted diets, and shouldn't be used on a long-term basis by anyone.

One other warning is worth your attention. If you have really overindulged—in other words, pigged out—*do not* reach for the baking soda to relieve the bloated, full feeling. A report from the FDA has warned of an unusual hazard associated with sodium bicarbonate. A man who had a gigantic Mexican meal took baking soda to relieve his discomfort. Instead, he experienced excruciating pain and passed out.

During emergency surgery the doctors discovered that his stomach had a hole in it, apparently caused by the extremely rapid buildup of carbon dioxide gas from the baking soda. Because his stomach had already been stretched to its limits, there was no room for the gas to escape. A miniexplosion actually blew a hole in his gut.

Fortunately, this fellow's life was saved, but it was a close call. FDA staffers immediately checked the scientific literature for similar events, and sure enough, they found about half a dozen cases reported since 1845. Clearly, this kind of reaction is a medical rarity, but it does serve to remind us to maintain moderation in all things. And if we do overindulge, we should at least

be cautious about how we seek relief. Nevertheless, for someone
with a rare attack of indigestion without any complicating problems, sodium bicarbonate will do the job without straining the
pocketbook.

Okay, you're tired of home remedies and you hate the taste of
baking soda. I don't blame you, it's not my idea of an antacid
taste treat either. Well what about r-e-l-i-e-f . . . is it really spelled
**Rolaids**?

**Rolaids** contains dihydroxyaluminum sodium carbonate.
Whew. Sounds like that ought to cure something, doesn't it? The
aluminum hydroxide is the key. It has less capacity to neutralize
acid than baking soda, but it will get the job done . . . eventually.
(Aluminum hydroxide takes a while to get to work, which may
be why we also see sodium carbonate in **Rolaids**. Which is also
its undoing. There is a high enough sodium level in **Rolaids** to
make its regular use questionable for those on low-salt diets. But
back to aluminum.) The problem with aluminum salts, which
also show up in antacids such as **AlternaGel, Aluminum Hydroxide Gel,** and **Amphojel,** is that they frequently cause constipation. Chances are pretty good that anyone who downs such
antacids regularly will be plugged up. This side effect can sometimes be put to good advantage if you have a bout with diarrhea.
As an antacid, though, pure aluminum salts do have their drawbacks.

Wait. Can this ingredient be saved? What would happen if we
combined it with another good antacid that had a tendency to
produce a laxative effect?

Magnesium hydroxide is that other antacid. Never heard of it?
Of course you have, except that you know it as **Milk of Magnesia.** While most people think of **Milk of Magnesia** for its justly
famed laxative qualities, the stuff is actually a fine antacid as
well. At least you won't have heartburn while you're sitting in
the john.

Mixing aluminum and magnesium yields products that, to a
greater or lesser degree, cancel out each other's unwanted gastric
consequences. So what you get is a long-lasting antacid with
relatively few side effects. Among these combination antacids are

Aludrox, Alurex, A.M.T., Creamalin, Delcid, Di-Gel, Estomul-M, Gaviscon tablets, Gelusil, Kessadrox, Kolantyl, Kudrox, Maalox, Magna Gel, Magnatril, Mylanta, Riopan, Silain-Gel, Simeco, Syntrogel, and WinGel.

With so many brands containing aluminum and magnesium, how do you pick the best buy for the money? Surprisingly, some of the most familiar brands appear to provide excellent acid-neutralizing action at a reasonable cost. These include **Maalox TC** (Therapeutic Concentrate), **Mylanta II**, and **Gelusil II**. Also scoring very high as good buys are **Delcid** and **Simeco**.[24, 25] One bonus with **Mylanta II** and **Maalox TC** is flavor. A tasting party conducted at the Oregon Health Sciences University found that volunteers preferred these two brands over the competition.[26] For a more complete evaluation of aluminum- and magnesium-containing antacids, see the table at the end of this chapter.

## Aluminum and Alzheimer's: Is There a Connection?

There's one additional question about aluminum that I would prefer not to tackle because the data are so murky. Let me warn you right off that trying to make sense out of the aluminum–Alzheimer's connection is at this moment almost impossible. There are no easy answers.

Given that, let me plunge ahead and at least try to present this controversy as objectively as possible. Several years ago researchers discovered that aluminum had accumulated in the tangled nerve cells of Alzheimer's disease patients.[27, 28] Investigators have also found that when aluminum is administered to animals it can produce pathological changes in brain tissue.[29, 30] And patients who require kidney dialysis sometimes develop "dialysis dementia" because aluminum accumulates in their brains.[31]

All this has led some scientists to speculate that aluminum may be somehow linked to Alzheimer's disease.[32, 33] One group of pharmacologists and toxicologists has gone so far as to caution that many people, especially older patients who may be susceptible to senility, should cut back on their aluminum exposure. They point out that this mineral is ubiquitous in the environment:

> Since there are no demonstrable consequences of aluminum deprivation, the prophylactic reduction of aluminum intake by many patients would appear prudent. . . . The most common foods that contain substantial amounts of aluminum-containing additives include some processed cheeses, baking powders, cake mixes, frozen doughs, pancake mixes, self-raising flours and pickled vegetables. The aluminum-containing non-prescription drugs include some antacids, buffered aspirins, antidiarrhoeal products, douches and haemorrhoidal medications.[34]

Wow! Little more than a decade ago most researchers didn't believe aluminum was even absorbed from antacids. Most people believed that it passed through the digestive tract virtually intact. But now we know that it can be absorbed into the body. Whether that's a problem, though, is up for grabs.

The Associated Pharmacologists and Toxicologists, who warned about aluminum exposure, have, in essence, recommended that older people reduce their intake of buffered aspirin (the buffers usually contain aluminum), aluminum-containing antacids, and many foods like processed cheese and cake mixes. Some folks have even gone so far as to suggest that you may want to consider throwing out your aluminum pots and pans or be extra cautious about not cooking anything acidic, such as tomatoes or tart applesauce in them.[35]

If all this scares the wits out of you, please don't panic. The truth is that we are faced with a puzzle: Is aluminum the chicken or the egg? At the time of this writing no one knows whether aluminum contributes to senility or whether the accumulation of this metal in brain tissue occurs as a consequence of Alzheimer's disease.

Dr. Katherine L. Bick, director of the National Institute of

Neurological and Communicative Disorders and Stroke, states that the "evidence concerning the role of aluminum has been contradictory. But it's clearly not the prime cause, because [people have been exposed to aluminum in] so many situations without any particular increase in the risk of Alzheimer's disease."[36]

Investigators at the National Institute of Mental Health who have been looking into this issue have reported that "there is no evidence that Alzheimer's disease patients are more likely to have taken aluminum-containing antacids" than anyone else.[37, 38] Other experts have also concluded that any aluminum accumulation in the brain is secondary to the Alzheimer's condition.[39]

So where does all this research leave us? Well, you pay your money and you take your chances. I warned you it would be inconclusive. And I sure don't have any answers. I seriously doubt that there is any risk from cooking with aluminum pots and pans as long as you do not cook anything highly acidic or salty, like tomato sauce or sauerkraut. I myself like those old-fashioned cast-iron pans that weigh a ton. They cook like crazy, and there is the added bonus that they supply some iron, something that is surely safe and often lacking in our diets.

As far as the safety of aluminum-containing antacids is concerned, I'm not worried, yet. There is certainly no evidence of danger at this point. But the final chapter hasn't been written, and it is hard to tell what the future holds.

## Sticks and Stones May Break Your Bones, but So Could Aluminum

Alzheimer's disease aside, there is growing concern that aluminum-containing antacids could be undesirable for another reason. Older women are at a higher risk of developing osteoporosis, which weakens the bones and makes them more susceptible to fractures. As many as fifteen million people may suffer some degree of osteoporosis. Every year, hundreds of thousands of older people break wrists, arms, legs, and hips because their bones have become thin and weakened. Such fractures are slow to heal, and complications are a leading cause of death in the elderly. We're talking about a very big problem here.

Anything that could increase the risk of weakened bones should naturally be avoided, and aluminum just may be a bad guy. A number of reports in the medical literature suggest a connection between aluminum and soft bones. One sixty-year-old woman had to be admitted to the hospital because of pain and weakness in her legs, which made it impossible for her to rise from a chair or walk without support.[40] X-rays suggested osteoporosis, which would have been hard to treat. But the doctors discovered something else when they looked at her lab results. She had very low blood-phosphate levels, and there was no phosphate in her urine.

Here was a mystery. But these physicians were on their toes. They realized that symptoms of bone pain and weakness in combination with similar metabolic changes "have been induced in normal volunteers by prolonged treatment with aluminum-containing antacids."[41] Checking the medical history, they found that:

The only notable incident in the patient's medical history was a "hiatus hernia" that was manifested as burning epigastric pain [heartburn], for which she had taken magnesium aluminum hydroxide liquid antacid (Maalox) for 12 years before admission. Initially, she had taken approximately 120 ml [4 oz] of antacid per day, but for at least six months before admission she had taken 360 ml [12 oz] or more daily.[42]

The doctors immediately stopped her antacid regimen, and by the end of one month,

the patient noted dramatic clinical improvement. She was able to rise unassisted from a chair and was only rarely using her walker. The pain in her legs had improved consid-

**erably. Three months after discharge she was ambulating
[doctor talk for walking] freely and without pain.**[43]

Phosphate, like calcium, is an essential element for healthy
bones. Large doses of aluminum grab on to phosphate found in
food, prevent its absorption into the body, and ultimately may
deplete phosphate from the system. This can lead to calcium loss,
which in turn may cause slow and insidious bone weakening.[44, 45] Recent reports in the medical literature suggest that men
as well as women may be at risk.[46-49]

Now of course we're talking big doses here, folks. The patients
that have shown up with bone pain, malaise, muscular weakness,
and bone problems were gorping down lots of aluminum-containing antacid over long periods of time. One poor fellow was
consuming seventy-two ounces of **Maalox** [over two quarts] a
week.[50]

So what does this mean for you? Well, if you have a rare bout
of indigestion and reach for the **Maalox, Mylanta,** or **Gelusil,** I
feel reasonably certain you have little to worry about. But if you
are one of those people who is in the habit of sucking on aluminum-containing antacids as if they were candy, you might be
asking for trouble. And older women who glug gallons of the
chalky glop to save their stomachs may increase the risk of
weakening already susceptible bones.

## Calcium to the Rescue

In the first edition of *The People's Pharmacy,* I was lukewarm
when it came to calcium carbonate, the primary antacid ingredient in **Tums** (for the tummy), **Tums E-X (extra strength), Alka-2
Chewable, Alkets, Amitone, Chooz, Dicarbosil, Glycate, Gustalac, Pama, Ratio,** and **Titralac.**

As an antacid, calcium carbonate is fast-acting and also capable of neutralizing stomach acidity. Even more promising, it is
cheap and keeps working for a relatively long time. Sounds great.
Why my earlier lack of enthusiasm? For one thing, gastroen-

terologists were pushing aluminum-magnesium antacids, and I bought their line. For another, there were lots of reports in the medical literature that calcium carbonate caused something called acid rebound. As a result of this information I unabashedly wrote the following drivel in 1974:

> Unluckily, we have to cross this otherwise great antacid off our list of beneficial drugs. It works, but it has the nasty habit of stimulating your own sad tummy to start producing acid. So the good acid-neutralizing effect of calcium carbonate is undone by its ability to simulate excessive acidity. You may find yourself consuming countless tablets and trapped, just like the nose-drop junkies who have to keep spraying their congested noses to relieve the stuffiness caused by the rebound effect of the drops. It also has the potential to make kidney-stone sufferers much worse with its high calcium level. So all you Tums-takers, just cool it.[51]

Well, baloney, I'm afraid. Of course, in those days I tended to believe what I read in medical textbooks. And since decent research on this question was lacking, I bought the party line. Well, I can now admit I was wrong. Calcium carbonate *is* an excellent antacid and does not have to be discarded for fear of acid rebound.

An editorial in the *Journal of the American Medical Association* discusses this issue, and I think it puts calcium in a much more favorable light.

> We may ask why calcium carbonate, a more potent antacid than aluminum magnesium, is no longer actively used in the treatment of peptic ulcer. Its form, palatability, frequency of administration, potency, and duration of action can be balanced with aluminum mangesium antacids. Many claim that calcium antacids cause "acid rebound," rendering them therapeutically untenable. Despite statements to the contrary, this partial truth persists.

These statements stem from studies employing double and quadruple the usual clinical dose of 2 g [grams] of calcium carbonate. Moreover, the experimental methods of these studies have been questioned. . . . Since then, others have shown that equivalent neutralizing doses of calcium, aluminum magnesium antacids, and sodium bicarbonate all produce acid rebound.[52]

So calcium carbonate doesn't seem to be worse than any other antacids when it comes to acid rebound. Almost anything can cause the stomach to stimulate acid production, including milk.

The moral of this tale is that calcium is an excellent acid neutralizer and can probably be used safely for occasional bouts of indigestion. Large doses for long periods of time may produce excessive calcium levels, and this could get you into metabolic trouble (alkalosis) and be dangerous for people with kidney problems. But overall, I now feel comfortable recommending such antacids as **Tums, Alka-2, Alkets, Titralac,** and any others containing calcium carbonate.

Well, that's good news, but there's another bonus with such products besides effective acid neutralization. As bad as aluminum may be for bones, calcium may be good. Remember that calcium plays an important role in keeping bones strong. Surveys have shown that as many as half of the women over thirty-five years of age have diets that provide far less than the recommended dietary allowance (RDA) for calcium (800 mg). And some experts now think the RDA itself is low. There is evidence that adults need at least 1.2 grams a day, not just to prevent bone loss but also to keep blood pressure down.[53-56] In recent years, some doctors have found signs of bone loss in women as young as twenty-five.[57]

Unfortunately, our eating habits don't come close to providing adequate calcium levels. Mothers are telling their children to "Drink your milk," while they themselves are sipping coffee, juice, or diet soda. Fess up. How often do you drink a quart of milk a day? And when is the last time you ate tofu? Cheese and yogurt are good sources of calcium, but cheese is also high in fat, and much of the yogurt sold today contains lots of sugar. Greens are rich in calcium, but few people eat enough collards, kale, or watercress to do much good.

In order to get close to 1,000 or 1,500 mg of calcium a day, most people need nutritional supplements. That's where your choice of antacid comes in. As strange as this may sound, antacids like **Tums** can provide extra calcium at a reasonable price.[58] After all, the primary ingredient in **Tums, Titralac, Chooz, or Alka-2** is calcium carbonate, the same kind of calcium found in vitamins and supplements.

To reach the RDA of 800 mg you would have to swallow four **Tums** a day, since only about 40 percent of each 500-mg tablet is pure calcium. This averages out to about fifteen cents per 800 mg, which is comparable to calcium supplements like **Caltrate 600** and is considerably less than the twenty-five or thirty cents you would pay for some calcium products.

Now I am not recommending that everyone past thirty-five should start popping antacids every day just to get extra calcium. But if you're worried about osteoporosis, you might want to talk to your doctor about diet and supplementation. You should also make sure you get a little Vitamin D and magnesium.

Most important of all, make regular exercise a habit. There is growing evidence that exercise is just as important as diet in maintaining healthy bones. Walking, running, tennis, and bike riding (even on a stationary bicycle) can all be helpful in preventing bone loss. And if you do need something for that occasional bout of indigestion, calcium-containing antacids seem to be your best bet, particularly if you are concerned about daily calcium intake.

Well, my friend, would you ever have imagined in your wildest dreams that selecting something as simple as an antacid could be so bewildering? For years you've been watching those commercials on TV for **Alka-Seltzer, Rolaids, Maalox,** and **Tums,** but all you saw was plopping and fizzing or sponges sopping up simulated acid.

Advertisers are not anxious to talk about aluminum and weak

bones, or about sodium and hypertension. Now you've had a crash course in antacids, and you can see that over-the-counter drugs can be complicated. And we haven't even discussed all the problems that can occur when you start mixing and matching. Antacids interact with many prescription drugs. So selecting the right brand is not as easy as you thought. Advertising is just about the last place to look for the information you need to make the right decisions.

## Mouthwash: Is It Good for Anything?

Mouthwash probably should be sold with lipstick and face powder, because its effects are entirely cosmetic. Millions upon millions of dollars have been spent trying to convince you that **Listerine, Lavoris,** or **Scope** will kill germs and prevent bad breath, as if the two ideas were somehow linked. And the American public, fearing social, sexual, or job failure, has bought in to the idea, to the tune of about $350 million a year.[59]

When the FDA Review Panel got around to mouthwashes, they didn't think these claims smelled so good. The experts concluded that there were few, if any, reasons to justify the use of over-the-counter mouthwashes, mouth rinses, and gargles containing antiseptics or antimicrobial agents.[60, 61]

There was a slight problem with the mouthwash claims, inasmuch as none—zero, zip, blank, void—*none* of the oral germ killers could substantiate its effectiveness. That was hardly a surprise to anyone familiar with oral health. First of all, lots of microbes live happily in every mouth, causing no problems at all. Second, any mouthwash would reach only a fraction of the throat and thus kill only a fraction of the bugs.

And third, any bacteria that succumbed would be replaced in almost no time. That's especially true if, as the ads imply, a given mouthwash made you so sexually appealing that someone just couldn't wait to kiss you. That's worth a few million germs right there.

Bad breath, like indigestion, is merely a catchall term for a symptom common to many varied and different problems. A normal healthy mouth will not have an offensive odor, though it is true that almost everyone experiences a furry, scuzzy mouth upon rising. Believe me, "morning mouth" is no big deal. It will disappear rapidly with talking or after breakfast, since it is due to the oral inactivity of sleeping, a period of time when bacteria can act freely on food particles.

While it is true that your mouth is loaded with germs (a normal adult probably has around ten million bugs in every drop of saliva), that is the way it is supposed to be. There are all sorts of beasties living in happy harmony in your oral cavity—from strep and staph to diplococci and spirochetes. But these microscopic flora and fauna are important in keeping everything in balance, and without some of them this equilibrium could become upset. Any disturbance in our natural germ population could leave us more sensitive to invading microorganisms.

Mouthwashes do upset our normal resident flora. Whether that's bad or good no one really knows. But some dental specialists I have consulted worry that "the depression of the normal bacterial flora by these mouthwashes leads to overabundance of *Candida albicans,* followed by the appearance of the white patches characteristic of moniliasis" (thrush).[62]

Okay, so I've got you a little nervous about overdosing on mouthwash. But I can almost hear you exclaim, "What about onion breath?" After all, drug companies have spent tens of millions of dollars trying to convince us that our indulgence in onions or garlic will turn us into social outcasts unless we gargle with their superbrand.

The makers of **Scope** took this one step further in their battle against the makers of **Listerine**. Ads in magazines showed a man and woman with the most rapturous look on their faces. What produced this nirvana? Why, the "onion test," of course. They have their noses jammed up to within an inch of a cut raw onion that has been dipped in **Scope**, and they look like they are in heaven. You the consumer are encouraged to capture this bliss by trying it yourself:

1. Cut a smelly onion in half and smell it.
2. Dip half the onion in Scope. Dip the other half in the leading antiseptic mouthwash.
3. Now smell them both. The half you dipped in Scope smells minty-fresh. The other half smells mediciney.

If Scope can make a smelly onion minty-fresh, imagine what it can do to your breath.[63]

Can you imagine anything less enticing than a "mediciney" *or* a "minty-fresh" onion? What nonsense! Such a test should be declared illegal on the grounds that it represents cruelty to dumb onions.

Have you ever wondered why a mouthwash doesn't really seem to take care of garlic and onion breath, graphically illustrated TV ads notwithstanding? Simple. The problem isn't in your mouth.

Garlic and onions contain highly volatile oils. Once swallowed, their odoriferous chemicals are absorbed from your stomach into your bloodstream. From there they circulate through your body, reaching your lungs, where they are exhaled with each breath. You would have to stop breathing in order to really block out onion breath. I've always felt that's a tad drastic for a minor dietary indiscretion, especially since I have a fondness for raw onion sandwiches myself. You might be able to overpower the smell for a very few minutes with the most strongly scented of the mouthwashes, but as for really doing anything about the problem—forget it.

Sound like we've been had again? You bet. But it's even worse than just wasted money. True bad breath—halitosis—is a symptom. It's nature's way of saying something has gone wrong in a system that normally takes care of itself pretty well. The problem might be a festering sinus or throat infection, a decaying tooth, or gum problems. All are potentially very serious, and covering them up with mouthwash is an invitation to disaster.

The American Dental Association's Council on Dental Therapeutics has this to say: "If marked breath odor persists after proper toothbrushing, the cause should be investigated."[64]

How about sore throats? Surely something as mediciney-tasting as **Listerine** must be good for a sore throat even if it doesn't do anything great for onion breath? Wrong again. In the first place, the infection responsible for your sore throat is in such a location that a brief gargle will not amount to much. Even if you bathe the affected tissue for many minutes, you could not kill the bugs responsible. Most sore throats are due to virus infections which will respond neither to antibiotics or mouthwashes.

There are other problems with mouthwashes. The FDA panel found that many popular brands contain ingredients for which safety and effectiveness data are lacking. Then there's the alcohol problem. Most popular mouthwash brands contain alcohol, and lots of it. Some of the numbers:

**Astring-O-Sol** (undiluted), 65 percent
**Listerine**, 26.9 percent
**Scope**, 18.5 percent
**K-Mart Amber**, 30 percent
**Oral Pentacresol**, 30 percent
**Cepacol**, 14 percent
**Isodine Mouthwash Gargle Concentrate**, 35 percent
**Odara**, 48 percent

Since most people don't drink their mouthwash, getting high isn't the problem. But getting dry could be. Alcohol acts to dry out tissues. If you go after a sore throat with a gargle of mouthwash, you can dry out and irritate throat tissues already dried and irritated by an infection. In fact, the drying effect of heating systems has been blamed for a large part of the rise in throat infections during the winter. The same bugs are around all year, but they have a better chance of finding a place to live when throat tissues are abnormally dry. Tossing something that's one-third or more alcohol into the back of your throat may up the risk.

Evidence has recently come to light that some mouthwashes could eventually justify their existence by reducing plaque, the buildup of bacteria on tooth surfaces which accounts for decay and some gum disease. Preliminary evidence suggests that some mouthwash ingredients, used in conjunction with brushing and flossing, can make a significant impact on the quantity of plaque in the mouth.

Results are preliminary, and mouthwashes have such a long history of making unsubstantiated claims that many wary observers are taking a "wait and see" attitude for the moment. There are specially formulated antiplaque mouthwashes already being used in Europe. Most contain the ingredient chlorhexidine. It's an effective plaque remover, but one not yet approved by the FDA for use in the United States.

For the moment, see mouthwashes for what they are—cosmetics. They can indeed produce a momentary freshness in the mouth, and that might be a real relief on a morning when a furry tongue and dragon-mouth seem too much to bear. But keep in mind that you're paying a high cost for a chore that could be equally well accomplished with a thorough brushing and flossing.

If you really have to gargle in order to satisfy some primeval urge, the best thing to use is what doctors always recommend: one-half teaspoon of salt (any stronger concentration may be irritating) in an eight-ounce glass of water. It will moisten your mucous membranes with a physiological solution, and the very act of gargling should make your mouth and throat feel better. If you have indulged in onions or garlic, you can chew on some gum or suck a breath mint, but why not accept your fate and just maintain an appropriate distance from friends and loved ones till this minor side effect wears off?

## In the Pits

We live in a sanitized society. Killing germs and stamping out odors is practically a national pastime. We have deodorant soaps, deodorant tampons, foot deodorants, underarm deodorants, and more recently, genital deodorants. The cost to the consumer for underarm deodorants alone is in excess of $800 million a year.

Now believe me, I am as offended by unpleasant smells as the
next guy, but enough is enough. Cleanliness may be next to
godliness, but this passion for sterilizing our skin and deodorizing body cavities has very little to do with personal hygiene. I
mean, seriously, folks, aren't genital deodorants carrying things
a BIT too far?

Body odor occurs when bacteria normally present on the skin
attach to and decompose organic material contained in perspiration. Since we all sweat to one degree or another, we all smell
sometimes. On the average we put out around one-half quart of
sweat a day (save that one for your next cocktail party). Perspir-
ing is a means of maintaining body temperature and is really an
important body process.

Nervous tension and emotional stress can contribute a significant amount of sweat above the normal level. This nervous sweat
comes from an entirely different set of pores, and seems to be
broken down much more readily by bacteria. There really is a
"smell of fear."

Obviously, good hygiene (lots of soap and water) will go a long
way toward keeping down both the bacterial level and the accumulation of sweat. But you can't shower five times a day, and
clearly there are times when you really do need that "all-day
protection." Since we cannot keep our underarms clean and dry
all the time, a deodorant is a handy thing to have around.

But what should you select? They all sound fantastic. There's
**Soft & Dri, Sure, Arrid Extra Dry, Ultra-Ban, 5-Day,** and
**Tickle,** to name just a few. How do you know which is the best
brand for the least money?

Some advertisers will try to lure you with claims of extra
long-lasting protection, while others will tell you that their product goes on dry. Since there are relatively few active ingredients
in most of the brands on the market, the companies spend incredible sums trying to come up with subtle variations so they can
create new and innovative advertising campaigns.

Take the Gillette Company, for example. A company official
bragged that "This company knows more about armpits" than
any of the competitors.[65] It also knew the power of the buck.

When Gillette launched **Dry Idea**, says the *Wall Street Journal,* it spent $18 million on promotion and advertising:

> **The company concedes that Dry Idea won't stop perspiration any better than at least five products on the market for some time, but no matter. For Gillette says its product "goes on dry," feels better—and thus leads the user to feel it is more effective. And the company is backing the stuff with more advertising and promotion than any other product in its 77-year history.**
>
> **The story of Dry Idea tells a lot about how and why such products are conceived, developed, tested and sold in a highly competitive industry. It is an industry in which what a so-called "emotional" product does is apt to be less important than what the public can be convinced it does.**[66]

That sounds familiar. Once again they seem to be selling the sizzle instead of the steak. Well, I'm going to do my best to give you the beef, not the B.S.

Take a long, careful look at the "deodorants" next time you're at the store. Some say they're an "antiperspirant" or an "antiperspirant deodorant," while others claim to be "deodorants."

What's the difference? The key is in the name, which tells you what the stuff will and won't do. An antiperspirant contains a chemical capable of reducing perspiration by decreasing its flow from one of the two types of sweat glands. Just how this is accomplished is, believe it or not, still something of a mystery.

It was once thought that antiperspirants worked because they were astringents—chemicals that caused shrinking and a closing off of the pores. However, we now know that many astringents aren't very effective antiperspirants, so scratch that theory. Some researchers think that the chemicals cause sweat ducts to swell. Others offer the hypothesis that the antiperspirants plug up the ducts through which perspiration travels. Suffice it to say, we still don't know what's going on.

One important fact to understand about antiperspirants is that *none* of them is capable of closing off the flow of sweat from the second, "nervous" set of sweat glands. If it's your first date with someone you really like, a speech in front of a big audience, or an important meeting with the boss, all the **Right Guard** or **Secret** in the world is not going to keep you dry.

In fact, all the antiperspirants can do is reduce—by an average of about 20 percent—the flow of moisture. Some are better at the job than that, and some will work better for a given person than another, so when it comes to dampening the flow, a bit of experimentation is in order.

So much for wetness. Now there's the problem of odor. Enter the second set of labels, for deodorants plain and simple. A deodorant is something that decreases odor. It can do that by reducing the bacteria, reducing the material they work on, or by simply sloshing on enough perfume to cover the whole problem up.

The antibacterial approach sounds very logical, just like it sounds as though a mouthwash that kills "millions of germs on contact" should be good for something. The problem in this instance is that nobody knows just which bacteria, in just what quantity, actually cause an odor problem. One study showed a variation of more than a hundredfold in the underarm bacterial count of healthy people without an odor problem.[67]

So if we don't know what to kill, or how much killing to do, how can the problem be solved? But you should realize by now that lack of information rarely stops drug companies. Undaunted, manufacturers put in various "germ killers," including benzethonium chloride and triclosan, presumably on the assumption that the more bacteria you kill, the better off you are. Balderdash!

Antibacterial agents are relatively benign, though some people do develop allergic reactions with continual use. More interesting, ingredients like benzethenium chloride (found in **Right Guard Deodorant**) become inactivated if applied after showering or washing, because of the soapy residue left on the skin. What this means is that the jock who showers vigorously with soap after a heavy workout and then immediately sprays on **Right Guard Deodorant** is not going to get the kind of protection he expects.

Perhaps for such reasons most people opt for antiperspirants or antiperspirant/deodorant combinations. Probably the major active ingredient in most antiperspirants is aluminum chlorohydrate. It can be found in **Almay, Arrid Extra Dry, Ban, Dial Aerosol, 5-Day** pads, **Mitchum aerosol, Old Spice Antiperspirant, Right Guard Anti perspirant aerosol, Soft & Dri, Tickle,** and **Tussy Roll-on.**

Certain other brands do contain other active ingredients. However, the biggest differences among brands are in price, especially if you compare the quantity in the dispenser. Personally, I recommend the house brands whenever possible. In my area you can buy 2.5 ounces of generic aluminum chlorohydrate for about $1.50, whereas a comparable amount of the leading brands can run well over $3.00.

No matter what antiperspirant/deodorant you select, be aware of the following:

1. These products will be rendered utterly useless if applied to pores that are already sweating.[68] Apply only to a clean, dry underarm.

2. Never apply any of these products immediately after shaving the area, or if there's any kind of a cut or open sore.

3. People differ remarkably in their responses to the various chemicals. If one doesn't work, try another.

4. No antiperspirant will shut off sweat from the "nervous" pores. Don't expect the impossible.

5. Antiperspirants reduce somewhat the normal volume of sweat. They will not do the trick if you are an incredibly profuse sweater.

Most people don't worry too much about sweating, but for some poor folks excessive perspiration can be a terrible problem. A reader of my newspaper column sent in the following question:

**I dread summer. The problem is, I perspire excessively, and in the summertime I have to take two or three extra shirts in to the office every day. Even then, it's not enough.**

As an executive, I can't afford to look sloppy or nervous,
but my underarms get drenched. Are there any antiperspirants which are more effective than the usual brands?

Almost anyone can sympathize with this poor fellow. In such
a severe case my best recommendation would be an antiperspirant containing an old-fashioned ingredient called aluminum
chloride. It can be found in several prescription products (**Drysol, Xerac AC**). Over-the-counter brands containing aluminum
chloride are less expensive, however.

Unfortunately, not all of these products are widely available.
**Certan-Dri** or **At Last** are hardly household names. They do
work quite well, however, and if not carried in a local pharmacy
can be ordered by writing to the manufacturers. For **Certan-Dri,**
contact Leon Products, Inc., P.O. Box 16537, Jacksonville, FL
32245. And for **At Last,** you can write to Professional Formulations, Inc., 3255 E. Livingston Ave., Columbus, OH 43227.

Here are some further tips on getting the most out of an
aluminum chloride antiperspirant: Apply it sparingly to DRY
skin. These products can be irritating, so it is important not to
aggravate that by putting them on wet or freshly shaved underarms. The best time to put any antiperspirant on is in the evening
before bed. Although most people include antiperspirant in their
morning ritual, these products do better if you give them a head
start. And don't worry about it washing off. You may find that
you only need to apply it two or three times a week. For people
with a big sweating problem, aluminum chloride comes closest
to a solution for soaked summertime shirts.

Now a word about "strength." The FDA panel of experts took
note of the tendency of some products to claim they contain
"extra strength," or "super strength," or some other such nonsense. (What's next, "industrial strength"?) Even if that were
literally true in terms of chemical contents (which it isn't, since
most products contain the maximum strength of active ingredient permitted by the rules), there is also no evidence of a direct
link between concentration and effectiveness. The panel proposed a prohibition on all such hype, permitting only "extra

effective" if a product produced an average 30 percent or greater reduction in sweat volume.

There are, by the way, some differences in effectiveness between how various forms of antiperspirants deliver their ingredients. Roll-ons vary from a 14 percent to a 70 percent reduction in sweating. The range for sprays is 20 percent to 33 percent; sticks, 35 percent to 40 percent; creams, 35 percent to 47 percent; and liquids, 15 percent to 54 percent.[69] Aerosols, on average, appear to be the least effective means of application.

Sprays present their own hazards, since they produce a fine aerosol mist, some of which is inevitably inhaled when you apply the antiperspirant/deodorant in the confines of a bathroom. If you can smell it, you are breathing it.

There has been considerable debate over the years about the safety of aluminum-containing aerosol antiperspirants. At one point the FDA considered requiring additional testing in animals to see if there was any danger of lung tumors, but in 1982 it decided that such experiments were unnecessary.[70] Instead, the FDA will probably require a warning on aerosols along the lines of *"Avoid Excessive Inhalation."*

I'll be damned if I know what that means. Since a lifetime of inhaling aluminum just plain sounds unhealthy to me, I'd recommend selecting either a stick or a roll-on as being the best combination of what's safe and effective. If you insist that the convenience of an aerosol is worth any potential risk, please try taking a deep breath before you start spraying. Then get your butt out of the bathroom before taking another breath.

Antiperspirants are a classic illustration of an OTC product with virtually no difference among dozens of competing brands in terms of the active ingredient. The only real differences are in meaningless things such as the packaging, the promotion, and whether the manufacturer makes it smell like musk or a meadow.

As a smart consumer, you'll first decide which of the two or three major deodorant ingredients consistently does the job for you and then shop for a product containing that ingredient at the lowest price per application.

## Flake Off, Dandruff

Dandruff isn't a disease, but you'd never know that if you watch television. Commercials are designed to make you feel as if you'd die of embarrassment if a few white flakes ever showed up on your collar.

But no matter how healthy your scalp may be, some scaling and flakiness is to be expected. About a third of the adult population suffers from dandruff at one time or another. Despite Herculean attempts, researchers have yet to find a "cause" for dandruff, in the sense of there being a particular bacterium, or virus, or anything else that sets in motion the flaking, scaling, and itching that are so uncomfortably familiar to the dandruff sufferer.

Dandruff is simply an acceleration of the normal process by which we shed external skin cells. Dandruff occurs when the rate of scalp shedding reaches two or three times normal, and when certain other changes lead to larger-than-normal clumps of cells. That makes what's normally invisible, visible.

While there is no cause, there are lots of "cures," which in the case of dandruff really means controlling the problem rather than making it go away completely. To some extent, most dandruff treatments on the OTC market can do the job of controlling dandruff pretty well. The choice of one product over another has to do largely with the makeup of your scalp and the severity of the dandruff.

The court of first resort would be to shampoo regularly with plain old ordinary shampoo. This has the virtues of being inexpensive, safe, and in many cases remarkably effective. By "regularly" I mean two to three times a week, or even once a day, with a mild shampoo.

Let's assume, for information's sake, that this doesn't do the trick to your satisfaction. The choice now comes down to two equally effective ingredients found in the majority of antidandruff shampoos: zinc pyrithione and selenium sulfide. The zinc pyrithione is the stuff of which **Head and Shoulders, Breck One,**

**Danex, Zincon,** and **Anti-Dandruff Brylcreem** are made. Selenium sulfide turns up in **Selsun Blue** and **Sul-Blue**.

Both chemicals are called cytostatic agents, which is a fancy way of saying they retard the rate at which cells reproduce themselves. Since dandruff is a problem of cells reproducing too quickly, reining in the reproduction rate should do the trick. And these shampoos *will* solve the problem for almost everyone *if* they're used properly.

And there's the rub, or rather, the lack of it. We're an impatient bunch at best, used to fast food, instant breakfast, and quick cures. Somewhere on the label of most dandruff shampoos it says to lather up and let the stuff sit there for quite a chunk of time —say, several minutes or more—at a *minimum*. But we're not a nation of careful label readers, either; and besides, five minutes can seem like a l-o-n-g time when you're standing there in the shower with your eyes closed knowing that if any of that stuff drips into an eyeball, it's going to hurt.

Now hear this—the effectiveness of dandruff shampoos is closely pegged to the amount of contact time. Anything under the recommended time and you might as well be using pig grease. After spending a lot of money (dandruff shampoos do not come cheap, as you already may have discovered), why wash it down the drain? Learn to sing a five-minute song, get a tape of a five-minute egg cooking, or wear a headband to keep the shampoo out of the eyes, and go on with your shower. By the time everything else is squeaky clean, the top will be done, too.

There is one important difference between the zinc and selenium shampoos. Selenium sulfide has a tendency to make the scalp oily. While the degree of oiliness has not been proved a factor in dandruff, if your scalp is naturally oily you may want to give a zinc shampoo first try.

Give these shampoos a couple of weeks to shake everything loose. Still have a problem? Then the next step is the keratolytic shampoos—those that break down keratin, the hard outer layer of scalp cells, and thus facilitate the removal of this detritus from the head.

The two major keratolytic agents are sulfur, in a concentration of 2 percent to 5 percent, and salicylic acid in a concentration of 2 percent to 3 percent. Among the shampoos containing one or both of these agents in some form are **Sebucare, Sebulex Medicated Shampoo, Sebutone, Vanseb, Sulpho-Lac, Cuticura Anti-Dandruff Shampoo, Diasporal, Meted, Neomark,** and **Sulfur-8 Hair and Scalp Conditioner.**

The keratolytic agents take some time to do their job, so don't expect to be cured the minute you step out of the shower. At the concentrations available in shampoos, it takes anywhere from one to two weeks for the cells to slow down their reproduction in response to regular treatment.

If all that has failed, it's probably past time to see a dermatologist. One thing to learn there is whether what's bothering you is really just simple dandruff, or is in fact something more complex such as seborrhea or psoriasis. These two diseases can mimic dandruff in that they cause scalp cells to flake, but each condition produces its own unique signs and symptoms.

The doctor will also be able to prescribe even other kinds of medicated shampoos, such as coal-tar concoctions, should the problem prove to simply be an irritatingly intractable case of dandruff.

As for regular old shampoos for "normal" hair, they've become almost as confusing as the medicated brands. If you've gone shopping for shampoo lately, you might have wondered whether you had wandered into a restaurant by mistake.

If you're in the mood for dessert, you could pick lemon, chocolate, or strawberry mousse. But if you'd rather begin with breakfast, how about eggs, apples, or apricots, wheat germ or honey? If you're a health-food purist seeking organic herbs, there's plenty to choose from: aloe vera with keratin, jojoba oil with biotin, henna, yarrow, coconut oil, almond oil, mistletoe, comfrey, rosemary, and ginseng, just for starters.

Shampoo labels also sport a wide range of vitamins, such as Vitamin D, Vitamin E, or panthenol, not to mention protein enricheners and minerals. Of course, if you're thirsty, you can look for a shampoo with milk, cocamilk, or beer.

Do you get a stomachache just thinking about these shampoos? Your troubles have just begun. Now you need to pick between a "pH balanced" product and one that's "nonalkaline," and decide whether your shampoo should contain DNA or RNA. And if you really want confusion, just turn the bottle over and look at the list of ingredients. It's hard to imagine anyone except a cosmetics chemist deciphering names like sodium hydroxymethane sulfonate, TEA-lauryl sulfate, FD&C Red Number 33, triethanolamine dimethicone, and guar hydroxypropyltrimonium chloride.

Confused? Ready to give up and grab the first bottle you find? You're not alone. It turns out that shampoo shoppers are notoriously fickle, ready to switch brands without turning a hair. And no wonder. Many products don't live up to expectations. For one thing, hair is dead. Vitamins, minerals, protein, DNA and RNA, eggs or beer can't be absorbed into the hair shaft and make it healthier. Most of those fancy additives will be rinsed away with the dirt and the suds anyway.

Even if you try to make it simple and just concentrate on whether your hair is dry or oily, you've still got problems. A *Consumer Reports* survey discovered that when people were not told what type of shampoo they were using, people with oily hair usually preferred shampoo formulated for dry hair and vice versa.

As one leading hair expert points out, most people have both oily and dry hair on different parts of their scalp. Some shampoos for oily hair strip too much oil out with strong astringents, so that after several uses the scalp starts making more oil to compensate. As a result, such shampoos may make the original problem worse.

So what is the answer to the shampoo stalemate? I'm afraid there are no rules that will work for everyone. Trial and error is unfortunately the only true test. For most people shampooing several times a week, the milder the shampoo, the better. Even baby shampoo may be a good bet.

So next time you go searching for a shampoo, don't be taken in by long lists of gourmet ingredients. Save the vitamins, minerals, wheat germ, and honey for your breakfast cereal and the chocolate mousse or raspberry delight for dessert.

## Athlete's Foot: An Itch That's Hard to Scratch

It's fun to report on categories of OTC remedies where there have been great strides (pardon the running gag) since the first edition of *The People's Pharmacy,* and this is certainly one of those areas.

Athlete's foot is nothing more than a fungus infection. Remember "there's a fungus among us" from grade-school days? Well, athlete's foot is a fungus among the toes, where it takes root and happily grows fully supplied with everything it needs —warmth, moisture, and a friendly surface to live on.

Though I say it's "just a fungus," don't underestimate athlete's-foot infections. They can be downright nasty, especially if you let them run wild before setting up a defense. At first the symptoms may just be a bit of redness between the toes, and a slight itch. Before long, there are deep cracks and fissures, raw, macerated skin, severe itching, burning, and pain.

Anyone who's ever fought the athlete's-foot battle knows that the fungus can be tough to eradicate. One of the reasons for that, scientists have learned, is that the infections are sometimes a mixture of fungus and bacteria, each contributing to the attack on and destruction of the skin between your toes. There is also speculation that our immune systems play an important defensive role. Why is it, for example, that some people can walk barefoot on a wet locker room floor day after day and never come down with athlete's foot, while someone else can pick the darn stuff up after only one exposure?

For a long, long time about the best science could offer (at least over the counter) were things like **Whitfield's Ointment**, a mixture of benzoic and salicylic acids. And they didn't exactly cause the fungus to run and hide.

There was also undecylenic acid and zinc undecylenate, which came to you as **Blis-To-Sol, Decylenes, Desenex, Deso-Creme,**

**Devine's Kool Foot, Cruex, Merlenate, NP-27, Pertinex, Ting Improved Shaker and Spray, Undoguent,** and many others.

The problem with undecylenic acid was that it could just about achieve a standoff. The fungal infection usually stopped getting worse, but for many, it never quite went away. Or if the athlete's foot did disappear, it often came back when the medicine was discontinued. Undecylenic acid was better at control than eradication, and it tended to work best on the more superficial infections.

Then along came tolnaftate, in the form of **Tinactin, Aftate, Pro Comfort,** and **Dr. Scholl's Athlete's Foot Powder/Gel/ Spray.** This chemical is much more adept at rooting out the stubborn fungal invaders, apparently by disrupting their means of reproduction. It was a major breakthrough in treating athlete's foot, something which was significantly better (and, of course, significantly more expensive) than its predecessors.

Once again there has been a breakthrough in nonprescription treatment for athlete's foot. You can now obtain the drug miconazole as **Micatin.** This is really a heavy-duty fungal fighter. It's been in use for many years to treat a variety of fungal infections. Many of our female readers might recognize miconazole as **Monistat,** a cream frequently prescribed for vaginal fungal infections.

Miconazole is a big improvement. Like any antifungal, it takes a while to get the job done. Fungi are much more tenacious than bacteria, which can often be killed in just hours. Still and all, miconazole works a lot quicker and a lot better than what's been available up to now, and it should allow most athlete's-foot sufferers to once again put their best foot forward . . . without having to scratch it.


## Warts, Corns, and Calluses

When I was a kid I would have given anything for a jar of spunk water. I didn't know what it was, but I knew Huck Finn and Tom Sawyer used it to get rid of warts.

No such luck for me. My mother dragged me off to the doctor, who burned, blistered, froze, or surgically removed the warts, depending on what kind of mood he was in that day. Spunk water sure would have been better.

No matter what you may have heard, warts don't come from frogs or toads. Warts are caused by a virus which can be spread from one part of the body to another or from one person to another. Although the pesky things have been around as long as we have records of people, they're still surrounded by much mystery and mystique.

And little wonder. Warts can pop up literally overnight, appearing out of nowhere to stick out their cauliflowery little noses at us in sheer defiance. Like some sort of guerrilla fighter, warts are tough, wily, and seemingly indestructible. Yet left well enough alone, about one third will disappear of their own free will within a year. Few linger forever.

It's this tendency to disappear as silently and quickly as they came that through the eons has tended to make believers of people who've applied all manner of disgusting material to their warts and then seen them go away. That's what's behind the "success" of spunk water, pennies, potatoes, and dead cats.

That and the power of the mind. Dr. Lewis Thomas, professor of pathology and medicine at Cornell University and president of the Memorial Sloan-Kettering Cancer Center, describes the process this way:

**It is one of the great mystifications of science: Warts can be ordered off the skin by hypnotic suggestion. Not everyone believes this, but the evidence goes back a long way and is persuasive. Generations of internists and dermatologists, and their grandmothers for that matter, have been convinced of the phenomenon.[71]**

How the unconscious mind can mobilize the body's immune system, wiping the wart from the body, is indeed one of medicine's mysteries. If it could be solved, we might be on our way to overcoming many of the most vexing problems related to the body's immune capabilities.

Even if we can't figure out how the process works, that doesn't mean we can't take advantage of the mind-over-matter technique, especially when treating children's warts. If you make up some outrageous but safe "cure," throwing in lots of hokey techniques, the chances are that the warts will disappear over the next several weeks or months.

Such magical techniques could include touching the wart with ice cubes, painting it with food coloring, or gently poking it with a chopstick while reciting a nonsensical incantation. The bigger the production, the better the chances for success.

If you don't want to wait until your mind makes itself up to will away your own warts, or if you just don't have the patience to wait a few months for them to get up and go, what does the friendly local pharmacy have to offer that might hasten the process?

Before applying anything, make certain you've got a do-it-yourself wart. The only two types safe for home treatment are common warts of the hands or fingers and plantar warts, which occur on the soles of the feet. If you have anything else, or have a simple wart anywhere else, take it to the doctor.

The choice of materials is easy, because in reviewing wart cures the FDA panel on miscellaneous external drug products found only one thing in the "safe and effective" category. That ingredient was salicylic acid in strengths from 5 percent to 17 percent. Some of the brand names are **Off-Ezy, Compound W Wart Remover, Wart-Off, Freezone,** and **Gets-It Liquid.**

A couple of things to know before slathering, slapping, dripping, or pasting any of this stuff on. First, it's basically skin eater. So don't get it anywhere you don't want skin eaten. Second, salicylic acid does the best job when the material is held in direct contact and covered with a waterproof material, to hold in moisture. A plaster of salicylic acid fills the bill and can be easily cut, placed over the wart and changed every few days. Plasters are available in much greater strengths (up to 40 percent) under names such as **Dr. Scholl's Fixo Corn Plaster** and **Mediplast.** This greater strength is necessary and acceptable in the plaster, especially for plantar warts on the foot.

Third, and most important, *do not treat yourself for warts (or any other foot problem) if you have diabetes or circulatory problems.*

Having read all about warts, you're probably sitting there with a corn or callus, wondering when I'll get to that. Well, I already did. Once again, products with salicylic acid are the drugs of choice with concentrations in the 5-percent-to-17-percent range. Some come as liquids, some as plasters, some as a flexible material known as colloidion. Among the names you'll see on the shelf are **Dr. Scholl's "2" Drop Corn-Callus Remover, Off-Ezy, Dr. Scholl's Zino-Pads, Dr. Scholl's Waterproof Corn Pads,** and **Calicylic Creme.**

It was the FDA panel's opinion that none of the zillions of other ingredients often thrown into these preparations has been clearly demonstrated as safe and effective, though the book is still open on things like glacial acetic acid (found in **Compound W Wart Remover**). Following the general principle that less is better, look for something with straight salicylic acid, apply it carefully as directed, and fall asleep dreaming of how the wart, corn, or callus will disappear. Something should work.

## For Women Only

For reasons best left to chroniclers of American society, women have been a major target audience for all sorts of "made-up" products. By that I mean products that exist much more by virtue of their advertising than anything else. First they were invented, then a "need" was created by intensive promotion.

Drug manufacturers have played on the fears and insecurities of generations of women to create such nonproducts as vaginal deodorants and menstrual pills. Perhaps the most blatant examples of made-up products are the "feminine hygiene sprays." At least that's what they were called when first marketed. The FDA finally awakened to the fact that there was nothing hygienic about these sprays and forced the manufacturers to drop all references to hygiene.

Undaunted, the hype masters convinced hundreds of thousands of women to pay millions of dollars out of fear that they were suddenly (after having survived many generations *without* such a product) desperately in need of deodorizing their vaginas.

This is such hogwash that it's unbelievable, but obviously a lot of women bought into the notion. A normal, healthy vagina doesn't need to be dosed and doused with a chemical spray containing perfumes, propellants, and solvents of various sorts. Such compounds could irritate sensitive skin, and there have indeed been reports of adverse reactions to vaginal-spray products.

The best "feminine deodorant" is still soap and water. If you have an offensive vaginal odor that soap and water can't get rid of, see a doctor. There's a good chance you've got an infection that should be treated medically, not cosmetically.

Menstrual problems have also been fertile ground for the OTC people. One reason for that, sadly, is that for years many doctors tended to dismiss complaints about menstrual cramps and premenstrual physical complaints as being "all in the mind." Deprived of sympathetic and efficacious medical help, women turned to nonprescription products that at least promised to help.

Since the exact causes of menstrual distress were (and to a large extent still are) unclear, it was of course a bit hard to say exactly what *would* help. That, as we've seen with so many other OTC drugs, hardly stopped the manufacturers from trying. After all, there are a *lot* of menstruating women out there. They must need something.

What women got was a veritable witch's brew with everything from diuretics (medications to help the body shed water) to a variety of herbs (function unknown).

Not much has changed. **Lydia E. Pinkham Tablets** still consist of extract of Jamaica dogwood, pleurisy root, licorice, and dried ferrous sulfate. **Fluidex-Plus with Diadax** contains buchu, couch grass, powdered corn silk, powdered hydrangea, and phenylpropanolamine (PPA). The latter ingredient is a major constituent of most OTC weight-reducing pills, and has been linked to episodes of high blood pressure.

And then there's **Pamprin, Sunril, Cardui**, and **Pursettes Pre-menstrual Tablets.** Among other things, these three contain pyrilamine maleate, an antihistamine. That's apparently in case a woman's menstrual cramps are all in her nose.

Actually, the antihistamine may be in there to make women sleepy on the principle that if you're feeling sluggish and spacey, your cramps won't be so bothersome. The makers of **Pursettes** have the audacity to promote their product as relieving "nervous tension, irritability, and anxiety." Although the FDA panel on menstrual products allowed antihistamines to be included for treating psychological complaints, another FDA panel (on day-time sedatives) said that such use was not effective and inappropriate. Contradictory? You bet. But don't forget, we're dealing with federal bureaucracy.

There is no doubt that many women suffer physical distress immediately preceding or during their period. Those who do have menstrual problems should seek relief. Some women may find that aspirin or acetaminophen (**Tylenol, Panadol, Datril, Anacin-3, APAP,** etc.), which are the principal ingredients in most OTC menstrual products, can help. But the really big news these days is ibuprofen (**Advil** and **Nuprin**).

Until recently ibuprofen was available only by prescription under the names **Motrin** and **Rufen**. It is one of the all-time big best-sellers for arthritis, pain, and inflammation of all varieties. A few years ago scientists discovered that women who suffer severe menstrual cramps have higher levels of hormonelike sub-stances circulating in their bodies. These compounds, known as prostaglandins, seem to be responsible for the problem, and drugs like ibuprofen are far more effective at shutting down prostaglandin production and relieving cramps than **Tylenol** or other OTC pain relievers.

## A Smart OTC Strategy

When the doctor is faced with a sick patient, he or she goes through an ordered process for determining what might or might not be causing the problem. If you're going to be your own doctor, using OTC remedies, you'll have to do the same thing. If you follow these hints from *The People's Pharmacy,* you may be able to take advantage of useful OTC aids without getting ripped off.

- *Be conservative*—Just as every car repair isn't a do-it-yourself project, lots of body ills will be beyond the reach of any OTC medicine. If you're in doubt, get professional assistance. Anything that doesn't get better quickly should be taken to the doctor, and so should anything that continues to get worse in spite of your treatment.

- *Think in terms of stepped care*—Stepped care is an important concept in medicine. It means treating a condition with the least possible force initially and escalating the potency or frequency of medication only when lesser things won't do the job. This helps minimize adverse drug reactions and drug interactions. The doctor's first rule is Do no harm. The same principle applies to your OTC efforts. Since most conditions are self-limiting and will go away fairly promptly all by themselves, think in terms of the *least* medication you can take to be comfortable. Two aspirin will still solve a lot of problems.

- *Beware of mixtures*—There is a tremendous tendency on the part of OTC drug makers to whip up complicated combinations of things. This happens partly because they want to be different, or appear to be different, from a competitor and partly because they're often taking a "shotgun" approach. Instead of killing the fly with a swatter, they prefer to pull both triggers and blow away the fly and the barn door he's sitting on.

  The problem for the patient is that each and every drug you take involves a risk. There's the risk you will have an adverse reaction to that drug, there's a risk it will interact with something else you take, and there's the risk that the combination of ingredients will affect you in a way no single ingredient would have.

It makes sense to try to treat your problem with a single effective ingredient whenever possible. Use this book and other resources to determine what ingredients really work for a specific problem, and then buy only what you need. As a bonus, you'll likely find it will result in savings to your pocketbook.

- *Shop comparatively*—Once you know what drug is needed, look for it in the lowest priced product available. This will frequently mean a generic or house brand, rather than the stuff you saw hawked on a clever TV commercial the night before. Good. You'll be getting more value for your money. What you want to purchase is the active ingredient, not the hype. Don't pay for what you don't need. For more information on saving money with generic drugs, turn to Chapter 12.

- *Follow directions*—If it says to leave the dandruff shampoo on for five minutes, make darn certain you've left it on a full five minutes. If the package says not to exceed eight tablets daily, don't gulp fifteen. Sometimes not following the directions can render the medication useless . . . and sometimes not following the directions can render you even sicker than you were to start with.

## OTC—The Real People's Pharmacy

If there was ever any doubt that people are ready, willing, and eager to self-medicate, it was set to rest by a study showing that 59 percent of the people questioned had used an OTC product the week before.[72] Pain relievers (used by 41 percent), vitamins (32 percent), and cold remedies (15 percent) were the leading items.

It is less clear that consumers have all the information they need to do the job of doctoring themselves properly. One study found that 8 percent of the people thought aspirin was an antibiotic, and 13 percent thought an antibiotic was a stronger form of aspirin.[73] We're going to have to do better than that.

The OTC drug review was a helpful step, since it set in motion changes that should eventually eliminate many useless and even dangerous OTC drugs. That should, in theory at least, leave us only with things whose safety and effectiveness have been tested in competent scientific research.

Along with that change we need to alter consumers' attitudes about OTC drugs. It's time we saw them for what they are—pharmacological agents with all the capacity for good and bad possessed by their by-prescription-only relatives. OTC medications *are* drugs, so we need to keep in mind the possibility of adverse reactions and interactions.

Most of all, we need to choose very carefully in order to protect both our bodies and our pocketbooks from unnecessary damage. To assist you, the following tables list some brand names to look for—and some to look out for.

## A Handy Guide to Nonprescription Products

### ANTACIDS

| Good Choice | Okay | Not Recommended† |
|---|---|---|
| ** Alka-2 Tablets | *** Alka-Seltzer Effervescent Antacid (Alka-Seltzer Gold) | Alka-Seltzer Effervescent Pain Reliever and Antacid |
| ** Alkets | | AlternaGel |
| * Aludrox | | Alu-Cap |
| * Alurex | | Aluminum Hydroxide Gel |
| ** Amitone | *** Baking soda (good value) | Alu-Tab |
| * A.M.T. | | Amphojel |
| ** Bisodol Tablets | *** Bell/ans | Basaljel |
| ** Calcilac (good value) | *** Bisodol Powder | Bromo-Seltzer |
| ** Camalox | *** Citro-carbonate | Dialume |
| ** Chooz | **** Di-Gel | Eno |
| * Creamalin | *** Gaviscon tablets | Phosphajel |
| * Delcid (very good value) | **** Gelusil II (good value) | Robalate |
| ** Dicarbosil | **** Mylanta II (good value) | |
| ** Equilet | **** Riopan Plus | |
| * Estomul-M | * Rolaids | |
| ** Eugel | | |
| ** Glycate | | |
| ** Gustalac | | |
| * Kolantyl Gel | | |

---

†"Not Recommended" does not mean that these products are unsafe or ineffective.

*Aluminum content may have an adverse effect on bone strength, especially in older people. Occasional use should not pose a problem.

**Contains calcium carbonate; recommended for women past forty and all others vulnerable to osteoporosis.

***High in sodium—occasional use only.

****In addition to effective antacids this product contains simethicone, which is of questionable effectiveness.

**ANTACIDS** *cont.*

| Good Choice | Okay | Not Recommended† |
|---|---|---|
| ** **Lo-Sal Tablets** | **** **Silain-Gel** | |
| * **Maalox TC** (very good value) | **** **Simeco** (very good value) | |
| * **Magnatril** | *** **Soda Mint** | |
| * **Magnesium-Aluminum Hydroxide Gel, USP** (good value) | | |
| ** **Mallamint** | | |
| ** **Marblen** | | |
| ** **Pama** | | |
| ** **Ratio** | | |
| * **Riopan** | | |
| ** **Titralac** | | |
| * **Trialka Liquid** | | |
| ** **Trialka** | | |
| ** **Tums** (good value) | | |
| ** **Tums E-X** (good value) | | |
| * **WinGel** | | |

†"Not Recommended" does not mean that these products are unsafe or ineffective.

*Aluminum content may have an adverse effect on bone strength, especially in older people. Occasional use should not pose a problem.

**Contains calcium carbonate; recommended for women past forty and all others vulnerable to osteoporosis.

***High in sodium—occasional use only.

****In addition to effective antacids this product contains simethicone, which is of questionable effectiveness.

**ATHLETE'S FOOT REMEDIES**

| Good Choice | Okay | Not Recommended† |
|---|---|---|
| **Aftate** | **Blis-To-Sol** | **Blis Foot Bath** |
| Aluminum chloride, 30 percent (especially for hard-to-treat athlete's foot— mixed bacterial/ fungal infection) | **Caldesene Medicated Powder** | **Bluboro Medicated Foot Powder** |
| | **Desenex** | **Neo-Castaderm** |
| | **NP-27 Aerosol or Liquid** | **NP-27 Powder** |
| **Burow's Solution** (for open blisters) | **Quinsana Plus Medicated Foot Powder** | **Rid-Itch Liquid** |
| | | **Ting Cream/ Powder** |
| **Dr. Scholl's Athlete's Foot Powder/Gel/ Spray** | **Verdefam** | |
| **Micatin** (excellent) | **Whitfield's Ointment** | |
| **Pro Comfort** | **Whitsphill Ointment** | |
| **Tinactin** | | |

†"Not Recommended" does not mean that these products are unsafe or ineffective.

## DANDRUFF SHAMPOOS

| Good Choice | Okay | Not Recommended† |
|---|---|---|
| **Anti-Dandruff Brylcreem** | **Cuticura Anti-Dandruff Shampoo** | **Ionil** |
| **Breck One Dandruff Shampoo** | **Meted Shampoo** | **Rinse-Away** |
| **Danex** | **Rezamid Shampoo** | **Sebucare** |
| **DHS Zinc** | **Sebaveen** | |
| **Head & Shoulders** | Sebulex Conditioning Shampoo with Protein | |
| **Sebulon** | **Sebulex Medicated Shampoo** | |
| **Selsun Blue** | Sebutone | |
| **Sul-Blue** | | |
| **Zincon** | | |

---

†"Not Recommended" does not mean that these products are unsafe or ineffective.

## DEODORANTS AND ANTIPERSPIRANTS

| Good Choice | Okay | Not Recommended† |
|---|---|---|
| * **Almay** | | ALL AEROSOLS |
| * **Arrid Extra Dry** | | |
| ** **At Last** (only for severe sweating problems) | | |
| * **Ban** | | |
| ** **Certan-Dri** (only for severe sweating problems) | | |
| * **5-Day Antiperspirant & Deodorant Pads** | | |
| * **Lady Speed Stick** | | |
| * **Mum Gentle Formula** | | |
| * **Right Guard Antiperspirant and Deodorant** | | |
| * **Soft & Dri** | | |
| * **Tickle** | | |
| * **Tussy Roll-on** | | |

†"Not Recommended" does not mean that these products are unsafe or ineffective.
*All these products are essentially equal, since they contain the same active ingredient, aluminum chlorohydrate. Shop comparatively for the best price.
**These products contain aluminum chloride, one of the most effective OTC antiperspirants available. Apply to dry skin before bedtime for maximum effect. Aluminum chloride is strong and may cause irritation. It can also destroy shirts.

## MENSTRUAL PRODUCTS

| Good Choice | Okay | Not Recommended† |
|---|---|---|
| Ibuprofen:<br>  **Advil**<br>  **Nuprin** | Acetaminophen:<br>  **Anacin-3**<br>  **APAP**<br>  **Datril**<br>  **Panadol**<br>  **Tylenol**<br>Aspirin | **Aqua-Ban**<br>**Cardui**<br>**Fluidex-Plus with Diadax**<br>**Humphrey's #11**<br>**Lydia E. Pinkham**<br>**Midol**<br>**Pamprin**<br>**Pursettes Premenstrual Tablets**<br>**Sunril Premenstrual Tablets**<br>**Tri-Aqua**<br>**Vanquish** |

†"Not Recommended" does not mean that these products are unsafe or ineffective.

## MOUTHWASH AND GARGLES

| *Good Choice* | *Not Recommended†* |
| --- | --- |
| Brushing and flossing your teeth daily | **Astring-O-Sol** |
| | **Cepacol** |
| | **Cepastat** |
| Salt water (1/2 teaspoon per 8-ounce glass of water) | **Chloraseptic** |
| | **Isodine** |
| | **Mouthwash** |
| | **Gargle** |
| | **Concentrate** |
| | **K-Mart Amber** |
| | **Lavoris** |
| | **Listerine** |
| | **Listermint** |
| | **Odara** |
| | **Oral Pentacresol** |
| | **Scope** |

†"Not Recommended" does not mean that these products are unsafe or ineffective.

## SLEEP MEDICATIONS AND AIDS

| Good Choice | Okay | Not Recommended† |
|---|---|---|
| Counseling | Compoz | Dormarex |
| Dr. Emmett Miller's | Nighttime | Excedrin P.M. |
| Audio Tapes: | Sleep Aid | Nervine |
| "Easing into | Nytol with | Nighttime Sleep |
| Sleep" | DPH | Aid |
| "Letting Go of | Sleep-Eze 3 | Quiet World |
| Stress" | Sleepy Now | Sominex |
| "Healing | Maximum | Somnicaps |
| Journey" | Strength | |
| Exercise during the | Capsules | |
| day | Sominex | |
| Hot bath | Formula 2 | |
| An instant | Twilite | |
| breakfast | Unisom | |
| drink made with | | |
| warm | | |
| milk and malt | | |
| Progressive muscle | | |
| relaxation | | |
| Stress reduction | | |
| Tryptophan | | |
| Warm milk with | | |
| honey, crackers, | | |
| or cookies | | |

†"Not Recommended" does not mean that these products are unsafe or ineffective.

**WART AND CORN REMOVERS**

| Good Choice | Okay | Not Recommended† |
| --- | --- | --- |
| **Calicylic Cream** | **Compound W** | Home surgery |
| **Compound W** | **Wart** | |
| **Dr. Scholl's "2"** | **Remover** | |
| **Drop** | Placebo | |
| **Corn-Callus** | treatments— | |
| **Remover** | spunk water, | |
| **Dr. Scholl's Fixo** | new pennies, | |
| **Corn Plaster** | etc. | |
| **Dr. Scholl's** | | |
| **(medicated)** | | |
| **Waterproof** | | |
| **Corn Pads** | | |
| **Dr. Scholl's** | | |
| **(medicated)** | | |
| **Zino Pads** | | |
| **Freezone** | | |
| **Gets-It** | | |
| **Mediplast** | | |
| **Off-Ezy** | | |
| Salicylic Acid | | |
| Plaster 10 | | |
| percent to 40 | | |
| percent | | |
| **Wart-Off** | | |

†"Not Recommended" does not mean these products are unsafe or ineffective.

# References

1. "Consumer Expenditure Study." *Product Marketing* 13(8):18–22, 1983.

2. "Best Selling OTCs." *Drug Store News* Mar. 19, 1984, pp. 59–67.

3. Caranasos, George, J., et al. "Drug-induced Illness Leading to Hospitalization." *JAMA* 228:713–717, 1974.

4. "OTC Review Milestone." *FDA Consumer* 18(1):32, 1984.

5. *Science Digest,* Apr. 1983, p. 86.

6. Pacific News Service. "The Perils of Sleeping Pills." *San Francisco Examiner* Aug. 7, 1982, p. A10.

7. "No OTC Sleep Aids Safe, Effective, FDA Claims." *Drug Topics* 122(14):24, 1978.

8. Lijinsky, William, et al. "Liver Tumors Induced in Rats by Oral Administration of the Antihistaminic Methapyrilene Hydrochloride." *Science* 209:817–819, 1980.

9. Kales, Joyce, and Kales, Anthony. "Are Over-the-Counter Sleep Medications Effective? All-Night EEG Studies." *Curr. Ther. Res.* 13:-143–151, 1971.

10. Reznik-Schuller, H. M., and Lijinsky, W. "Morphology of Early Changes in Liver Carcinogenesis Induced by Methapyrilene." *Arch. Toxicol.* 49(1):79–83, 1981.

11. Althaus, F. R., et al. "DNA Damage Induced by the Antihistaminic Drug Methapyrilene Hydrochloride." *Mutat. Res.* 103:213–18, 1982.

12. Couri, D., et al. "Methapyrilene Effects on Initiation and Promotion of Gamma-glutamyl-transpeptidase Positive Foci in Rat Liver." *Res. Commun. Chem. Pathol. Pharmacol.* 35:51–61, 1982.

13. Ohshima, M. "A Sequential Study of Methapyrilene Hydrochloride-induced Liver Carcinogenesis in Male F344 Rats." *JNCI* 72:759–768, 1984.

14. Lijinsky, William. "Chronic Toxicity Tests of Pyrilamine Maleate and Methapyrilene Hydrochloride in F344 Rats." *Food. Chem. Toxicol.* 22:27–30, 1984.

15. Hartman, Ernest. "Effects of L-tryptophan on Sleepiness and on Sleep." *J. Psychiatr. Res.* 17(2):107–113, 1982.

16. Lindsley, J. G., et al. "Selectivity in Response to L-tryptophan among Insomniac Subjects: A Preliminary Report." *Sleep* 6(3):247–256, 1983.

17. Schneider-Helmert, D. "Interval Therapy with L-tryptophan in

Severe Chronic Insomniacs. A Predictive Laboratory Study." *Int. Pharmacopsychiatry* 16(3):162–173, 1981.

18. Hartmann, Ernest. "L-Tryptophan: A Possible Natural Hypnotic Substance." *JAMA* 230:1680–1681, 1974.

19. Karacan, I. "New Approaches to the Evaluation and Treatment of Insomnia." *Psychosomatics* 12:81–88, 1971.

20. "Consumer Expenditure Study," op. cit.

21. Personal communication, Arthur W. Weil, Dec. 3, 1984.

22. Lamy, Peter. "Over-the-Counter Medication: The Drug Interactions We Overlook." *J. Am. Ger. Soc.* 30(11) Suppl. S69–S75, 1982.

23. Kannel, W. B., and Abbott, R. D. "Incidence and Prognosis of Unrecognized Myocardial Infarction: An Update on the Framingham Study." *N. Engl. J. Med.* 311:1144–1147, 1984.

24. "Antacids." *Medical Letter* 24:61–62, 1982.

25. Garnett, William R. "Antacid Products" in *Handbook of Nonprescription Drugs*. 7th ed. Washington, D.C.: American Pharmaceutical Association, 1982, p. 31.

26. Klein, Kenneth, and Lieberman, David. "A Good Little Antacid." *N. Engl. J. Med.* 306:1492, 1982.

27. Perl, Daniel P., and Brody, Arnold R. "Alzheimer's Disease: X-ray Spectrometric Evidence of Aluminum Accumulation in Neurofibrillary Tangle-bearing Neurons." *Science* 208:297–299, 1980.

28. Perl, Daniel P., et al. "Intraneuronal Aluminum Accumulation in Amyotrophic Lateral Sclerosis and Parkinsonism-Dementia of Guam." *Science* 217:1053–1055, 1982.

29. Crapper, D. R., et al. "Intranuclear Aluminum Content in Alzheimer's Disease, Dialysis Encephalopathy, and Experimental Aluminum Encephalopathy." *Acta Neuropathol.* 50:19–24, 1980.

30. Banks, W. S., and Kastin, A. J. "Aluminum Increases Permeability of the Blood-Brain Barrier to Labelled DSIP and Beta-Endorphin: Possible Implications for Senile and Dialysis Dementia." *Lancet* 2:1227–1229, 1983.

31. Treichel, J. A. "Aluminum Linked with Dialysis Dementia." *Science News* 122:292–293, 1982.

32. King, R. G. "Do Raised Brain Aluminum Levels in Alzheimer's Dementia Contribute to Cholinergic Neuronal Deficits?" *Med. Hypotheses* 14:301–306, 1984.

33. King, S. W., et al. "The Clinical Biochemistry of Aluminum." *CRC Crit. Rev. Clin. Lab. Sci.* 14:1–20, 1981.

34. Lione, A. "The Prophylactic Reduction of Aluminum Intake." *Food Chem. Toxicol.* 21:103–109, 1983.

35. Levick, Stephen E. "Dementia from Aluminum Pots?" *N. Engl. J. Med.* 303:164, 1980.

36. Trubo, Richard. "The Growing Problem of Alzheimer's Disease." *Medical World News* 25(17):54–63, 1984.

37. Shore, D., and Wyatt, R. J. "Aluminum and Alzheimer's Disease." *J. Nerv. Ment. Dis.* 171:553–558, 1983.

38. Brody, J. A., and White, L. R. "An Epidemiological Perspective on Senile Dementia." *Psychopharmacol. Bull.* 18:222–225, 1982.

39. Hixson, Joseph. "Dementia Key Not Aluminum" *Med. Trib.* 25(28):3, 1984.

40. Insogna, Karl L., et al. "Osteomalacia and Weakness from Excessive Antacid Ingestion." *JAMA* 244:2544–2546, 1980.

41. Ibid.

42. Ibid.

43. Ibid.

44. Lotz, M., et al. "Evidence for a Phosphate Depletion Syndrome in Man." *N. Engl. J. Med.* 278:409–415, 1968.

45. Lotz, M., et al. "Osteomalacia and Debility Resulting from Phosphorous Depletion." *Trans. Assoc. Am. Physicians* 77:281–295, 1964.

46. Carmichael, Kim A., et al. "Osteomalacia and Osteitis Fibrosa in a Man Ingesting Aluminum Hydroxide Antacid." *Am. J. Med.* 76:-1137–1142, 1984.

47. Sebes, J. I., et al. "Radiographic Manifestations of Aluminum-induced Bone Disease." *AJR* 142:424–426, 1984.

48. Spencer, Herta, and Kramer, Lois. "Antacid-induced Calcium Loss." *Arch. Intern. Med.* 143:657–659, 1983.

49. Herzog, P., and Holtermuller, K. H. "Antacid Therapy—Changes in Mineral Metabolism." *Scand. J. Gastroenterol. Suppl.* 17(75):56–62, 1982.

50. Carmichael, op. cit.

51. Graedon, Joe. "Over-the-Counter Medication" in *The People's Pharmacy,* 1st ed. New York: St. Martin's Press, 1976, pp. 85–86.

52. Clayman, Charles B. "The Carbonate Affair: Chalk One Up." *JAMA* 244:2554, 1980.

53. Prescott, Lawrence M. "Stay with Calcium." *Medical Tribune,* Feb. 15, 1984, p. 16.

54. Williamson, David. "Bone Study Underscores Value of Calcium, Exercise." *Durham Morning Herald,* Jul. 15, 1984, p. 4A.

55. Ince, Susan. "Authority Answers Questions on Calcium Supplementation." *Medical Tribune,* Nov. 7, 1984, p. 4.

56. McCarron, David A., et al. "Hypertension and Calcium." *Science* 226:386–389, 1984.

57. Findlay, Steve, and Liebman, Bonnie. "Brittle Bones: Insufficient Calcium One of Many Culprits." *Nutrition Action* 9(5):12–13, 1982.

58. "Calcium: Which Supplements Are Best?" *Nutrition Action* Jul.–Aug., 1984, p. 12.

59. "Mouthwashes." *Consumer Reports,* Mar. 1984, pp. 143–146.

60. "Over-the-Counter Oral Health Care and Discomfort Drugs; Establishment of a Monograph." *Federal Register* 47(101):22711–22930, 1982.

61. Hecht, Annabel. "Some Medicine for Toothache . . . But None for Bad Breath." *FDA Consumer* 16(7):10–12, 1982.

62. Personal communication, Jeff Mazza, Oct. 18, 1980.

63. Scope advertisement. *People,* Mar. 19, 1979.

64. *Accepted Dental Therapeutics.* 37th ed. Chicago: American Dental Assn., 1979, pp. 340–343.

65. Ulman, Neil. "Time, Risk, Ingenuity All Go into Launching New Personal Product." *Wall Street Journal,* Nov. 17, 1978, p. 1.

66. Ibid.

67. *Federal Register* 43:46694, 1978.

68. Holzle, E., and Kligman, A. "Mechanism of Action of Aluminum Salts." *J. Soc. Cosmet. Chem.* 30:279–295, 1979.

69. *Federal Register,* 43:46694, 1978.

70. "Aerosol Aluminum Chlorohydrate Antiperspirants Get Bu-Drugs Category I Recommendation; Two-Year Rat Carcinogenicity Study No Longer Necessary." *F-D-C Reports* 44(20):9–10, 1982.

71. Thomas, Lewis. In *The Medusa and the Snail.* New York: Viking, 1979.

72. Vener, A.; Krupka, L.; and Climo, J. "Drugs (Prescription, Over-the-Counter, Social) and the Young Adult: Use and Attitudes." *Int. J. of the Addictions* 17(3):399–415, 1982.

73. Chandler, D. and Dugdale, A. "What Do Patients Know about Antibiotics?" *Lancet* 2:422, 1976.

## Table References

Covington, Timothy R., ed. *Drug Facts and Comparisons* St. Louis: Lippincott, 1985.

*Handbook of Nonprescription Drugs.* 7th ed. Washington, D.C.: American Pharmaceutical Association, 1982.

Kaufman, Joel, et al. *Over the Counter Pills That Don't Work.* New York: Pantheon, 1983.

Zimmerman, David R. *The Essential Guide to Nonprescription Drugs.* New York: Harper & Row, 1983.

# 6

# Drug Interactions: When 1+1 May Equal 3

---

*Who's in charge? • How to protect yourself from your doctor • Hospitals can be hazardous to your health • Drug-induced depression and disorientation • What is a drug interaction? • Problems with Tagamet, tetracycline, Fiorinal, and Coumadin • Avoiding drug interactions • Watch out for Dalmane • Table of Drug Interactions.*

---

"The time has come," the Walrus said,
"To talk of many things:
Of shoes—and ships—and sealing-wax—
Of cabbages—and kings—
And why the sea is boiling hot—
And whether pigs have wings."

—*Through the Looking-Glass*

"Drug interactions are the Achilles heel of the medical profession. The laws of nature no longer hold true. This is a crazy world where one plus one equals three, where down may very well be up and surely pigs have wings. In fact, mixing medicines is very much like playing Russian roulette. You never know when a particular combination will produce a lethal outcome."

When I wrote those words almost a decade ago in the first edition of this book, I had no idea how many people would be interested in this issue. Drug interactions seemed like a pretty esoteric topic, and I was surprised when thousands of letters started pouring in about the various combinations of drugs people were being given.

All of a sudden, what had been of only theoretical concern became all too real. Readers related horror stories that sent chills up and down my spine. One woman from Orlando, Florida, wrote about her sister:

> My sister was taking Valium, Lanoxin, Enduron and Emfaseem every day. When her ankles swelled her doctor prescribed Lasix and Inderal.
>
> I was with her when she asked the doctor what medication she should stop while she took these new prescriptions. He told her just to add them to the others.
>
> She became extremely weak and lost ten pounds of fluid very suddenly, so she went back to the doctor. He just told her to keep taking all the medicine. When she complained that all the drugs were making her feel weak and tired, he answered, "If playing bridge and going to the hairdresser means more to you than getting well, then do whatever you like."
>
> Naturally, she did what her doctor told her to. She died a month later, a senile old lady, though she had been an active, outgoing person before. The death certificate just read "cardiac arrest." That only means her heart stopped beating, but I think all those medications killed her.

Of course there is no way to know whether this woman did indeed die from drug interactions, but the medications she was taking could easily have been responsible for her symptoms of fatigue, disorientation, and confusion. The diuretics **Lasix**

(furosemide) and **Enduron** (methyclothiazide) could have depleted her body of potassium, a life-threatening situation for
anyone taking the heart medicine **Lanoxin** (digoxin). Low potassium levels predispose people taking digitalis to potentially fatal
irregular heart rhythms. As if that weren't enough, **Inderal** may
have removed what little reserve was left in a heart already
failing.

This is only one case, but we have received so many other
heart-wrenching letters it makes you want to cry. I'll never
forget the story of the young mother who was put on **Reglan**
(metoclopramide) for her heartburn, **Asendin** (amoxapine) for
depression, **Halcion** (triazolam) for insomnia, and **Valium**
(diazepam) for anxiety.

This combination turned her into a zombie, barely able to
walk or talk. One of her drugs (**Reglan**) could have brought on
insomnia, anxiety, and depression by itself, and could also have
produced drowsiness and dizziness. The other medications prescribed to treat the insomnia, depression, and anxiety only added
to the problem by increasing her sedation, disorientation, fatigue, and faintness. When a new doctor advised her to stop all
medications abruptly, she went through hell and even weeks
later was having a terrible time sleeping.

## Who's in Charge?

How does this sort of thing happen? Why do people end up
receiving prescriptions for numerous medications that should
never be taken together? Several factors are responsible. First, of
course, there is an enormous number of medications available by
prescription, with more being added all the time. Add to that the
hundreds of thousands of over-the-counter remedies, all of
which also have the potential to interact with each other and
with prescription medications, and you begin to grasp the im-
mensity of the situation.

Another part of the problem may be arrogance. Too many
doctors either assume they know all the essential information

about the drugs they prescribe or wish to appear knowledgeable in front of their patients. Just how would it look, they think, to have to flip through a "crib sheet" like the PDR (Physicians' Desk Reference) while a patient watches?

But that's just plain foolishness and false pride. It's impossible for any human being to remember all the relevant side effects and cautions associated with the tens of thousands of prescription drugs on the market, let alone know how all of them interact with one another. It would take a computer to keep track of all the possible permutations and combinations. Most people would be delighted if their doctor took a few extra minutes to look up drug-interaction precautions.

The risk of experiencing an adverse reaction increases astronomically as the number of drugs a person takes goes up. Aspirin alone interacts with dozens of other drugs to produce unexpected and occasionally serious results. Beta blockers such as **Blocadren** (timolol), **Corgard** (nadolol), **Inderal** (propranolol), **Lopressor** (metoprolol), **Normodyne** (labetolol), **Tenormin** (atenolol), **Trandate** (labetolol), and **Visken** (pindolol) are prescribed in huge quantities and can also react with dozens of other medications. So does the ulcer drug **Tagamet** (cimetidine), the epilepsy medication **Dilantin** (phenytoin), and the heart medicine **Lanoxin** (digoxin). Certainly not all drugs interact with this many other medications, but whenever you take more than one medicine at a time, the potential exists for a drug–drug interaction.

There are several other reasons why this problem has become so severe in recent years. When I was growing up we had a family doctor—the good old GP, or general practitioner. He took care of every member of the family for just about everything that ailed us. He even made house calls. Since he prescribed all our medicines, he could keep track of everything we were taking. When he gave us prescriptions, we always took them to the neighborhood pharmacy, where old Doc Sidon filled them and took a few minutes to chat and discuss family health matters.

Today we're in the era of specialty medicine. It sometimes seems there's a specialist for each body part, external and inter-

nal. If we have a stomachache, we are referred to the gastroenterologist. If our head hurts, it's off to the neurologist. Trouble
peeing? See a urologist. It's not at all unusual for a person to be
seeing two or more physicians, and that's where the worst drug
interaction dangers often lurk.

Unless Doctor B has reason to get your medical records from
Doctor A, he or she will have only one way of knowing what
medications you're taking. That's right, patient, it's show-and-
tell time for you.

Of course, a careful doctor will always ask, but if you count
on that to protect you it's likely you'll eventually get hurt. Some
doctors are very aware of drug interaction problems; others
don't give it a lot of thought. Some doctors might never think
you'd even consider seeing anyone else.

If your doctor—or any doctor—prescribes something but does
not ask what other medications you may be taking, tell him
anyway. Of course, this means that you have to be aware of all
the drugs you take. Knowing that you take "a little white heart
pill" or "a water pill" isn't enough.

Make sure you know the names and strengths of all the drugs
you take and how often you take them. Make a list if necessary,
and keep it in your wallet or purse at all times. Oh, and don't
forget to mention things like cigarettes. Turns out that people
who smoke metabolize drugs differently, and that may also affect
prescribed medication. Pin your doctor down about the chances
of a drug interaction. If he doesn't know it automatically, he may
be prompted to look it up.

This may not only prevent dangerous interactions but *duplica-
tions* as well. I am constantly amazed at how many readers will
write in with a list of the drugs they are taking and on that list
will be the same medicine twice. For example, someone might
have received the minor tranquilizer **Equanil** from one doctor
and meprobamate from another. Different names, but the same,
identical drug (one is the brand name, the other its generic
equivalent). I have received letters from people who were simultaneously taking the heart medicine **Lanoxin** as well as digoxin

—again, the same drug. Such duplication can lead to dangerous overdoses and toxic reactions.

Perhaps it's time to look for a neighborhood pharmacy again. There are so many drugstores these days, many of them chains with the druggist squirreled away in back behind a partition, that it is hard to form a personal relationship with a pharmacist. But today's pharmacists are better trained than ever before and in many cases know even more about drug interactions than the doctor. In fact, many pharmacies now have computers that immediately red-flag potentially hazardous drug combinations.

If you can find a pharmacist who cares and is willing to communicate valuable health information, it could be worth your while to buy all medicines from that person. And that includes over-the-counter remedies. Cold remedies, pain relievers (especially new and more potent products like ibuprofen—**Advil** and **Nuprin**), antacids, and even vitamins can interact with prescription drugs.

And don't forget alcohol. It can interact with over 150 other drugs or chemicals, and you'll find it not just in beer, wine, and liquor. Alcohol is often a "hidden" ingredient in many nonprescription medications such as **Nyquil** (50 proof), **Halls Mentho-Lyptus** (44 proof), **Comtrex** (40 proof), **Formula 44-D** (40 proof), **Romilar CF** (40 proof), and **Viromed Liquid** (33 proof).

If the pharmacist keeps a patient profile that lists all the prescriptions, over-the-counter medications, and vitamins you are taking, she can prevent duplication and drug–drug interactions. Of course a good rule of thumb is to try and limit all drug consumption to as few things as possible. In the event you must take more than one medicine at a time, check with your doctor *and* your pharmacist about possible complications.

## Hospitals Can Be Hazardous to Your Health

If you have to go into a hospital, this whole crazy drug interaction situation becomes even more serious. Studies show the average hospital patient will gulp an astounding nine drugs in the course of his or her visit.[1] Many poor souls will get the dubious benefits of more than twenty types of pills and potions while hospitalized.

It's hardly a surprise to learn that about one third of those hospitalized suffer some sort of adverse drug reaction.[2] According to one report, "Patients in nursing homes take an average of 7 to 10 drugs each day, and a Tennessee study showed that one patient in 10 received powerful tranquilizers, keeping them in 'chemical straitjackets.' "[3]

Nothing brings this home better than a personal example. Let me tell you about William. At seventy he is one of the most active, capable people I know. He still works eight-hour days, cuts his own lawn (with a push mower), and has a mind that is sharp as a tack. Normally William is a cautious person who thinks twice and asks plenty of good questions before he'll take any medicine.

William's doctor wanted him to go into the hospital for some tests. It was not supposed to be a big deal—some X-rays and blood work—but in the hospital William almost died because of a series of mistakes leading to drug complications. Almost from the moment he walked in the door, hospital policy undermined his confidence.

Wanting to be a good patient, William did not complain, even though he suspected all was not right. Not only did the nurses insist that he take sleeping medicine he did not need, they kept making him swallow all sorts of other pills without telling him what they were or why he had to take them. If he had been less reluctant to protest, he might not have received the wrong medications and suffered a life-threatening drug reaction.

What happened to William is not an isolated event. An analysis of medication errors at forty hospitals uncovered a startling 3,427 mistakes in a year.[4] The wrong medicine was given in the wrong way for the wrong reasons. Sometimes the right drug was administered too often, while other times the right drug wasn't given at all.

Even when the medicine is given correctly—that is, according to the doctor's instructions—there can be problems. Dr. Marion Friedman, writing in the journal *Postgraduate Medicine,* relates the following:

> In the past several years I have seen several cases in my own practice which I feel involved iatrogenic problems [problems induced by the physician or by the care prescribed]. One was a sudden death which I attributed to interaction of digoxin and quinidine. Another involved a patient with daily fever spiking to 104° F, evidence of newly acquired liver damage, severe leukopenia, and marked lymphadenopathy, all produced by tetracycline. The patient rapidly recovered after discontinuing tetracycline use.[5]

Dr. Friedman also found that increasing confusion and eventual coma in one elderly man were at first attributed to a stroke but actually resulted from the ulcer drug **Tagamet**. When this drug was stopped the patient "regained complete alertness within 24 hours."[6]

Adverse psychological or behavioral reactions to drugs are far more common than most physicians realize. People taking high-blood-pressure medications containing reserpine (**Diupres, Diutensen, Hydromox, Hydropres, Metatensin, Naquival, Regroton, Renese-R, Salutensin, Ser-Ap-Es, Serpasil, Unipres,** etc.) can experience severe psychological depression. Beta blockers like **Inderal** or **Lopressor** can produce the same kind of reaction.

Patients who complain about feeling down in the dumps may be given antidepressants like **Elavil** (amitriptyline) or **Triavil** (amitriptyline and perphenazine) to counteract the side effects of their blood pressure medications. Then they may become confused and disoriented from the drug combinations.

An article in the *Journal of the American Medical Association (JAMA)* has provided some startling statistics. When thirty-four people diagnosed as having delirium from "unknown causes" were reexamined, 38 percent of them were found to be having a toxic reaction to prescribed drugs. Add to that group the 17 percent of the diagnosed "major depression" cases and the nearly one third of the "adjustment disorder" patients who also were having delirium due to drug reactions, and you get a pretty significant percentage of patients whose problem was their "cure."[7]

A lot of people were just sick of their drugs, and a lot of doctors didn't realize the cause of the problem. Dr. Friedman admits quite candidly that one patient he witnessed "almost died from the effects of tetracycline, and the other from those of procainamide, even when each had been seen by a number of physicians and was under hospital supervision."[8]

There are ways you can help protect yourself against drug errors and interactions when in the hospital:

- *Number one*—Never swallow any tablet, capsule, or liquid, or accept any shot or suppository without knowing exactly what you are being given and why. This is especially important if you've been moved to a new room, or the nursing shift has just changed. If you've been put in Mrs. Smith's bed, someone could be giving you Mrs. Smith's medication.
- *Number two*—Make sure you know what the risks and benefits of the medication are, and never forget that you have the right to refuse any medicine. Just because they have taken your clothes away in the hospital doesn't mean you have given up your rights, too. If you feel intimidated by the nurse or doctor, get a family member to stand up for you. When in doubt, say no. I know of one man who almost died because the nurse insisted he take a penicillin-type antibiotic although he told her he was allergic to penicillin.
- *Number three*—Always tell the doctor, nurse, medical student, pharmacist, or any other health worker you see, what medications you're taking. Do not assume that the information is in your chart or that it has necessarily been seen and remembered.
- *Number four*—Most important, report *any* side effects so it can be determined whether what's supposed to be making you better isn't in fact making you sick. Don't leave home without a healthy dose of skepticism to swallow with the

medications you will almost inevitably be offered while in a hospital.

## What Is a Drug Interaction?

What is a drug interaction, anyway? Here we've been rambling on about all sorts of scary cases and you still don't know what exactly we're talking about. A drug–drug interaction is simply a situation in which two or more compounds, finding themselves together in your body, produce unwanted, unpredictable, or unfortunate complications.

When two drugs are taken simultaneously they may go about their pharmacologic business without affecting each other in the least. That would be the best of all possible worlds, but don't count on it working that way, because you are literally betting your life on the outcome.

A more likely possibility is that one medication will give an extra kick to either the therapeutic or toxic effects of the other. This is where 1 + 1 starts to add up to trouble very quickly. For example, someone who's taking tranquilizers can get quite dead by drinking too much. The two drugs together (remember, alcohol *is* a drug) sedate more heavily than either alone.

That's an example you have read about over and over, ad nauseam. Here is one I'll bet you've never heard of. And dollars to donuts your doctor hasn't heard about it either. Say you develop an ulcer. Chances are good that your physician will prescribe **Tagamet**. What he probably won't tell you is that the drug might make you drunker if you drink. There are several reports in the medical literature suggesting that **Tagamet** increases blood alcohol levels.[9-11]

It is not clear exactly how **Tagamet** boosts the buzz. Researchers speculate that the drug may speed up absorption of alcohol from the stomach, which means it gets into your bloodstream faster. Then again the ulcer medicine may delay elimination of alcohol by mucking up the metabolism in the liver. No matter how it works, I doubt seriously that the judge will accept a

**Tagamet** defense if you are arrested DWI (driving while intoxicated).

Sometimes drugs interact in the opposite way—they cancel each other out. Lots of folks actually try this gambit on New Year's Eve when they down lots of coffee in an attempt to reverse the sedative and reflex-slowing effects of too much booze. Unfortunately, this tactic doesn't work very well. You may end up a little more awake, but you'll still be drunk as a skunk. Driving could be more hazardous than ever, since you may be left with a false sense of confidence.

A better example of the $1 + 1 = 0$ scenario happens when the antibiotic tetracycline is prescribed simultaneously with penicillin. Tetracycline can reduce the effectiveness of penicillin and thus prolong an infection. Tetracycline can also have its benefits wiped out if you take antacid tablets or consume milk products (yogurt, cream in your coffee, cottage cheese, ice cream, etc.) along with the drug. This is one of the most common drug interactions.

While less dangerous than the life-threatening type of mix-up, this kind of interaction can prolong an illness or lead to the prescribing of more toxic medications since the doctor probably won't understand why the original medicine wasn't working.

Less common but no less significant is the interaction between barbiturates (pentobarbital, phenobarbital, secobarbital, etc.) and oral contraceptives. Imagine a woman who suffers from tension headaches. She could easily receive a prescription for **Fiorinal**, which contains the barbiturate butalbital along with aspirin and caffeine. Do you think the doctor will warn her that this headache remedy could interact with her contraceptive to reduce its effectiveness? How many *Rs* are there in fat chance?

But butalbital, as well as other barbiturates, may increase the rate of metabolism of oral contraceptives, thereby reducing their effectiveness. This could lead to spotting and breakthrough bleeding, not to mention an unwanted pregnancy.[12]

Sometimes interactions can be predicted based on knowledge of the drug's expected behavior in the body. At other times the interactions come as quite a surprise. New drugs are often the biggest problem because it may take several years and hundreds of thousands of human "guinea pigs" before physicians realize through trial and error that certain combinations of drugs are dangerous.

Even something as simple as a laxative can indirectly interfere with another drug. The speeding up of gastric motion can hinder normal absorption. That means less of what you need winds up getting into the blood where it can go to work.

Most times a drug interaction is unwanted and harmful, but on occasion it can be exploited to a patient's advantage. Giving an antidote for a particular poison is a beneficial drug interaction. When a person overdoses on a narcotic such as heroin or morphine, the first thing the emergency room physician does is administer Narcan (naloxone), a narcotic "antagonist." Within seconds a patient who is comatose and on the verge of croaking from respiratory depression will wake up and start breathing normally.

Sometimes doctors use one drug to make another more effective. When Benemid (probenecid) is given at the same time as penicillin or some of the newer cephalosporin antibiotics, the medicine reaches much higher levels in the bloodstream and remains in the body for a longer time. This greatly increases the bacteria-killing power of a dose of penicillin. In fact, probenecid was developed for just this purpose way back when penicillin was a rare and costly item. Today it's used primarily to decrease uric acid levels in patients with gout.

Drug interactions can affect many different parts of the body, but one of the most important sites is the liver. This organ is responsible for the detoxification and elimination of a great many of the chemicals we put into our bodies. If the liver doesn't work well enough, these chemicals can build up to toxic levels in the bloodstream. On the other hand, if the liver does its job a bit too energetically, a drug can be zapped out of existence before getting the job done.

Many drugs have the power to speed up the rate at which the liver breaks down other drugs. Hormones, alcohol, nicotine, sleeping pills, insecticides, tuberculosis drugs, and sedatives are but a few of the hundreds of chemicals that possess this property. But some medications may impair the liver's ability to metabolize other drugs.

Confused? How about an example to help straighten out this mess. Meet Mr. Deagan. Except for a little high blood pressure, he has had the blessing of good health almost his whole life. But at age sixty-four Mr. Deagan developed a painful case of thrombophlebitis as a result of several blood clots forming in the veins of his legs. His doctor prescribed an anticoagulant called **Coumadin** (warfarin) to thin his blood and prevent more clots from developing.

Mr. Deagan did just fine on the **Coumadin**. Periodically he went in for a blood test to make sure the drug was working all right. Everyone was happy. But then Mr. Deagan started complaining of indigestion and stomach pain. He had been under a lot of stress at work, and having had an ulcer once before, he figured he'd better get in to see his ulcer doc pronto. Sure enough, an ulcer it was, and out came a prescription for **Tagamet**. Mr. Deagan didn't think to mention he was also taking **Coumadin**, and the gastroenterologist didn't ask if he was taking any other medicine.

Mr. Deagan was delighted to find that his stomach pain disappeared almost as soon as he started taking the **Tagamet**, but within several days he noticed that his gums were beginning to bleed after brushing his teeth. That was disturbing, but not scary. Then his stools turned black and tarry. Now Mr. Deagan was worried.

He immediately went to the doctor's office and while there had a routine blood checkup. The doctor was amazed. Mr. Deagan's blood wasn't clotting as expected, because it was far too "thin." He had been hemorrhaging into his digestive tract (showing up as black, tarry stools) because the anticoagulant **Coumadin** had reached a dangerously toxic level in his blood. What could have gone wrong?

What happened was **Tagamet**. Remember, this ulcer medicine can affect liver enzymes and slow metabolism of other drugs. Mr. Deagan was no longer able to eliminate **Coumadin** the way he had before, so the drug began building up in his body. If he hadn't gotten in to the doctor and had his dosage reduced, he might have died from abdominal hemorrhaging or bleeding into the brain.

Mr. Deagan's case is purely hypothetical, but it could have happened just this way. There are reports in the medical literature of people who did in fact hemorrhage because they were taking **Tagamet** and **Coumadin** simultaneously.[13]

Other drugs that may also raise **Coumadin**'s blood levels to potentially toxic levels include aspirin, **Antabuse** (disulfiram), **Anturane** (sulfinpyrazone), **Atromid-S** (clofibrate), **Butazolidin** (phenylbutazone), **Chloromycetin** (chloramphenicol), **Choloxin** (dextrothyroxine), **Dolobid** (diflunisal), **Flagyl** (metronidazole), sulfa antibiotics, thyroid hormones, and possibly antidepressants. Even a flu shot (influenza vaccine) may raise blood levels of **Coumadin**.[14]

## Avoiding Drug Interactions

Let's get down to brass tacks. How can you or your doctor predict the potential for an adverse drug combination before getting caught with your chemical defenses down? Well, there are no ironclad guarantees, but there are a lot of steps to take, each of which greatly reduces the risk of suffering needlessly.

The first thing to do is write down exactly what you are taking, including all nonprescription drugs. I cannot stress this enough. The list may be bigger than you think. It was for Jane. At thirty-two she had recently separated from her husband. This had left her feeling incredibly depressed. Not only did she have trouble sleeping, but just dragging herself to work had become an almost impossible task. Jane's doctor prescribed **Nardil** (phenelzine) for her depression and **Dalmane** (flurazepam) for the insomnia.

Jane also suffered from hay fever and asthma. Not too serious, mind you, but whenever she caught a cold, she usually developed a bronchial wheeze. Jane was also a sucker for cats. Whenever

her neighbor's Persian came calling, Jane had a hard time resisting the urge to pet her. Usually within minutes she would start
sneezing and sniffling and later she would begin to wheeze.
Whenever that happened Jane would dig up some **Allerest** allergy pills for the sneezes and stuffy nose and **Primatene M**
tablets for her lungs. These nonprescription remedies generally
calmed things down within twenty or thirty minutes.

Jane was also slightly overweight. Having a marriage go down
the tubes was incredibly stressful, and Jane had taken to gorging
on ice cream and Oreo cookies when she was feeling particularly
bummed out.

As Jane started feeling less down with the help of the antidepressant **Nardil**, she resolved to shed those extra pounds. She
picked up a package of over-the-counter diet pills called **Dexatrim**, figuring they would suppress her appetite and make dieting
easier.

Every once in a while Jane developed a urinary-tract infection.
Her gynecologist prescribed **Achromycin V** (tetracycline), which
usually cleared up the problem in a few days. Jane always kept
some of the antibiotic on hand just in case a new infection flared
up.

Jane also averaged several drinks a day. If she went out to
lunch, she would usually have a glass or two of white wine.
When work was particularly grueling she might indulge in a
Bloody Mary or a Scotch on the rocks in the evening. Oh, and
let's not forget the vitamins. Jane wouldn't think of starting the
day without a vitamin and mineral complex plus some extra
vitamins E and C, not to mention **Os-Cal**, a calcium supplement.

If a doctor ever asked Jane how many medications she was
taking, she would probably have mentioned only **Nardil**. Jane
did not like to think of herself as a drug taker. Oh sure, she did
take the **Dalmane** for sleep now and again, but not *every* night.
And as for the over-the-counter drugs, she rationalized that they
didn't really count.

But the truth is that Jane had eight different drugs in her
medicine cabinet, not to mention the vitamins and minerals and

the alcohol. If you think that all sounds like a prescription for problems, you're right. Let's take a look at some of them.

Jane's over-the-counter allergy remedy **Allerest** contains the antihistamine chlorpheniramine and the decongestant **PPA** (phenylpropanolamine). Interestingly, her diet pill **Dexatrim** also contains **PPA**. That's because **PPA** is supposed to be able to suppress appetite as well as shrink swollen sinuses. But Jane rarely reads drug labels and wasn't aware that **Dexatrim** and **Allerest** both had the same ingredient.

If she were to take the diet pills and the hay-fever medicine on the same day, Jane could double her dose of **PPA**, which might lead to serious side effects, including headache, dizziness, nausea, heart palpitations, increased blood pressure, and tremor.

But far more dangerous would be the effect of taking either **Allerest** or **Dexatrim** in combination with the antidepressant **Nardil**. Blood pressure could skyrocket. And were Jane also to swallow her asthma medicine **Primatene M** (ephedrine, theophylline, and pyrilamine), she could experience a hypertensive crisis. Such a reaction, characterized by headache, neck stiffness, sweating (possibly with fever), palpitations, and chest pain, can produce such a serious increase in blood pressure that a person might have a stroke.

Jane is also in big trouble every time she has a drink. The problem here is that easily forgotten sleeping pill, **Dalmane**. This drug tends to accumulate in the body over several days. As a result, the sedative effects may linger, even during waking hours. Since many people may not realize that this is happening, they go ahead and have some white wine at lunch or a Bloody Mary after work. The combination of booze and **Dalmane** can be lethal if you try to drive. Coordination and reaction reflexes can be markedly slowed.

The package insert supplied to physicians and pharmacists has a very clear warning about this problem:

**Warnings: Patients receiving Dalmane should be cautioned about possible combined effects with alcohol and other CNS depressants. Also, caution patients that an additive effect**

may occur if alcoholic beverages are consumed during the day following the use of **Dalmane** for nighttime sedation. The potential for this interaction continues for several days following discontinuance of flurazepam . . .

Patients should also be cautioned about engaging in hazardous occupations requiring complete mental alertness such as operating machinery or driving a motor vehicle after ingesting the drug, including potential impairment of the performance of such activities which may occur the day following ingestion of **Dalmane**.[15]

The antihistamines in Jane's allergy and asthma medicine could also interact with **Dalmane** to increase the drug's sedative potential.

A less dangerous interaction occurs every time Jane swallows the antibiotic **Achromycin V** at breakfast. Remember that she also regularly downs her **Os-Cal** calcium supplement around mealtime. The calcium grabs onto the tetracycline in **Achromycin V** and renders it useless. Thus it is unlikely Jane's urinary-tract infection will clear up as quickly as it should.

As you can see, Jane is at risk for a number of serious drug interactions. Now Jane is actually a composite of a number of different newspaper column readers. Nevertheless, this theoretical example is really more typical than you think. Millions of people consume aspirin, alcohol, antacids, high-blood-pressure pills, sedatives, ulcer medicine, and heart pills at the same time. The "walking drugstore" phenomenon is extremely common, and doctors often fail to warn patients that certain chemical combinations can be dangerous.

Even scarier is the fact that many people never think the symptoms they experience can be directly related to the drugs they are taking. Doctors are sometimes reluctant to admit to themselves or their patients that the problem could be the cure. It's almost always the last possibility they consider, and then often reluctantly.

What commonly happens is that the side effects encountered with one drug are treated with another. Drug number two may produce an adverse reaction, or interact with drug number one. The "answer," of course, is often to prescribe something else, which has its own problems.

The answer for you, as a patient, is to take an active role in seeing that drug interaction problems don't become *your* problem. Here are some of the steps you can take to protect yourself:

- *Make certain the doctor is aware of all drugs—prescription and OTC—you are taking or are* likely *to take.* This is essential if he or she is to properly assess the possibilities of a drug interaction.

- *Always ask about possible interactions when getting a prescription.* Ask the doctor if the drug interacts with alcohol, any foods, OTC drugs, etcetera. And after you've asked the doctor, ask the pharmacist. This is an excellent means of double-checking information, and in many cases you will find the pharmacist a much more current and aware source of interaction information than the harried doctor. After all, drugs are the pharmacist's sole concern. Make no apologies for double-checking. It's *you* who will suffer from any mistakes.

- *Become your own best expert.* Check out the tables at the end of this chapter or those in *The People's Pharmacy-2* and *The New People's Pharmacy-3* to see what drugs don't mix. If you really want to get into this, you could check your local medical library or invest in a drug-interaction reference book. Although most are written in medicalese for physicians, pharmacists, and pharmacologists, you can still benefit, especially if you have a medical dictionary handy. My favorite resource is *Drug Interaction Facts* published by J. B. Lippincott Company (111 West Port Plaza, Suite 423, St. Louis, MS 63146). Unfortunately, like all medical books these days, this one is outrageously expensive. At the time of this writing it costs about $50, and that is bound to rise.

- *Reduce or eliminate alcoholic beverages while taking prescription drugs.* Booze can interact with an incredible num-

ber of drugs or chemicals in a potentially harmful way. A
good rule of thumb is to try to limit all drug consumption
to one thing at a time. If you must take more than one
medicine, check with your doctor or pharmacist about complications.

- *Don't mix drugs unnecessarily.* Be aware that if any drug
has some risk, any two taken together are probably more
than twice as risky. Ask the doctor whether you can do
without something you're already taking, if it's not absolutely essential. And don't reach for an OTC preparation
casually. Remember that it, just like a prescription drug,
will multiply your risk of suffering from a drug interaction.
In fact, the risk may be greater because you'll be proceeding
without trained advice.

- *Watch out for food–drug interactions.* The classic example
of this is the inactivation of tetracycline by milk or dairy
products. Another example is the antibiotic erythromycin.
This drug should never be taken with fruit juice or any
other acid drink because much of its antibacterial activity
could be destroyed by the acidity. (See *The People's Phar-
macy-2* for a list of food–drug, food–drink interactions.)

On the other hand, vitamins A, C, and E, and the mineral
selenium could interact with certain chemicals to our benefit rather than our detriment. These naturally occurring
substances may inhibit the cancer-causing properties of dietary chemicals, natural as well as man-made.[16] What the
proper cancer-preventing doses of these food supplements is
remains unclear, so don't start gobbling them in megadoses,
at least not yet. Hypervitaminosis (taking too many vitamins) can be a serious problem.

- *Be aware of the relative risk of various drugs.* Some common
drugs are frequently implicated in drug interactions, but the
dangers posed by each vary considerably. Drug interactions
with acetaminophen (Tylenol) are rarely very severe. Those
with anticoagulants (like Coumadin) often are.

Among the frequent-interaction drugs are aspirin and aspirin-
like pain relievers, alcohol, antacids, antibiotics, anticoagulants

(blood thinners), antihistamines, asthma medications, barbiturates, birth-control pills, blood-pressure medications, cough and cold preparations, diuretics (water pills), hay-fever remedies, sleeping pills, tranquilizers, and ulcer medications.

Other drugs, while less frequently involved in interactions, must be used with great caution, because when interactions *do* occur they're very often dangerous ones. Taking one of the following should wave a red flag of caution at both you and the doctor: anticoagulants (**Coumadin**), theophylline-type asthma medications (**Bronitin, Bronkaid, Bronkotabs, Elixophyllin, Marax, Primatene, Quibron, Slo-Phyllin, Somophyllin, Tedral, Thalfed, Theobid, Theo-Dur, Verquad**, etcetera), heart medicine like **Lanoxin** (digoxin), the antiseizure drug **Dilantin** (phenytoin), and all manner of sedating drugs.

This is not to say that other drugs and drug combinations are not potentially dangerous. Some important drug interactions are listed in the following table. Bear in mind that this list is, of necessity, incomplete. A complete treatment of the subject requires a text, and a thick one at that.

The very best protection is your own heightened sense of caution and awareness of the problem. Just keep in mind how often 1 + 1 adds up to something more (or less) than two.

# DRUG INTERACTIONS

## ORAL ANTICOAGULANTS (BLOOD-THINNING DRUGS)*

The following drugs antagonize and diminish the effectiveness of oral anticoagulant medication. In order to maintain therapeutic blood-thinning effects, your doctor may increase the dosage of anticoagulant. Conversely, any sudden discontinuation of the following drugs could precipitate a severe bleeding episode if the anticoagulant dosage is not reduced beforehand. It should be stressed that being under-anticoagulated can be just as dangerous as being over-anticoagulated. Oral anticoagulants are usually prescribed in an attempt to prevent a potentially life-threatening blood clot from forming, and an adequate dose of the medication is necessary to achieve this result:

**Alurate, Amytal, Butisol, Gemonil, Lotusate, Mebaral, Mysoline, Nembutal, Phenobarbital, Seconal, Tuinal** (all barbiturates), **Dilantin, Doriden, Fulvicin, Grifulvin V, Gris-Peg, Grisactin, Rimactane, Placidyl, Tegretol**

Because oral anticoagulant drugs interact in such a dangerous way with so many different types of medications, care should always be exercised if another drug is prescribed simultaneously.

*Any dosage alterations *must* be supervised by a physician!

## Oral Anticoagulants *cont.\**

**If a person who is consuming** oral anticoagulants: **Coumadin, Coufarin, Panwarfin** (warfarin sodium), **Athrombin-K** (warfarin potassium), **Liquamar** (phenprocoumon), **Dicumarol** (dicumarol or bishydroxycoumarin), **Hedulin** (phenindione), **Miradon** (anisindione)

| Also Uses | This Could Result |
|---|---|
| Analgesic Pain-relievers, Including Many Arthritis Preparations | This is a good way to die unexpectedly. For starters, many pain and arthritis medications not only enhance the anticoagulant's blood-thinning ability, but have some anticlotting activity of their own. Also, these drugs tend to irritate the stomach lining and can cause bleeding or even ulcers. |

**Also Uses**

Analgesic Pain-relievers, Including Many Arthritis Preparations

**Alka-Seltzer, Anacin, Ascriptin, Aspergum, Bayer Aspirin, Bufferin, Cope, Coricidin D, Ecotrin, Empirin, Excedrin, Vanquish,** etc. (all aspirin or aspirin-containing combination products) **Arthrolate, Arthropan, Disalcid, Durasal, Trilisate, Uracel 5,** etc. (related salicylate products) **Butazolidin, Clinoril, Dolobid, Indocin, Meclomen, Ponstel, Tandearil,** and probably others (nonsteroidal anti-inflammatory medications)

**This Could Result**

This is a good way to die unexpectedly. For starters, many pain and arthritis medications not only enhance the anticoagulant's blood-thinning ability, but have some anticlotting activity of their own. Also, these drugs tend to irritate the stomach lining and can cause bleeding or even ulcers.

Put all of these effects together, and your chances of seriously hemorrhaging have increased substantially. For minor pain acetaminophen (**Tylenol, Datril, Anacin-3, Panadol,** etc.) may be safer than aspirin, but even this drug can lead to the same trouble if used regularly. For arthritis, ibuprofen (**Motrin, Rufen, Advil, Nuprin**) and tolmetin (**Tolectin**), may be a little safer. Your physician

---

*\*Any dosage alterations *must* be supervised by a physician!*

## Oral Anticoagulants *cont.**

**If a person who is consuming** oral anticoagulants: **Coumadin, Coufarin, Panwarfin** (warfarin sodium), **Athrombin-K** (warfarin potassium), **Liquamar** (phenprocoumon), **Dicumarol** (dicumarol or bishydroxycoumarin), **Hedulin** (pheinindione), **Miradon** (anisindione)

|  | **This Could Result** *cont.* |
|---|---|
|  | should monitor your blood's clotting ability carefully and regularly no matter what pain or arthritis medicine you take. |
| **Also Uses** | **This Could Result** |
| Oral Antibiotics | *Note:* Many antibiotics, given by injection only, also interact with oral anticoagulants. As they are mostly restricted to hospital use, they are not listed here. |
|    **Achromycin, Azo-Gantanol, Azo-Gantrisin, Azotrex, Azulfidine, Bactrim, Chloromycetin, Declomycin, Erythromycin, Fansidar, Flagyl, Fulvicin, Gantanol, Gantrisin, Humatin, Ilosone, Kantrex, Minocin, Mycifradin, NegGram, Neomycin, Quinine, Renoquid, Rondomycin, Septra, Sulfadiazine, Sulfapyridine, Sumycin,** | Broad-spectrum antibiotics kill not only the bad-guy bugs, but some good ones as well, including those bacterial residents of our intestines that do us a favor by making Vitamin K. By the way, we need Vitamin K if we don't want to bleed to death. It is crucial for proper blood coagulation. |

*Any dosage alterations *must* be supervised by a physician!

## Oral Anticoagulants *cont.**

**If a person who is consuming** oral anticoagulants: **Coumadin, Coufarin, Panwarfin** (warfarin sodium), **Athrombin-K** (warfarin potassium), **Liquamar** (phenprocoumon), **Dicumarol** (dicumarol or bishydroxycoumarin), **Hedulin** (pheinindione), **Miradon** (anisindione)

| Also Uses *cont.* | This Could Result *cont.* |
|---|---|
| **Terfonyl, Terramycin,** Tetracycline, **Thiosulfil, Urobiotic-250, Vibramycin,** and other similar antibiotics | Oral anticoagulants act in part by suppressing the activity of Vitamin K. It is obvious that if the vitamin-making bacteria are killed off by antibiotics, the blood-thinning effects of the anticoagulants will be exaggerated. In addition, some sulfa antibiotics can enhance the anticoagulant's effects by increasing the levels of active drug in the bloodstream. The bottom line is an increased susceptibility to bleeding and hemorrhaging when these antibiotics are administered at the same time as oral anticoagulants. |
| **Also Uses** | **This Could Result** |
| Oral Antidiabetic Medications | See table listing *Diabetes Medicine.* |

*Any dosage alterations *must* be supervised by a physician!

## Oral Anticoagulants *cont.**

If a person who is consuming oral anticoagulants: **Coumadin, Coufarin, Panwarfin** (warfarin sodium), **Athrombin-K** (warfarin potassium), **Liquamar** (phenprocoumon), **Dicumarol** (dicumarol or bishydroxycoumarin), **Hedulin** (pheinindione), **Miradon** (anisindione)

| Also Uses | This Could Result |
|---|---|
| Cholesterol-lowering Medications<br><br>**Atromid-S, Choloxin** | **Atromid-S** (clofibrate) will increase blood-thinning responses to the point of serious hemorrhage, and deaths have occurred due to this interaction. **Choloxin** (dextrothyroxine) can also increase the risk of bleeding and the dose of the oral anticoagulant should be decreased by a doctor to compensate for this effect. Close blood-test monitoring is essential. |
| **Colestid, Questran** | **Questran** and **Colestid** both prevent the oral anticoagulant from being absorbed into the bloodstream and therefore an increased anticoagulant dose may be necessary to achieve the desired effect. |

| Also Uses | This Could Result |
|---|---|
| Anticonvulsants (Antiepilepsy Medications) | See table listing *Anticonvulsant Medications*. |

*Any dosage alterations *must* be supervised by a physician!

## Oral Anticoagulants *cont.*＊

**If a person who is consuming** oral anticoagulants: **Coumadin, Coufarin, Panwarfin** (warfarin sodium), **Athrombin-K** (warfarin potassium), **Liquamar** (phenprocoumon), **Dicumarol** (dicumarol or bishydroxycoumarin), **Hedulin** (pheinindione), **Miradon** (anisindione)

| Also Uses | This Could Result |
|---|---|
| Antidepressants<br><br>**Adapin, Asendin, Aventyl, Elavil, Janimine, Norpramin, Pamelor, Sinequan, Surmontil, Tofranil, Triavil, Vivactil** | These "tricyclic antidepressants" have been reported to increase the blood levels of **Dicumarol** and **Liquamar**, but don't seem to be affected by warfarin. |
| **Also Uses** | **This Could Result** |
| Foods<br><br>Green Leafy Vegetables, (Asparagus, Broccoli, Kale, Lettuce, Spinach, Watercress), Onions | Though probably not too important, onions, if consumed in large quantities, could intensify the anticoagulant effect. Green leafy vegetables, which are sources of Vitamin K, could do just the opposite and antagonize the blood-thinning effect. |

＊Any dosage alterations *must* be supervised by a physician!

## Oral Anticoagulants *cont.**

If a person who is consuming oral anticoagulants: **Couma-din, Coufarin, Panwarfin** (warfarin sodium), **Athrombin-K** (warfarin potassium), **Liquamar** (phenprocoumon), **Dicuma-rol** (dicumarol or bishydroxycoumarin), **Hedulin** (pheinind-ione), **Miradon** (anisindione)

| Also Uses | This Could Result |
|-----------|-------------------|
| Gout Medication<br><br>    **Anturane, Zyloprim** | **Zyloprim** (allopurinol) can enhance the anticoagulant effects of **Dicumarol** and **Liquamar,** but apparently not of warfarin. **Anturane** (sulfinpyrazone) has a similar interaction with warfarin and **Dicumarol,** but not with **Liquamar.** |

*Any dosage alterations *must* be supervised by a physician!

## Oral Anticoagulants *cont.**

**If a person who is consuming** oral anticoagulants: **Couma-din, Coufarin, Panwarfin** (warfarin sodium), **Athrombin-K** (warfarin potassium), **Liquamar** (phenprocoumon), **Dicuma-rol** (dicumarol or bishydroxycoumarin), **Hedulin** (pheinind-ione), **Miradon** (anisindione)

| Also Uses | This Could Result |
|---|---|
| Thyroid Medications<br><br>propylthiouracil,<br>**Tapazole** (taken for overactive thyroids),<br>**Armour Thyroid, Cytomel, Euthroid, Levothroid, Noroxine, Proloid, S-P-T, Synthroid, Thyrar, Thyroid USP, Thyrolar, Westhroid**<br>(thyroid-replacement hormones taken for underactive thyroids) | Therapy with thyroid-active medication is aimed at keeping the thyroid gland operating at a normal, or "euthyroid" state. As long as you remain euthyroid, no adverse effects or interactions should occur while taking oral anticoagulants. The problems arise when you take too much or too little medication. Taking an excess of propylthiouracil or of **Tapazole,** or not taking enough of the thyroid-replacement hormones, will leave you effectively hypothyroid ("hypo" = not enough). In this condition you will need more anticoagulant than usual.<br>  If you take too much thyroid-replacement hormone or not enough of the other two, you will become hyperthyroid ("hyper" = too |

*Any dosage alterations *must* be supervised by a physician!

## Oral Anticoagulants *cont.*\*

**If a person who is consuming** oral anticoagulants: **Couma-din**, **Coufarin**, **Panwarfin** (warfarin sodium), **Athrombin-K** (warfarin potassium), **Liquamar** (phenprocoumon), **Dicuma-rol** (dicumarol or bishydroxycoumarin), **Hedulin** (pheinind-ione), **Miradon** (anisindione)

|  | **This Could Result** *cont.* |
|---|---|
|  | much), and you will need to reduce the dosage of the anticoagulant or face possible bleeding problems. Your physician should take extra pains to make sure you are kept euthyroid and properly anticoagulated. |
| **Also Uses** | **This Could Result** |
| Ulcer Medicine | See table listing **Tagamet** (cimetidine). |

\*Any dosage alterations *must* be supervised by a physician!

## Oral Anticoagulants *cont.**

**If a person who is consuming** oral anticoagulants: **Couma-din, Coufarin, Panwarfin** (warfarin sodium), **Athrombin-K** (warfarin potassium), **Liquamar** (phenprocoumon), **Dicuma-rol** (dicumarol or bishydroxycoumarin), **Hedulin** (pheinind-ione), **Miradon** (anisindione)

| Also Uses | This Could Result |
|---|---|
| Vitamin Supplements<br><br>  Vitamins C, E, and<br>  especially K | The interactions between oral anticoagulants and vitamins C and E are controversial. Massive doses of Vitamin C have been reported to interfere with blood-thinning activity and moderate amounts of Vitamin E have been implicated in enhancing oral anticoagulant activity. The evidence for both interactions is pretty slim, but I mention it because vitamin popping is so common and the potential for trouble exists.<br><br>On the other hand, the case for an interaction with Vitamin K is crystal clear. Oral anticoagulants and Vitamin K act in direct opposition to each other. In fact, in cases of severe anticoagulant overdose, Vitamin K is given as an antidote. Do not take any vitamin supplements containing Vitamin K while on oral anticoagulants. |

*Any dosage alterations *must* be supervised by a physician!

## ANTICONVULSANT MEDICATIONS (FOR EPILEPSY)*

**If a person who is consuming** anticonvulsants **Clonopin** (clonazepam), **Depakene** (valproic acid), **Depakote** (divalproex sodium), **Dilantin** (phenytoin), **Gemonil** (metharbital), **Luminal** (phenobarbital), **Mebaral** (mephobarbital), **Mesantoin** (mephenytoin), **Mysoline** (primidone), **Peganone** (ethotoin), **Phenurone** (phenacemide), **Tegretol** (carbamazepine), **Tranxene** (clorazepate), **Valium** and **Valrelease** (diazepam)

| Also Uses | This Could Result |
|---|---|
| Oral Anticoagulants (Blood Thinners)<br><br>**Athrombin-K, Coumadin, Coufarin, Panwarfin** (all forms of warfarin), **Dicumarol, Liquamar** | The interactions between the "hydantoin" drugs **(Dilantin, Mesantoin,** and **Peganone)** and the oral anticoagulants are myriad and complex. **Dicomarol** (dicumarol or bishydroxycoumarin) and **Liquamar** (phenprocoumon) can interfere with the metabolism of **Dilantin** and the other hydantoins, causing increased blood levels of the anticonvulsant, leading to severe toxicity. On the other hand, **Dilantin** may reduce or even soup up warfarin's horsepower and can cause bleeding problems. If you must take these two types of drugs together, your doctor should monitor the blood levels of *both* drugs. |

*Any dosage alterations *must* be supervised by a physician!

## Anticonvulsant Medications *cont.* *

**If a person who is consuming** anticonvulsants **Clonopin** (clonazepam), **Depakene** (valproic acid), **Depakote** (divalproex sodium), **Dilantin** (phenytoin), **Gemonil** (metharbital), **Luminal** (phenobarbital), **Mebaral** (mephobarbital), **Mesantoin** (mephenytoin), **Mysoline** (primidone), **Peganone** (ethotoin), **Phenurone** (phenacemide), **Tegretol** (carbamazepine), **Tranxene** (clorazepate), **Valium** and **Valrelease** (diazepam)

### This Could Result *cont.*

When the barbiturate anticonvulsants **(Gemonil, Luminal, Mebaral,** and **Mysoline)** are mixed with oral anticoagulants, the blood levels of the anticoagulant decrease. The real problem comes if you stop taking the barbiturate. The inhibiting effect disappears and the levels of anticoagulant increase, possibly leading to bleeding problems. The same interaction can occur with **Tegretol.** Again, your physician should carefully monitor the blood levels of the anticoagulant.

*Any dosage alterations *must* be supervised by a physician!

## Anticonvulsant Medications *cont.*\*

**If a person who is consuming** anticonvulsants **Clonopin** (clonazepam), **Depakene** (valproic acid), **Depakote** (divalproex sodium), **Dilantin** (phenytoin), **Gemonil** (metharbital), **Luminal** (phenobarbital), **Mebaral** (mephobarbital), **Mesantoin** (mephenytoin), **Mysoline** (primidone), **Peganone** (ethotoin), **Phenurone** (phenacemide), **Tegretol** (carbamazepine), **Tranxene** (clorazepate), **Valium** and **Valrelease** (diazepam)

| Also Uses | This Could Result |
|---|---|
| Other Anticonvulsants<br><br>**Depakene, Depakote, Dilantin, Luminal Mesantoin, Mysoline, Peganone, Phenurone** | **Depakene** and **Depakote** can increase the toxicity of **Dilantin, Mesantoin,** and **Peganone** without altering the hydantoin's blood levels. Since these two classes of anticonvulsant medications are frequently given together, extra care must be taken, and the dosage of the hydantoin will likely have to be decreased. **Luminal** (phenobarbital) blood levels are increased by **Depakene** and **Depakote** and side effects such as sedation and loss of balance may occur. |

\*Any dosage alterations *must* be supervised by a physician!

## Anticonvulsant Medications *cont.**

If a person who is consuming anticonvulsants **Clonopin** (clonazepam), **Depakene** (valproic acid), **Depakote** (divalproex sodium), **Dilantin** (phenytoin), **Gemonil** (metharbital), **Luminal** (phenobarbital), **Mebaral** (mephobarbital), **Mesantoin** (mephenytoin), **Mysoline** (primidone), **Peganone** (ethotoin), **Phenurone** (phenacemide), **Tegretol** (carbamazepine), **Tranxene** (clorazepate), **Valium** and **Valrelease** (diazepam)

| Also Uses *cont.* | This Could Result *cont.* |
|---|---|
| **Mesantoin, Mysoline, Peganone, Phenurone** | **Mysoline** toxicity is enhanced when one of the hydantoins are added to the anticonvulsant regimen. The **Mysoline** dose should probably be decreased to compensate for the interaction. Doses of **Dilantin, Mesantoin,** and **Peganone** should likewise be reduced if **Phenurone** (phenacemide) is also given. Although no direct evidence links the two classes of drugs, other drugs similar to phenacemide, although not available in this country, have been proven to cause increased **Dilantin** levels when given concurrently. In this case it is best to play it safe and monitor the blood levels of the hydantoin. |

*Any dosage alterations *must* be supervised by a physician!

## Anticonvulsant Medications *cont.**

**If a person who is consuming** anticonvulsants **Clonopin** (clonazepam), **Depakene** (valproic acid), **Depakote** (divalproex sodium), **Dilantin** (phenytoin), **Gemonil** (metharbital), **Luminal** (phenobarbital), **Mebaral** (mephobarbital), **Mesantoin** (mephenytoin), **Mysoline** (primidone), **Peganone** (ethotoin), **Phenurone** (phenacemide), **Tegretol** (carbamazepine), **Tranxene** (clorazepate), **Valium** and **Valrelease** (diazepam)

| Also Uses | This Could Result |
|---|---|
| Arthritis Drugs (Nonsteroidal Anti-Inflammatories) | See table listing *Arthritis Medication.* |

| Also Uses | This Could Result |
|---|---|
| Oral Contraceptives | See table listing *Birth-control Pills.* |

| Also Uses | This Could Result |
|---|---|
| Beta Blockers<br><br>  **Inderal, Lopressor** | The barbiturate anticonvulsants **Gemonil, Luminal, Mebaral, Mesantoin,** and **Mysoline** can stimulate the liver's metabolism of these two beta blockers. A higher dose of the latter may be necessary. Another option is to switch to another noninteracting beta blocker. |

*Any dosage alterations *must* be supervised by a physician!

## Anticonvulsant Medications *cont.*\*

**If a person who is consuming** anticonvulsants **Clonopin** (clonazepam), **Depakene** (valproic acid), **Depakote** (divalproex sodium), **Dilantin** (phenytoin), **Gemonil** (metharbital), **Luminal** (phenobarbital), **Mebaral** (mephobarbital), **Mesantoin** (mephenytoin), **Mysoline** (primidone), **Peganone** (ethotoin), **Phenurone** (phenacemide), **Tegretol** (carbamazepine), **Tranxene** (clorazepate), **Valium** and **Valrelease** (diazepam)

| Also Uses | This Could Result |
|---|---|
| Steroid Medications | See table listing *Cortisone-type Anti-Inflammatory Medication.* |

| Also Uses | This Could Result |
|---|---|
| Sulfa Antibiotics, Miscellaneous Antibiotics<br><br>**Azo-Gantanol, Azo-Gantrisin, Azotrex, Azulfidine, Bactrim, Fansidar, Gantanol, Gantrisin, Renoquid, Septra, Sulfadiazine, Sulfapyridine, Terfonyl, Thiosulfil, Urobiotic-250** (all sulfa antibiotics or combinations containing sulfa) | The sulfa antibiotics can prevent the normal elimination of the hydantoin anticonvulsants **(Dilantin, Mesantoin, and Peganone).** The increased levels of the epilepsy drugs can lead to a whole series of alarming reactions. Blood levels of the anticonvulsant should be monitored by your doctor if you need to take these drugs together. |

\*Any dosage alterations *must* be supervised by a physician!

## Anticonvulsant Medications *cont.**

**If a person who is consuming** anticonvulsants **Clonopin** (clonazepam), **Depakene** (valproic acid), **Depakote** (divalproex sodium), **Dilantin** (phenytoin), **Gemonil** (metharbital), **Luminal** (phenobarbital), **Mebaral** (mephobarbital), **Mesantoin** (mephenytoin), **Mysoline** (primidone), **Peganone** (ethotoin), **Phenurone** (phenacemide), **Tegretol** (carbamazepine), **Tranxene** (clorazepate), **Valium** and **Valrelease** (diazepam)

| Also Uses *cont.* | This Could Result *cont.* |
|---|---|
| **Proloprim, Trimpex** (trimethoprim), **Nydrazid** (isoniazid), **Chloromycetin** (chloramphenicol), **E-Mycin, Ilosone** (erythromycin), **Tao** (troleandomycin), **Vibramycin** (doxycycline) | **Bactrim** and **Septra** pack a double whammy. Both are combinations of a sulfa antibiotic, sulfamethoxazole, and another antibiotic, trimethoprim. You've already seen what the sulfa drug can do, but trimethoprim interacts in just the same manner. The net result can lead to toxic levels of **Dilantin** and, presumably, **Mesantoin** and **Peganone.** Trimethoprim also comes as a single drug in **Proloprim** and **Trimpex.** |
| | Isoniazid, a drug used to treat tuberculosis, blocks the metabolism of **Dilantin** and the other hydantoins as well as **Tegretol.** The chances of toxicity due to too much an- |

*Any dosage alterations *must* be supervised by a physician!

## Anticonvulsant Medications *cont.**

**If a person who is consuming** anticonvulsants **Clonopin** (clonazepam), **Depakene** (valproic acid), **Depakote** (divalproex sodium), **Dilantin** (phenytoin), **Gemonil** (metharbital), **Luminal** (phenobarbital), **Mebaral** (mephobarbital), **Mesantoin** (mephenytoin), **Mysoline** (primidone), **Peganone** (ethotoin), **Phenurone** (phenacemide), **Tegretol** (carbamazepine), **Tranxene** (clorazepate), **Valium** and **Valrelease** (diazepam)

**This Could Result *cont.***

ticonvulsant are thereby increased. **Tegretol** toxicity is also seen when given with erythromycin and the related antibiotic troleandomycin. Similarly, **Dilantin** toxicity can occur when taken concurrently with **Chloromycetin.**

**Tegretol, Dilantin, Mesantoin, Peganone, Gemonil, Luminal, Mebaral,** and **Mysoline** decrease the blood levels of **Vibramycin** and probably its effectiveness as well. Play it safe and use plain old tetracycline instead (it's also a lot cheaper!).

*Any dosage alterations *must* be supervised by a physician!

## Anticonvulsant Medications *cont.*\*

**If a person who is consuming** anticonvulsants **Clonopin** (clonazepam), **Depakene** (valproic acid), **Depakote** (divalproex sodium), **Dilantin** (phenytoin), **Gemonil** (metharbital), **Luminal** (phenobarbital), **Mebaral** (mephobarbital), **Mesantoin** (mephenytoin), **Mysoline** (primidone), **Peganone** (ethotoin), **Phenurone** (phenacemide), **Tegretol** (carbamazepine), **Tranxene** (clorazepate), **Valium** and **Valrelease** (diazepam)

| Also Uses | This Could Result |
|---|---|
| Ulcer Medication | See table listing **Tagamet** (cimetidine). |

| Also Uses | This Could Result |
|---|---|
| Miscellaneous Other Medicines<br><br>**Antabuse, Butazolidin** | **Antabuse** (disulfiram) and **Butazolidin** (phenylbutazone) can both increase the pharmacologic effects of the hydantoin epilepsy drugs **Dilantin, Mesantoin,** and **Peganone.** The potential for side effects increases as well. |
| Folic Acid | Folic acid, a vitamin, can antagonize the effects of the hydantoins, leading to poor seizure control. Conversely, **Dilantin** and the other hydantoins can induce a state of folic acid deficiency, requiring folic acid supplementation. |

\*Any dosage alterations *must* be supervised by a physician!

## Anticonvulsant Medications *cont.**

**If a person who is consuming** anticonvulsants **Clonopin** (clonazepam), **Depakene** (valproic acid), **Depakote** (divalproex sodium), **Dilantin** (phenytoin), **Gemonil** (metharbital), **Luminal** (phenobarbital), **Mebaral** (mephobarbital), **Mesantoin** (mephenytoin), **Mysoline** (primidone), **Peganone** (ethotoin), **Phenurone** (phenacemide), **Tegretol** (carbamazepine), **Tranxene** (clorazepate), **Valium** and **Valrelease** (diazepam)

| Also Uses *cont.* | This Could Result |
|---|---|
| Antacids | Although controversial, there is the possibility that taking your **Dilantin** at the same time as an antacid can reduce the absorption of the epilepsy medicine. Play it safe and don't take the two together. |
| **Darvon**<br>Alcohol | **Darvon** (propoxyphene) can increase the effects of **Tegretol** and a decrease in anticonvulsant dose may be necessary. Since many of these anticonvulsant medications can make you drowsy, especially when first taking them, avoid alcohol to prevent oversedation. |

*Any dosage alterations *must* be supervised by a physician!

## ANTIDEPRESSANTS (TRICYCLIC AND RELATED COMPOUNDS)*

*Note:* It usually takes from two to four weeks before the beneficial effects of antidepressant medication become apparent. It may also take this long for the drug to disappear from a patient's system once it has been discontinued. This time lag must be considered if additional drugs are consumed. If you are taking an MAO inhibitor and your doctor wants to switch you to a tricyclic antidepressant, allow at least two weeks after you have stopped taking the former before beginning the latter.

**If a person who is consuming** antidepressants **Asendin** (amoxapine), **Aventyl** and **Pamelor** (nortriptyline), **Elavil** and **Endep** (amitriptyline), **Norpramin** and **Pertofrane** (desipramine), **Sinequan** and **Adapin** (doxepin), **Surmontil** (trimipramine), **Tofranil** and **Janimine** (imipramine), **Vivactil** (protriptyline) (all tricyclic antidepressants)

*or*

**Desyrel** (trazodone), **Ludiomil** (maprotiline) (related antidepressants)

| Also Uses | This Could Result |
|---|---|
| Alcohol<br><br>Beer, Hard Stuff, Wine | Help! This is a hazardous combination. Excessive sedation may occur, especially with **Elavil, Sinequan, Surmontil,** and **Ludiomil,** which tend to be fairly sedating even by themselves. "Beware the Jabberwock, my son!" |

*Any dosage alterations *must* be supervised by a physician!

## Antidepressants *cont.*\*

*Note:* It usually takes from two to four weeks before the beneficial effects of antidepressant medication become apparent. It may also take this long for the drug to disappear from a patient's system once it has been discontinued. This time lag must be considered if additional drugs are consumed. If you are taking an MAO inhibitor and your doctor wants to switch you to a tricyclic antidepressant, allow at least two weeks after you have stopped taking the former before beginning the latter.

---

**If a person who is consuming** antidepressants **Asendin** (amoxapine), **Aventyl** and **Pamelor** (nortriptyline), **Elavil** and **Endep** (amitriptyline), **Norpramin** and **Pertofrane** (desipramine), **Sinequan** and **Adapin** (doxepin), **Surmontil** (trimipramine), **Tofranil** and **Janimine** (imipramine), **Vivactil** (protriptyline) (all tricyclic antidepressants)

*or*

**Desyrel** (trazodone), **Ludiomil** (maprotiline) (related antidepressants)

| Also Uses | This Could Result |
|---|---|
| Oral Anticoagulants (Blood Thinners) **Athrombin-K, Coumadin, Coufarin, Panwarfin** (all forms of warfarin), **Dicumarol, Liquamar** | Watch out for increased anticoagulant action when **Dicumarol** or **Liquamar** is mixed with any of the tricyclic antidepressants. Bleeding could occur. The dose of oral anticoagulant should probably be decreased and the blood levels monitored if it is necessary to mix these two drugs. This interaction probably does not occur with warfarin. |

\*Any dosage alterations *must* be supervised by a physician!

## Antidepressants *cont.*\*

*Note:* It usually takes from two to four weeks before the beneficial effects of antidepressant medication become apparent. It may also take this long for the drug to disappear from a patient's system once it has been discontinued. This time lag must be considered if additional drugs are consumed. If you are taking an MAO inhibitor and your doctor wants to switch you to a tricyclic antidepressant, allow at least two weeks after you have stopped taking the former before beginning the latter.

If a person who is consuming antidepressants **Asendin** (amoxapine), **Aventyl** and **Pamelor** (nortriptyline), **Elavil** and **Endep** (amitriptyline), **Norpramin** and **Pertofrane** (desipramine), **Sinequan** and **Adapin** (doxepin), **Surmontil** (trimipramine), **Tofranil** and **Janimine** (imipramine), **Vivactil** (protriptyline) (all tricyclic antidepressants)

*or*

**Desyrel** (trazodone), **Ludiomil** (maprotiline) (related antidepressants)

| Also Uses | This Could Result |
|---|---|
| Blood-pressure Medications **Diupres, Enduronyl, Harmonyl, Hydromox, Hydropres, Moderil, Naquival, Raudixin, Rau-Sed, Rauwiloid, Rauzide,** Reserpine, **Ser-Ap-Es, Serpasil, Sandril** (all derivatives of rauwolfia) | The tricyclic antidepressants may counteract the blood-pressure-lowering effects of **Catapres** (clonidine), **Hylorel** (guanadrel), **Ismelin** (guanethidine), and **Combipres** and **Esimil** (combination products). Since there are other effective blood-pressure medications out on the market, this interaction |

\*Any dosage alterations *must* be supervised by a physician!

## Antidepressants *cont.**

*Note:* It usually takes from two to four weeks before the beneficial effects of antidepressant medication become apparent. It may also take this long for the drug to disappear from a patient's system once it has been discontinued. This time lag must be considered if additional drugs are consumed. If you are taking an MAO inhibitor and your doctor wants to switch you to a tricyclic antidepressant, allow at least two weeks after you have stopped taking the former before beginning the latter.

---

**If a person who is consuming** antidepressants **Asendin** (amoxapine), **Aventyl** and **Pamelor** (nortriptyline), **Elavil** and **Endep** (amitriptyline), **Norpramin** and **Pertofrane** (desipramine), **Sinequan** and **Adapin** (doxepin), **Surmontil** (trimipramine), **Tofranil** and **Janimine** (imipramine), **Vivactil** (protriptyline) (all tricyclic antidepressants)

*or*

**Desyrel** (trazodone), **Ludiomil** (maprotiline) (related antidepressants)

| Also Uses *cont.* | This Could Result *cont.* |
|---|---|
| Catapres, Combipres, Esimil, Hylorel, Ismelin | can easily be avoided. At the very least, increasing the dose of the blood pressure medication and taking frequent blood-pressure readings seems warranted. Paradoxically, **Desyrel** can cause low blood pressure on its own, and in combination with blood-pressure medications (other than **Catapres**) can |

---

*Any dosage alterations *must* be supervised by a physician!

## Antidepressants *cont.**

*Note:* It usually takes from two to four weeks before the beneficial effects of antidepressant medication become apparent. It may also take this long for the drug to disappear from a patient's system once it has been discontinued. This time lag must be considered if additional drugs are consumed. If you are taking an MAO inhibitor and your doctor wants to switch you to a tricyclic antidepressant, allow at least two weeks after you have stopped taking the former before beginning the latter.

**If a person who is consuming** antidepressants **Asendin** (amoxapine), **Aventyl** and **Pamelor** (nortriptyline), **Elavil** and **Endep** (amitriptyline), **Norpramin** and **Pertofrane** (desipramine), **Sinequan** and **Adapin** (doxepin), **Surmontil** (trimipramine), **Tofranil** and **Janimine** (imipramine), **Vivactil** (protriptyline) (all tricyclic antidepressants)

*or*

**Desyrel** (trazodone), **Ludiomil** (maprotiline) (related antidepressants)

**This Could Result *cont.***

cause excessively low blood pressure.

The interactions with the reserpine-type drugs are less clear. Since these high-blood-pressure medicines can cause depression in the first place, their use in a depressed patient is questionable.

*Any dosage alterations *must* be supervised by a physician!

## Antidepressants *cont.**

*Note:* It usually takes from two to four weeks before the beneficial effects of antidepressant medication become apparent. It may also take this long for the drug to disappear from a patient's system once it has been discontinued. This time lag must be considered if additional drugs are consumed. If you are taking an MAO inhibitor and your doctor wants to switch you to a tricyclic antidepressant, allow at least two weeks after you have stopped taking the former before beginning the latter.

**If a person who is consuming** antidepressants **Asendin** (amoxapine), **Aventyl** and **Pamelor** (nortriptyline), **Elavil** and **Endep** (amitriptyline), **Norpramin** and **Pertofrane** (desipramine), **Sinequan** and **Adapin** (doxepin), **Surmontil** (trimipramine), **Tofranil** and **Janimine** (imipramine), **Vivactil** (protriptyline) (all tricyclic antidepressants)

*or*

**Desyrel** (trazodone), **Ludiomil** (maprotiline) (related antidepressants)

| Also Uses | This Could Result |
|---|---|
| MAO Inhibitors (Used for Depression or High Blood Pressure)<br><br>**Eutonyl, Eutron, Furoxone** (an antibiotic!), **Marplan, Nardil, Parnate** | Beware! This may be an extremely serious interaction, especially with **Norpramin** and **Pertofrane** (desipramine) and **Tofranil** and **Janimine** (imipramine). Excitation, delirium, heart problems, elevated body temperature, and convulsions are but a few of the dangerous side effects of |

*Any dosage alterations *must* be supervised by a physician!

## Antidepressants *cont.** 

*Note:* It usually takes from two to four weeks before the beneficial effects of antidepressant medication become apparent. It may also take this long for the drug to disappear from a patient's system once it has been discontinued. This time lag must be considered if additional drugs are consumed. If you are taking an MAO inhibitor and your doctor wants to switch you to a tricyclic antidepressant, allow at least two weeks after you have stopped taking the former before beginning the latter.

**If a person who is consuming** antidepressants **Asendin** (amoxapine), **Aventyl** and **Pamelor** (nortriptyline), **Elavil** and **Endep** (amitriptyline), **Norpramin** and **Pertofrane** (desipramine), **Sinequan** and **Adapin** (doxepin), **Surmontil** (trimipramine), **Tofranil** and **Janimine** (imipramine), **Vivactil** (protriptyline) (all tricyclic antidepressants)

*or*

**Desyrel** (trazodone), **Ludiomil** (maprotiline) (related antidepressants)

**This Could Result *cont.***

this combination. Under carefully controlled conditions, some of the other antidepressants have been safely used in conjunction with an MAO inhibitor, but this is surely risky business.

*Any dosage alterations *must* be supervised by a physician!

## Antidepressants *cont.*\*

*Note:* It usually takes from two to four weeks before the beneficial effects of antidepressant medication become apparent. It may also take this long for the drug to disappear from a patient's system once it has been discontinued. This time lag must be considered if additional drugs are consumed. If you are taking an MAO inhibitor and your doctor wants to switch you to a tricyclic antidepressant, allow at least two weeks after you have stopped taking the former before beginning the latter.

**If a person who is consuming** antidepressants **Asendin** (amoxapine), **Aventyl** and **Pamelor** (nortriptyline), **Elavil** and **Endep** (amitriptyline), **Norpramin** and **Pertofrane** (desipramine), **Sinequan** and **Adapin** (doxepin), **Surmontil** (trimipramine), **Tofranil** and **Janimine** (imipramine), **Vivactil** (protriptyline) (all tricyclic antidepressants)

*or*

**Desyrel** (trazodone), **Ludiomil** (maprotiline) (related antidepressants)

| Also Uses | This Could Result |
|---|---|
| Thyroid Medications<br><br>**Armour Thyroid, Cytomel, Euthroid, Levothroid, Noroxine, Proloid, S-P-T, Synthroid, Thyrar, Thyroid USP, Thyrolar, Westhroid**<br>(thyroid-replacement hormones taken for underactive thyroids) | Thyroid hormones can potentiate both the beneficial and harmful effects of the tricyclic antidepressants. Side effects such as an abnormally fast heart rate and abnormal heart rhythms seem to make this combination tricky. |

\*Any dosage alterations *must* be supervised by a physician!

## ARTHRITIS MEDICATION (NONSTEROIDAL ANTI-INFLAMMATORY AGENTS)*

**If a person who is consuming** arthritis medication **Anaprox** and **Naprosyn** (naproxen), **Azolid** and **Butazolidin** (phenylbutazone), **Clinoril** (sulindac), **Dolobid** (diflunisal), **Feldene** (piroxicam), **Indocin** (indomethacin), **Meclomen** (meclofenamate), **Motrin** and **Rufen** (ibuprofen), **Nalfon** (fenoprofen), **Ponstel** (mefenamic acid), and **Tolectin** (tolmetin)

| Also Uses | This Could Result |
|---|---|
| Anticancer, Antipsoriasis Medication<br><br>**Methotrexate, Mexate** | The toxic effects of this anticancer/antipsoriasis drug may be intensified by **Butazolidin.** Your doctor should monitor blood methotrexate levels carefully if you need to combine these drugs. |

*Any dosage alterations *must* be supervised by a physician!

## Arthritis Medication *cont.**

**If a person who is consuming** arthritis medication **Anaprox** and **Naprosyn** (naproxen), **Azolid** and **Butazolidin** (phenylbutazone), **Clinoril** (sulindac), **Dolobid** (diflunisal), **Feldene** (piroxicam), **Indocin** (indomethacin), **Meclomen** (meclofenamate), **Motrin** and **Rufen** (ibuprofen), **Nalfon** (fenoprofen), **Ponstel** (mefenamic acid), and **Tolectin** (tolmetin)

| Also Uses | This Could Result |
|---|---|
| Oral Anticoagulants (Blood Thinners)<br><br>**Athrombin-K, Coumadin, Coufarin, Dicumarol, Liquamar, Panwarfin** | This interaction crops up again and again. Many of the nonsteroidal anti-inflammatory agents can increase the effects of the coumarin-type oral anticoagulants (**Coumadin, Coufarin, Panwarfin, Athrombin-K, Liquamar,** and **Dicumarol**). This serious drug interaction can lead to severe bleeding problems. **Tolectin, Motrin,** and **Naprosyn** are probably safer to use with oral anticoagulants, but your doctor should closely monitor your blood's clotting ability if you need to combine these medicines. |

*Any dosage alterations *must* be supervised by a physician!

## Arthritis Medication *cont.**

**If a person who is consuming** arthritis medication **Anaprox** and **Naprosyn** (naproxen), **Azolid** and **Butazolidin** (phenylbutazone), **Clinoril** (sulindac), **Dolobid** (diflunisal), **Feldene** (piroxicam), **Indocin** (indomethacin), **Meclomen** (meclofenamate), **Motrin** and **Rufen** (ibuprofen), **Nalfon** (fenoprofen), **Ponstel** (mefenamic acid), and **Tolectin** (tolmetin)

| Also Uses | This Could Result |
|---|---|
| Anticonvulsant Medication<br><br>  **Dilantin, Mesantoin, Peganone** | **Butazolidin** (and perhaps others) can markedly increase the toxic effects of these seizure medicines. Loss of balance, mental confusion, slurred speech, and other disturbing side effects can occur from this drug interaction. |

*Any dosage alterations *must* be supervised by a physician!

## Arthritis Medication *cont.**

**If a person who is consuming** arthritis medication **Anaprox** and **Naprosyn** (naproxen), **Azolid** and **Butazolidin** (phenylbutazone), **Clinoril** (sulindac), **Dolobid** (diflunisal), **Feldene** (piroxicam), **Indocin** (indomethacin), **Meclomen** (meclofenamate), **Motrin** and **Rufen** (ibuprofen), **Nalfon** (fenoprofen), **Ponstel** (mefenamic acid), and **Tolectin** (tolmetin)

| Also Uses | This Could Result |
|---|---|
| Aspirin and Other Salicylate-containing Pain Relievers | Mixing arthritis medicines can be messy. If you can get by with aspirin, stick with it, but if you have to use one of the nonsteroidal anti-inflammatories, don't take aspirin too. Taken together you are asking for bad stomach trouble, maybe ulcers. |
| **Alka-Seltzer, Anacin, Ascriptin, Aspergum, Bayer Aspirin, Bufferin, Cope, Coricidin D, Ecotrin, Empirin, Excedrin, Vanquish**, etc. (aspirin-containing products) **Arthrolate, Arthropan, Disalcid, Durasal, Trilisate, Uracel 5**, etc. (other related salicylates) | |

*Any dosage alterations *must* be supervised by a physician!

## Arthritis Medication *cont.*\*

**If a person who is consuming** arthritis medication **Anaprox** and **Naprosyn** (naproxen), **Azolid** and **Butazolidin** (phenyl-butazone), **Clinoril** (sulindac), **Dolobid** (diflunisal), **Feldene** (piroxicam), **Indocin** (indomethacin), **Meclomen** (me-clofenamate), **Motrin** and **Rufen** (ibuprofen), **Nalfon** (feno-profen), **Ponstel** (mefenamic acid), and **Tolectin** (tolmetin)

| Also Uses | This Could Result |
|---|---|
| Oral Diabetes Medications<br><br>**Diabinese, Dymelor, Orinase, Tolinase** | The nonsteroidal anti-inflam-matory medications may cause these antidiabetic drugs to lower blood sugar excessively. This could lead to serious metabolic com-plications. **Butazolidin** (phe-nylbutazone) and **Tandearil** (oxyphenbutazone) seem to be the worst offenders. |

\*Any dosage alterations *must* be supervised by a physician!

## ASPIRIN, ASPIRIN-CONTAINING PRODUCTS, AND RELATED SALICYLATES*

**If a person who is consuming** salicylates **Alka-Seltzer, Anacin, Ascriptin, Aspergum, Bayer Aspirin, Bufferin, Cope, Coricidin D, Ecotrin, Empirin, Excedrin, Midol, Percodan, Vanquish,** etc. (all aspirin or aspirin-containing combination products)

*or*

**Arthrolate, Arthropan, Disalcid, Durasal, Trilisate, Uracel 5,** etc. (all salicylate products related to aspirin)

| Also Uses | This Could Result |
|---|---|
| Alcohol<br><br>  Beer, Hard Stuff, Wine | Ouch! **Alka-Seltzer** ads to the contrary, please don't ever mix booze and aspirin. Alcohol makes your stomach supersensitive to the irritating effects of salicylates. Significant bleeding from the stomach lining has been noted after this combination. |

*Any dosage alterations *must* be supervised by a physician!

**Aspirin, Aspirin-containing Products, and Related Salicylates** *cont.**

If a person who is consuming salicylates **Alka-Seltzer, Anacin, Ascriptin, Aspergum, Bayer Aspirin, Bufferin, Cope, Coricidin D, Ecotrin, Empirin, Excedrin, Midol, Percodan, Vanquish,** etc. (all aspirin or aspirin-containing combination products)

*or*

**Arthrolate, Arthropan, Disalcid, Durasal, Trilisate, Uracel 5,** etc. (all salicylate products related to aspirin)

| Also Uses | This Could Result |
|---|---|
| Oral Anticoagulants<br><br>**Athrombin-K, Coumadin, Coufarin, Panwarfin** (all forms of warfarin), **Dicumarol, Liquamar** | Very scary. This could be a terrible interaction. Aspirin taken in the presence of an oral anticoagulant could lead to very serious hemorrhaging. Anticoagulant dosage *must* be reduced in the presence of aspirin or aspirin-containing products. The effects of the other salicylates are unclear at this point, but it is probably best to stay away from them all if you are taking oral anticoagulants. |

*Any dosage alterations *must* be supervised by a physician!

## Aspirin, Aspirin-containing Products, and Related Salicylates *cont.**

**If a person who is consuming** salicylates **Alka-Seltzer, Anacin, Ascriptin, Aspergum, Bayer Aspirin, Bufferin, Cope, Coricidin D, Ecotrin, Empirin, Excedrin, Midol, Percodan, Vanquish,** etc. (all aspirin or aspirin-containing combination products)

*or*

**Arthrolate, Arthropan, Disalcid, Durasal, Trilisate, Uracel 5,** etc. (all salicylate products related to aspirin)

| Also Uses | This Could Result |
|---|---|
| Anticancer, Antipsoriasis Medication<br><br>**Methotrexate, Mexate** | The toxic effects of this anticancer/antipsoriasis drug may be intensified by aspirin and the other salicylates. Your physician should monitor blood methotrexate levels carefully and watch for adverse reactions if you combine these drugs. |
| **Also Uses** | **This Could Result** |
| Arthritis Medication (Nonsteroidal Anti-Inflammatories) | See table listing *Arthritis Medication.* |

*Any dosage alterations *must* be supervised by a physician!

**Aspirin, Aspirin-containing Products, and Related Salifylates** *cont.*\*

**If a person who is consuming** salicylates **Alka-Seltzer, Anacin, Ascriptin, Aspergum, Bayer Aspirin, Bufferin, Cope, Coricidin D, Ecotrin, Empirin, Excedrin, Midol, Percodan, Vanquish,** etc. (all aspirin or aspirin-containing combination products)

*or*

**Arthrolate, Arthropan, Disalcid, Durasal, Trilisate, Uracel 5,** etc. (all salicylate products related to aspirin)

| Also Uses | This Could Result |
|---|---|
| Oral Diabetes Medications<br><br>**Diabinese, Dymelor, Orinase, Tolinase** | If your doctor prescribes one of these diabetes medicines for you, do not make matters worse by taking aspirin or other salicylate too. Aspirin, in moderately high doses, can interact with these drugs, causing a too drastic reduction in blood sugar (hypoglycemia). Frequent blood-sugar tests are a must. |
| **Also Uses** | **This Could Result** |
| Gout Medications<br><br>**Benemid, Anturane** | Aspirin and the other salicylates can block the beneficial effects of these drugs, which may lead to a worsening of gout. Never combine them. |

\*Any dosage alterations *must* be supervised by a physician!

## BIRTH-CONTROL PILLS (ORAL CONTRACEPTIVES)*

**If a person who is consuming** oral contraceptives **Brevicon, Demulen, Enovid, Loestrin, Lo/Ovral, Modicon, Nordette, Norinyl, Norlestrin, Ortho-Novum, Ovcon, Ovral, Ovulen**

| Also Uses | This Could Result |
|---|---|
| Drugs That Alter Metabolism | *"Beware the Jubjub bird, and shun* |
| **Alurate, Amytal, Butisol, Fiorinal, Gemonil, Lotusate, Luminal, Mebaral, Mysoline, Nembutal, Seconal, Tuinal** (all barbiturates or contain barbiturates) | *The frumious Bandersnatch!"* Mixing any of these medications, on a long-term basis, with your birth-control pills could lead to trouble. These drugs can speed up the metabolism of your oral contraceptive, decreasing its effectiveness. The result could be breakthrough bleeding or possible unwanted pregnancy. Consider an alternate form of birth control if you must take these medicines. Many other drugs have been reported to have the same type of drug interaction with oral contraceptives, but the evidence is still pretty slim. Just to be on the safe side, ask your doctor or pharmacist about possible adverse drug interactions whenever you start taking a new drug. |
| **Ampicillin, Dilantin, Rifadin, Rifamate, Rimactane** | |

*Any dosage alterations *must* be supervised by a physician!

## Birth-Control Pills (Oral Contraceptives) *cont.**

**If a person who is consuming** oral contraceptives **Brevicon, Demulen, Enovid, Loestrin, Lo/Ovral, Modicon, Nordette, Norinyl, Norlestrin, Ortho-Novum, Ovcon, Ovral, Ovulen**

| Also Uses | This Could Result |
|---|---|
| Asthma Medication<br><br>Aminophylline, **Bronkodyl, Choledyl,** Oxtriphylline, **Respbid, Slo-phyllin, Somophyllin, Theobid, Sustaire, Synophylate, Theo-dur,** Theophylline, etc. | Birth-control pills may slow the metabolism and increase the blood levels of these asthma medications, all derivatives of theophylline. Since theophylline can be dangerous in only moderate excess, a lower dose of theophylline may have to be used and blood levels should be closely monitored. |

| Also Uses | This Could Result |
|---|---|
| Beta Blockers<br><br>**Inderal, Lopressor** | Birth-control pills can inhibit the metabolism of these two beta blockers, causing a build up of the medication and possibly increased side effects. The dose of these drugs may have to be decreased in compensation or another, noninteracting beta blocker should be chosen. |

*Any dosage alterations *must* be supervised by a physician!

## Birth-Control Pills (Oral Contraceptives) *cont.*\*

**If a person who is consuming** oral contraceptives **Brevicon, Demulen, Enovid, Loestrin, Lo/Ovral, Modicon, Nordette, Norinyl, Norlestrin, Ortho-Novum, Ovcon, Ovral, Ovulen**

| Also Uses | This Could Result |
|---|---|
| Minor Tranquilizers (Benzodiazepines)<br><br>**Ativan, Centrax, Dalmane, Halcion, Librium, Paxipam, Restoril, Serax, Tranxene, Valium, Xanax** | Oral contraceptives change the way the body metabolizes and eliminates minor tranquilizers. Depending on the particular sedative involved, birth-control pills may either increase or slow down its metabolism. If you are taking **Valium** (diazepam), **Librium** (chlordiazepoxide), **Paxipam** (halazepam), **Dalmane** (flurazepam), or **Xanax** (alprazolam), the sedative effects of the tranquilizer will likely be increased and therefore the dose may have to be decreased.<br><br>On the other hand, if you are taking **Serax** (oxazepam), **Ativan** (lorazepam), or **Restoril** (temazepam), you might actually need an increased dose. At the time of this writing the data are murky at best and |

\*Any dosage alterations *must* be supervised by a physician!

## Birth-Control Pills (Oral Contraceptives) *cont.*\*

**If a person who is consuming** oral contraceptives **Brevicon, Demulen, Enovid, Loestrin, Lo/Ovral, Modicon, Nordette, Norinyl, Norlestrin, Ortho-Novum, Ovcon, Ovral, Ovulen**

| | **This Could Result *cont.*** |
|---|---|
| | you may be your own best judge as to whether you are getting an overdose or an underdose. Discuss this confusion with your physician. |
| **Also Uses** | **This Could Result** |
| Smoking<br><br>    Cigarettes, Cigars, Pipes | Why worsen your already increased chances of developing a blood clot or having a heart attack? Smokers who are on the pill are ten to twelve times more likely to have a fatal heart attack than women who use neither tobacco nor oral contraceptives. |

\*Any dosage alterations *must* be supervised by a physician!

## CORTISONE-TYPE ANTI-INFLAMMATORY MEDICATION (STEROIDS)*

**If a person who is consuming** steroids **Alphadrol** (fluprednisolone), **Aristocort** and **Kenacort** (triamcinolone), **Celestone** (betamethasone), **Cortef** and **Hydrocortone** (hydrocortisone or cortisol), **Cortone** (cortisone), **Decadron** and **Hexadrol** (dexamethasone), **Delta-Cortef** and **Sterane** (prednisolone), **Deltasone** and **Meticorten** (prednisone), **Haldrone** (paramethasone), **Medrol** (methylprednisolone)

| Also Uses | This Could Result |
|---|---|
| Anticonvulsant (Epilepsy) Medication  **Dilantin, Mesantoin, Peganone** | These hydantoin drugs can increase the body's ability to deactivate and get rid of the steroid. This same interaction occurs with the barbiturates (see below), many of which are also used for seizure control. An increased dose of the steroid may be necessary to control the disease that the steroid is being given for. |

*Any dosage alterations *must* be supervised by a physician!

## Cortisone-type Anti-Inflammatory Medication *cont.*\*

**If a person who is consuming** steroids **Alphadrol** (fluprednisolone), **Aristocort** and **Kenacort** (triamcinolone), **Celestone** (betamethasone), **Cortef** and **Hydrocortone** (hydrocortisone or cortisol), **Cortone** (cortisone), **Decadron** and **Hexadrol** (dexamethasone), **Delta-Cortef** and **Sterane** (prednisolone), **Deltasone** and **Meticorten** (prednisone), **Haldrone** (paramethasone), **Medrol** (methylprednisolone)

| Also Uses | This Could Result |
|---|---|
| Antituberculosis Medication<br><br>**Nydrazid, Rifadin, Rifamate, Rimactane** | Rifampin **(Rimactane** and **Rifadin)** soups up the body's metabolism of steroid drugs. The result is less effect and possibly a worsening of the steroid-treated condition. It may be necessary to increase the dose of steroid to reestablish adequate control.<br><br>Steroids may increase the excretion of isoniazid **(Nydrazid),** which could lead to lessened benefit from this antituberculosis medication. An increase in the isoniazid dose might be necessary. The balance between steroids and tuberculosis medication is a difficult balancing act that requires careful supervision. |

\*Any dosage alterations *must* be supervised by a physician!

## Cortisone-type Anti-Inflammatory Medication *cont.*\*

**If a person who is consuming** steroids **Alphadrol** (flupred-nisolone), **Aristocort** and **Kenacort** (triamcinolone), **Cele-stone** (betamethasone), **Cortef** and **Hydrocortone** (hy-drocortisone or cortisol), **Cortone** (cortisone), **Decadron** and **Hexadrol** (dexamethasone), **Delta-Cortef** and **Sterane** (prednisolone), **Deltasone** and **Meticorten** (prednisone), **Haldrone** (paramethasone), **Medrol** (methylprednisolone)

| Also Uses | This Could Result |
|---|---|
| Aspirin and Other Salicylates | The steroids reduce the blood levels of aspirin and the other salicylates. This may be especially important if you take large regular doses of aspirin for arthritis. |
| **Alka-Seltzer, Anacin, Ascriptin, Aspergum, Bayer Aspirin, Bufferin, Cope, Coricidin D, Ecotrin, Empirin, Excedrin, Vanquish,** etc. (all aspirin or aspirin-containing products) | |
| **Arthrolate, Arthropan, Disalcid, Dolobid, Durasal, Pepto-Bismol, Trilisate, Tracel 5,** etc. (other related salicylates) | |

\*Any dosage alterations *must* be supervised by a physician!

## Cortisone-type Anti-Inflammatory Medication *cont.*\*

**If a person who is consuming** steroids **Alphadrol** (fluprednisolone), **Aristocort** and **Kenacort** (triamcinolone), **Celestone** (betamethasone), **Cortef** and **Hydrocortone** (hydrocortisone or cortisol), **Cortone** (cortisone), **Decadron** and **Hexadrol** (dexamethasone), **Delta-Cortef** and **Sterane** (prednisolone), **Deltasone** and **Meticorten** (prednisone), **Haldrone** (paramethasone), **Medrol** (methylprednisolone)

| Also Uses | This Could Result |
|---|---|
| Barbiturates<br><br>    **Alurate, Amytal, Butisol, Gemonil, Fiorinal, Lotusate, Luminal, Mebaral, Mysoline, Nembutal, Seconal, Tuinal** | Barbiturates put the enzymes responsible for the metabolism and deactivation of many drugs into overdrive. The result can be faster elimination of steroids and less therapeutic benefit. A higher dose of the steroid may be necessary if someone is also taking barbiturates. |

\*Any dosage alterations *must* be supervised by a physician!

## Cortisone-type Anti-Inflammatory Medication *cont.*\*

**If a person who is consuming** steroids **Alphadrol** (fluprednisolone), **Aristocort** and **Kenacort** (triamcinolone), **Celestone** (betamethasone), **Cortef** and **Hydrocortone** (hydrocortisone or cortisol), **Cortone** (cortisone), **Decadron** and **Hexadrol** (dexamethasone), **Delta-Cortef** and **Sterane** (prednisolone), **Deltasone** and **Meticorten** (prednisone), **Haldrone** (paramethasone), **Medrol** (methylprednisolone)

| Also Uses | This Could Result |
|---|---|
| Diuretics<br><br>**Anhydron, Aquatag, Bumex, Diuril, Edecrine, Enduron, HydroDIURIL, Hydromox, Hygroton, Lasix, Lozol, Naqua, Naturetin, Renese, Saluron, Zaroxolyn** | The combination of a cortisone-type drug and one of these diuretics often leads to excessive depletion of potassium from the body (hypokalemia). This low-potassium state can be especially dangerous if you are taking the heart medicine **Lanoxin** (digoxin). Special care must be taken to supplement potassium in the diet and blood-potassium levels should be checked periodically. |

\*Any dosage alterations *must* be supervised by a physician!

**Cortisone-type Anti-Inflammatory Medication** *cont.**

**If a person who is consuming** steroids **Alphadrol** (fluprednisolone), **Aristocort** and **Kenacort** (triamcinolone), **Celestone** (betamethasone), **Cortef** and **Hydrocortone** (hydrocortisone or cortisol), **Cortone** (cortisone), **Decadron** and **Hexadrol** (dexamethasone), **Delta-Cortef** and **Sterane** (prednisolone), **Deltasone** and **Meticorten** (prednisone), **Haldrone** (paramethasone), **Medrol** (methylprednisolone)

| Also Uses | This Could Result |
|---|---|
| Oral Contraceptives<br><br>**Brevicon, Demulen, Enovid, Loestrin, Lo/Ovral, Modicon, Nordette, Norinyl, Norlestrin, Ortho-Novum, Ovcon, Ovral, Ovulen** | Although all the returns aren't in yet, recent evidence indicates that birth-control pills can decrease the metabolism of the steroids. This interaction may result in steroid toxicity if the dose of the steroid isn't reduced in compensation. |

*Any dosage alterations *must* be supervised by a physician!

## Cortisone-type Anti-Inflammatory Medication *cont.*\*

**If a person who is consuming** steroids **Alphadrol** (fluprednisolone), **Aristocort** and **Kenacort** (triamcinolone), **Celestone** (betamethasone), **Cortef** and **Hydrocortone** (hydrocortisone or cortisol), **Cortone** (cortisone), **Decadron** and **Hexadrol** (dexamethasone), **Delta-Cortef** and **Sterane** (prednisolone), **Deltasone** and **Meticorten** (prednisone), **Haldrone** (paramethasone), **Medrol** (methylprednisolone)

| Also Uses | This Could Result |
|---|---|
| Vaccines (Live Attenuated)<br><br>B.C.G., German measles (rubella), Measles (rubeola), Mumps, Polio (oral), Smallpox, Yellow fever | Careful—this one could do you in! Cortisone-type drugs lower immunologic resistance to disease. If you receive a live-virus vaccine while your immune system is being suppressed by large doses of a steroid, a serious (if not fatal) illness might result.<br><br>This danger is not present with other types of vaccinations, but it is probably a good idea to be extracautious anyway. Your body cannot respond properly and the vaccination might not be effective. |

\*Any dosage alterations *must* be supervised by a physician!

## DIABETES MEDICATION (ORAL)*

**If a person who is consuming Diabinese** (chlorpropamide), **Dymelor** (acetohexamide), **Orinase** (tolbutamide), **Tolinase** (tolazamide)

| Also Uses | This Could Result |
|---|---|
| Alcohol<br><br>  Beer, Hard Stuff, Wine | Two types of drug interaction are possible here. If you drink while taking one of these drugs (especially **Diabinese**), you run the risk of becoming unpleasantly sick (flushing, headache, general Yuck City). This type of interaction is well known to alcoholics taking **Antabuse** (disulfiram) in order to help themselves stop drinking.<br><br>Alcohol can also affect your blood-sugar levels, either raising or lowering them. Since the whole point of taking an oral diabetes agent is to stabilize the blood sugar, this interaction is truly counterproductive. Try real hard to stay off the sauce! |

*Any dosage alterations *must* be supervised by a physician!

## Diabetes Medication *cont.**

**If a person who is consuming Diabinese** (chlorpropamide), **Dymelor** (acetohexamide), **Orinase** (tolbutamide), **Tolinase** (tolazamide)

| Also Uses | This Could Result |
|---|---|
| Antibiotics (Sulfa) and Others | This one can be very tricky. Antibiotics may increase the effect of oral diabetes medication. As a result, it may be necessary to lower the dose of the diabetes drug. Blood sugar levels should also be checked, as the possibility of low blood sugar (hypoglycemia) is increased because of this interaction. |
| **Azo-Gantanol, Azo-Gantrisin, Azotrex, Azulfidine, Bactrim, Fansidar, Gantanol, Gantrisin, Renoquid, Septra, Sulfadiazine, Sulfapyridine, Terfonyl, Thiosulfil, Urobiotic-250** (all sulfa antibiotics or combinations containing sulfa) | |
| **Chloromycetin** | |

*Any dosage alterations *must* be supervised by a physician!

## Diabetes Medication *cont.** 

**If a person who is consuming Diabinese** (chlorpropamide), **Dymelor** (acetohexamide), **Orinase** (tolbutamide), **Tolinase** (tolazamide)

| Also Uses | This Could Result |
|---|---|
| Arthritis Medication<br><br>**Butazolidin, Tandearil** | When this anti-inflammatory medicine is mixed with oral diabetes drugs excessively low blood sugar levels may result. The dose of the diabetes medication may have to be decreased, or it may be necessary to switch to a different arthritis treatment. The blood sugar should be carefully monitored if this combination is necessary. |

*Any dosage alterations *must* be supervised by a physician!

## Diabetes Medication *cont.**

**If a person who is consuming Diabinese** (chlorpropamide), **Dymelor** (acetohexamide), **Orinase** (tolbutamide), **Tolinase** (tolazamide)

| Also Uses | This Could Result |
|---|---|
| Aspirin and Other Salicylates | Large doses of aspirin or any of the salicylates can add to the blood-sugar-lowering properties of an oral diabetes drug, resulting in hypoglycemia. Blood-sugar levels should be checked and the dose of the diabetes medication decreased if necessary. |
| **Alka-Seltzer, Anacin, Ascriptin, Aspergum, Bayer Aspirin, Bufferin, Cope, Coricidin D, Ecotrin, Empirin, Excedrin, Vanquish,** etc. (all aspirin or aspirin-containing combination products) | |
| **Arthrolate, Arthropan, Disalcid, Dolobid, Durasal, Pepto-Bismol, Trilisate, Uracel 5,** etc. (related salicylate products) | |

*Any dosage alterations *must* be supervised by a physician!

## Diabetes Medication cont.*

**If a person who is consuming Diabinese** (chlorpropamide), **Dymelor** (acetohexamide), **Orinase** (tolbutamide), **Tolinase** (tolazamide)

| Also Uses | This Could Result |
|---|---|
| Oral Anticoagulant<br><br>**Dicumarol** | **Dicumarol** (but not the other oral anticoagulants) can increase the power of the diabetes drug. Dangerously low blood-sugar levels may be the result of this interaction. A switch to another anticoagulant such as **Coumadin** may eliminate this risk. |
| **Also Uses** | **This Could Result** |
| Diuretics<br><br>**Anhydron, Aquatag, Bumex, Diuril, Edecrine, Enduron, HydroDIURIL, Hydromox, Hygroton, Lasix, Lozol, Naqua, Naturetin, Renese, Saluron, Zaroxolyn** | These diuretics can raise blood-sugar levels, counteracting the effects of the oral diabetes medication. An increased dose of the diabetes drug plus careful blood-sugar monitoring may be necessary to take care of this relatively minor interaction. |

*Any dosage alterations *must* be supervised by a physician!

## Diabetes Medication *cont.*\*

**If a person who is consuming Diabinese** (chlorpropamide), **Dymelor** (acetohexamide), **Orinase** (tolbutamide), **Tolinase** (tolazamide)

| Also Uses | This Could Result |
|---|---|
| Gout Medication<br><br>**Anturane** | **Anturane** (sulfinpyrazone) can magnify the blood-sugar-lowering effects of **Orinase** and probably the other diabetes medications as well. The dose of **Orinase** may have to be reduced to prevent low blood sugar (hypoglycemia). |
| **Also Uses** | **This Could Result** |
| MAO Inhibitors (Used for Depression or High Blood Pressure)<br><br>**Eutonyl, Eutron, Furoxone** (an antibiotic!), **Marplan, Nardil, Parnate** | These antidepressants and other MAO inhibitors can decrease blood-sugar levels. Since insulin and oral antidiabetes drugs do the same thing, the combination is additive. To avoid possible low blood sugar (hypoglycemia), use another form of antidepressant or high blood pressure medication. If you must use an MAO inhibitor with your diabetes medicine, the latter will probably need to be trimmed back. |

\*Any dosage alterations *must* be supervised by a physician!

## DIURETICS*

**If a person who is consuming** diuretics **Aldactazide** (hydrochlorothiazide plus spironolactone), **Aldactone** (spironolactone), **Anhydron** (cyclothiazide), **Aquatag** (benzthiazide), **Aquatensin** and **Enduron** (methyclothiazide), **Diulo** and **Zaroxolyn** (metolazone), **Diupres** (chlorothiazide plus reserpine), **Diuril** (chlorothiazide), **Dyazide** (hydrochlorothiazide plus triamterene), **Dyrenium** (triamterene), **Esidrix** and **HydroDIURIL** (hydrochlorothiazide), **Hydromox** (quinethazone), **Hygroton** (chlorthalidone), **Lozol** (indapamide), **Midamor** (amiloride), **Moduretic** (hydrochlorothiazide plus amiloride), **Naqua** (trichlormethiazide), **Naturetin** (bendroflumethiazide), **Renese** (polythiazide), **Saluron** (hydroflumethiazide), etc., considered mild to moderate diuretics, and **Bumex** (bumetanide), **Edecrine** (ethacrynic acid), and **Lasix** (furosemide), the more potent diuretics

| **Also Uses** | **This Could Result** |
|---|---|
| Alcohol<br>    Beer, Hard Stuff, Wine | You really don't have to worry very much about this one. What happens is that booze and diuretics decrease blood pressure. If you stand up too quickly after downing a few, you may find yourself flat on your back. Caution is all that's necessary. |

| **Also Uses** | **This Could Result** |
|---|---|
| Oral Antidiabetic Agents | See table listing *Diabetes Medication (Oral)*. |

*Any dosage alterations *must* be supervised by a physician!

## Diuretics *cont.**

**If a person who is consuming** diuretics **Aldactazide** (hydrochlorothiazide plus spironolactone), **Aldactone** (spironolactone), **Anhydron** (cyclothiazide), **Aquatag** (benzthiazide), **Aquatensin** and **Enduron** (methyclothiazide), **Diulo** and **Zaroxolyn** (metolazone), **Diupres** (chlorothiazide plus reserpine), **Diuril** (chlorothiazide), **Dyazide** (hydrochlorothiazide plus triamterene), **Dyrenium** (triamterene), **Esidrix** and **HydroDIURIL** (hydrochlorothiazide), **Hydromox** (quinethazone), **Hygroton** (chlorthalidone), **Lozol** (indapamide), **Midamor** (amiloride), **Moduretic** (hydrochlorothiazide plus amiloride), **Naqua** (trichlormethiazide), **Naturetin** (bendroflumethiazide), **Renese** (polythiazide), **Saluron** (hydroflumethiazide), etc., considered mild to moderate diuretics, and **Bumex** (bumetanide), **Edecrine** (ethacrynic acid), and **Lasix** (furosemide), the more potent diuretics

| Also Uses | This Could Result |
|---|---|
| Blood-Pressure-Lowering Drugs | Hold your horses. Before you get nervous because your doctor has prescribed a diuretic along with a different high-blood-pressure medication, listen carefully. Often, it becomes necessary to decrease blood pressure significantly, and the combination of a "water pill" and one of the drugs listed may do the job. In fact, some of these combinations are quite common. However, the combination may decrease blood |
| **Aldoclor, Aldomet, Aldoril, Apresoline, Blocadren, Capoten, Catapres, Corgard, Esimil, Eutonyl, Eutron, Harmonyl, Hylorel, Inderal, Ismelin, Loniten, Lopressor, Minipress, Moderil, Raudixin, Rauwiloid, Reserpine, Ser-Ap-Es, Serpasil, Tenormin, Visken, Wytensin** | |

*Any dosage alterations *must* be supervised by a physician!

## Diuretics *cont.*\*

**If a person who is consuming** diuretics **Aldactazide** (hydrochlorothiazide plus spironolactone), **Aldactone** (spironolactone), **Anhydron** (cyclothiazide), **Aquatag** (benzthiazide), **Aquatensin** and **Enduron** (methyclothiazide), **Diulo** and **Zaroxolyn** (metolazone), **Diupres** (chlorothiazide plus reserpine), **Diuril** (chlorothiazide), **Dyazide** (hydrochlorothiazide plus triamterene), **Dyrenium** (triamterene), **Esidrix** and **HydroDIURIL** (hydrochlorothiazide), **Hydromox** (quinethazone), **Hygroton** (chlorthalidone), **Lozol** (indapamide), **Midamor** (amiloride), **Moduretic** (hydrochlorothiazide plus amiloride), **Naqua** (trichlormethiazide), **Naturetin** (bendroflumethiazide), **Renese** (polythiazide), **Saluron** (hydroflumethiazide), etc., considered mild to moderate diuretics, and **Bumex** (bumetanide), **Edecrine** (ethacrynic acid), and **Lasix** (furosemide), the more potent diuretics

### This Could Result *cont.*

pressure too far and it may be necessary to decrease the dose of one or the other drugs. This seems to be especially true with **Capoten.** Frequent blood-pressure tests are a good idea.

---

\*Any dosage alterations *must* be supervised by a physician!

## Diuretics *cont.*\*

**If a person who is consuming** diuretics **Aldactazide** (hydrochlorothiazide plus spironolactone), **Aldactone** (spironolactone), **Anhydron** (cyclothiazide), **Aquatag** (benzthiazide), **Aquatensin** and **Enduron** (methyclothiazide), **Diulo** and **Zaroxolyn** (metolazone), **Diupres** (chlorothiazide plus reserpine), **Diuril** (chlorothiazide), **Dyazide** (hydrochlorothiazide plus triamterene), **Dyrenium** (triamterene), **Esidrix** and **HydroDIURIL** (hydrochlorothiazide), **Hydromox** (quinethazone), **Hygroton** (chlorthalidone), **Lozol** (indapamide), **Midamor** (amiloride), **Moduretic** (hydrochlorothiazide plus amiloride), **Naqua** (trichlormethiazide), **Naturetin** (bendroflumethiazide), **Renese** (polythiazide), **Saluron** (hydroflumethiazide), etc., considered mild to moderate diuretics, and **Bumex** (bumetanide), **Edecrine** (ethacrynic acid), and **Lasix** (furosemide), the more potent diuretics

| Also Uses | This Could Result |
|---|---|
| Cholesterol-lowering Drugs<br><br>**Colestid, Questran** | **Colestid** (colestipol) and **Questran** (cholestyramine) both tend to grab onto thiazide-type diuretics in the gut and prevent the absorption of the blood-pressure medication. Just don't take them at the same time and you shouldn't have a problem. |
| **Also Uses**<br><br>Cortisone-type Drugs | **This Could Result**<br><br>See table listing *Cortisone-type Anti-Inflammatory Medication.* |

\*Any dosage alterations *must* be supervised by a physician!

## Diuretics *cont.**

**If a person who is consuming** diuretics **Aldactazide** (hydrochlorothiazide plus spironolactone), **Aldactone** (spironolactone), **Anhydron** (cyclothiazide), **Aquatag** (benzthiazide), **Aquatensin** and **Enduron** (methyclothiazide), **Diulo** and **Zaroxolyn** (metolazone), **Diupres** (chlorothiazide plus reserpine), **Diuril** (chlorothiazide), **Dyazide** (hydrochlorothiazide plus triamterene), **Dyrenium** (triamterene), **Esidrix** and **HydroDIURIL** (hydrochlorothiazide), **Hydromox** (quinethazone), **Hygroton** (chlorthalidone), **Lozol** (indapamide), **Midamor** (amiloride), **Moduretic** (hydrochlorothiazide plus amiloride), **Naqua** (trichlormethiazide), **Naturetin** (bendroflumethiazide), **Renese** (polythiazide), **Saluron** (hydroflumethiazide), etc., considered mild to moderate diuretics, and **Bumex** (bumetanide), **Edecrine** (ethacrynic acid), and **Lasix** (furosemide), the more potent diuretics

| Also Uses | This Could Result |
|---|---|
| Digitalis Heart Medications<br><br>**Cedilanid, Cedilanid-D, Crystodigin, Digiglusin,** Digitalis, Digitoxin, Digoxin, **Gitaligin, Lanoxin** | DANGER! This could well be the most significant drug interaction listed in this book. Digitalis-type heart medication can be quite dangerous all by itself. Add a diuretic (except potassium preservers like **Aldactone, Dyazide, Dyrenium, Maxzide, Moduretic,** and **Midamor**) in order to diminish fluid accumulation or reduce high blood pressure and you could be in a risky situation. Most diuretics deplete the |

*Any dosage alterations *must* be supervised by a physician!

## Diuretics *cont.**

**If a person who is consuming** diuretics **Aldactazide** (hydrochlorothiazide plus spironolactone), **Aldactone** (spironolactone), **Anhydron** (cyclothiazide), **Aquatag** (benzthiazide), **Aquatensin** and **Enduron** (methyclothiazide), **Diulo** and **Zaroxolyn** (metolazone), **Diupres** (chlorothiazide plus reserpine), **Diuril** (chlorothiazide), **Dyazide** (hydrochlorothiazide plus triamterene), **Dyrenium** (triamterene), **Esidrix** and **HydroDIURIL** (hydrochlorothiazide), **Hydromox** (quinethazone), **Hygroton** (chlorthalidone), **Lozol** (indapamide), **Midamor** (amiloride), **Moduretic** (hydrochlorothiazide plus amiloride), **Naqua** (trichlormethiazide), **Naturetin** (bendroflumethiazide), **Renese** (polythiazide), **Saluron** (hydroflumethiazide), etc., considered mild to moderate diuretics, and **Bumex** (bumetanide), **Edecrine** (ethacrynic acid), and **Lasix** (furosemide), the more potent diuretics

### This Could Result *cont.*

body's potassium. Lowered potassium levels will make the heart supersensitive to digitalis side effects. Fatal heart rhythm disturbances are possible.

We have always known that a sudden emotional crisis or a stressful event can cause the body to release epinephrine (adrenalin) into the bloodstream. What we have recently learned is that such a situation can produce a very rapid decrease in po-

*Any dosage alterations *must* be supervised by a physician!

## Diuretics cont.*

**If a person who is consuming** diuretics **Aldactazide** (hydrochlorothiazide plus spironolactone), **Aldactone** (spironolactone), **Anhydron** (cyclothiazide), **Aquatag** (benzthiazide), **Aquatensin** and **Enduron** (methyclothiazide), **Diulo** and **Zaroxolyn** (metolazone), **Diupres** (chlorothiazide plus reserpine), **Diuril** (chlorothiazide), **Dyazide** (hydrochlorothiazide plus triamterene), **Dyrenium** (triamterene), **Esidrix** and **HydroDIURIL** (hydrochlorothiazide), **Hydromox** (quinethazone), **Hygroton** (chlorthalidone), **Lozol** (indapamide), **Midamor** (amiloride), **Moduretic** (hydrochlorothiazide plus amiloride), **Naqua** (trichlormethiazide), **Naturetin** (bendroflumethiazide), **Renese** (polythiazide), **Saluron** (hydroflumethiazide), etc., considered mild to moderate diuretics, and **Bumex** (bumetanide), **Edecrine** (ethacrynic acid), and **Lasix** (furosemide), the more potent diuretics

### This Could Result cont.

tassium. If someone is already starting with lowered potassium levels caused by a diuretic, the potential for "sudden death" caused by heart arrhythmias may be increased.

The moral of this tale is to have frequent serum potassium tests done (normal potassium levels range roughly between 3.5 and 5.0 mEq/L). If you stray too far beyond these boundaries (on *either* side) you could be in very big trouble.

*Any dosage alterations *must* be supervised by a physician!

## Diuretics *cont.**

**If a person who is consuming** diuretics **Aldactazide** (hydrochlorothiazide plus spironolactone), **Aldactone** (spironolactone), **Anhydron** (cyclothiazide), **Aquatag** (benzthiazide), **Aquatensin** and **Enduron** (methyclothiazide), **Diulo** and **Zaroxolyn** (metolazone), **Diupres** (chlorothiazide plus reserpine), **Diuril** (chlorothiazide), **Dyazide** (hydrochlorothiazide plus triamterene), **Dyrenium** (triamterene), **Esidrix** and **HydroDIURIL** (hydrochlorothiazide), **Hydromox** (quinethazone), **Hygroton** (chlorthalidone), **Lozol** (indapamide), **Midamor** (amiloride), **Moduretic** (hydrochlorothiazide plus amiloride), **Naqua** (trichlormethiazide), **Naturetin** (bendroflumethiazide), **Renese** (polythiazide), **Saluron** (hydroflumethiazide), etc., considered mild to moderate diuretics, and **Bumex** (bumetanide), **Edecrine** (ethacrynic acid), and **Lasix** (furosemide), the more potent diuretics

| Also Uses | This Could Result |
|---|---|
| Other Diuretics | The combination of two different diuretics isn't necessarily bad; in fact **Aldactazide, Dyazide,** and **Moduretic** are combinations of diuretics designed to minimize potassium loss. However, some combinations such as **Diulo** or **Zaroxolyn** plus one of the stronger diuretics such as **Lasix** can lead to profound water loss and severe disturbances in blood chemistry (potassium, magnesium, uric acid, etc.). Diu- |
| **Aldactazide, Aldactone, Anhydron, Aquatag, Aquatensin, Bumex, Diulo, Diupres, Diuril, Dyazide, Dyrenium, Edecrine, Enduron, Esidrix, HydroDIURIL, Hydromox, Hygroton, Lasix, Lozol, Midamor, Moduretic, Naqua, Naturetin, Renese, Saluron, Zaroxolyn,** etc. | |

*Any dosage alterations *must* be supervised by a physician!

## Diuretics *cont.**

**If a person who is consuming** diuretics **Aldactazide** (hydrochlorothiazide plus spironolactone), **Aldactone** (spironolactone), **Anhydron** (cyclothiazide), **Aquatag** (benzthiazide), **Aquatensin** and **Enduron** (methyclothiazide), **Diulo** and **Zaroxolyn** (metolazone), **Diupres** (chlorothiazide plus reserpine), **Diuril** (chlorothiazide), **Dyazide** (hydrochlorothiazide plus triamterene), **Dyrenium** (triamterene), **Esidrix** and **Hy-droDIURIL** (hydrochlorothiazide), **Hydromox** (quinethazone), **Hygroton** (chlorthalidone), **Lozol** (indapamide), **Midamor** (amiloride), **Moduretic** (hydrochlorothiazide plus amiloride), **Naqua** (trichlormethiazide), **Naturetin** (bendroflumethiazide), **Renese** (polythiazide), **Saluron** (hydroflumethiazide), etc., considered mild to moderate diuretics, and **Bumex** (bumetanide), **Edecrine** (ethacrynic acid), and **Lasix** (furosemide), the more potent diuretics

### This Could Result *cont.*

retics should usually be combined with other types of blood-pressure medicines if single drug therapy isn't effective.

*Any dosage alterations *must* be supervised by a physician!

## Diuretics *cont.*\*

**If a person who is consuming** diuretics **Aldactazide** (hydrochlorothiazide plus spironolactone), **Aldactone** (spironolactone), **Anhydron** (cyclothiazide), **Aquatag** (benzthiazide), **Aquatensin** and **Enduron** (methyclothiazide), **Diulo** and **Zaroxolyn** (metolazone), **Diupres** (chlorothiazide plus reserpine), **Diuril** (chlorothiazide), **Dyazide** (hydrochlorothiazide plus triamterene), **Dyrenium** (triamterene), **Esidrix** and **HydroDIURIL** (hydrochlorothiazide), **Hydromox** (quinethazone), **Hygroton** (chlorthalidone), **Lozol** (indapamide), **Midamor** (amiloride), **Moduretic** (hydrochlorothiazide plus amiloride), **Naqua** (trichlormethiazide), **Naturetin** (bendroflumethiazide), **Renese** (polythiazide), **Saluron** (hydroflumethiazide), etc., considered mild to moderate diuretics, and **Bumex** (bumetanide), **Edecrine** (ethacrynic acid), and **Lasix** (furosemide), the more potent diuretics

| Also Uses | This Could Result |
|---|---|
| Licorice | Don't eat your heart out, licorice lover. Too much of this delicacy (and I do mean gobs and gobs) can give you trouble. A little now and then won't hurt. I am talking about truly porcine quantities. Licorice and water pills kick too much potassium out of your body. It could be dangerous, especially if you are taking a digitalis-type drug for your heart. |

---

\*Any dosage alterations *must* be supervised by a physician!

## Diuretics *cont.**

**If a person who is consuming** diuretics **Aldactazide** (hydrochlorothiazide plus spironolactone), **Aldactone** (spironolactone), **Anhydron** (cyclothiazide), **Aquatag** (benzthiazide), **Aquatensin** and **Enduron** (methyclothiazide), **Diulo** and **Zaroxolyn** (metolazone), **Diupres** (chlorothiazide plus reserpine), **Diuril** (chlorothiazide), **Dyazide** (hydrochlorothiazide plus triamterene), **Dyrenium** (triamterene), **Esidrix** and **HydroDIURIL** (hydrochlorothiazide), **Hydromox** (quinethazone), **Hygroton** (chlorthalidone), **Lozol** (indapamide), **Midamor** (amiloride), **Moduretic** (hydrochlorothiazide plus amiloride), **Naqua** (trichlormethiazide), **Naturetin** (bendroflumethiazide), **Renese** (polythiazide), **Saluron** (hydroflumethiazide), etc., considered mild to moderate diuretics, and **Bumex** (bumetanide), **Edecrine** (ethacrynic acid), and **Lasix** (furosemide), the more potent diuretics

| Also Uses | This Could Result |
|---|---|
| Potassium Supplements<br><br>Potassium, **Kaon, KCL, K-Lor, Klorvess, Klotrix, K-Lyte, K-Tab, Micro-K, Slow-K** | **Aldactone, Dyrenium,** and **Midamor:** These mild diuretics are considered to be "potassium-sparing" drugs in the sense that they do not cause the body to excrete excess amounts of potassium like the other diuretics do.<br><br>**Aldactazide, Dyazide, Maxzide,** and **Moduretic** are combination products containing potassium-sparing diuretics. It is important not to add supplemental po- |

*Any dosage alterations *must* be supervised by a physician!

## Diuretics *cont.**

**If a person who is consuming** diuretics **Aldactazide** (hydrochlorothiazide plus spironolactone), **Aldactone** (spironolactone), **Anhydron** (cyclothiazide), **Aquatag** (benzthiazide), **Aquatensin** and **Enduron** (methyclothiazide), **Diulo** and **Zaroxolyn** (metolazone), **Diupres** (chlorothiazide plus reserpine), **Diuril** (chlorothiazide), **Dyazide** (hydrochlorothiazide plus triamterene), **Dyrenium** (triamterene), **Esidrix** and **HydroDIURIL** (hydrochlorothiazide), **Hydromox** (quinethazone), **Hygroton** (chlorthalidone), **Lozol** (indapamide), **Midamor** (amiloride), **Moduretic** (hydrochlorothiazide plus amiloride), **Naqua** (trichlormethiazide), **Naturetin** (bendroflumethiazide), **Renese** (polythiazide), **Saluron** (hydroflumethiazide), etc., considered mild to moderate diuretics, and **Bumex** (bumetanide), **Edecrine** (ethacrynic acid), and **Lasix** (furosemide), the more potent diuretics

### This Could Result *cont.*

tassium to a diuretic regimen containing any of these drugs unless under constant medical supervision, because hyperkalemia (too much potassium) may result.

Blood levels of potassium should be checked periodically on all persons taking ANY diuretic, and potassium supplements should be prescribed ONLY if these tests show they are needed.

*Any dosage alterations *must* be supervised by a physician!

## MAJOR TRANQUILIZERS*

**If a person who is consuming** tranquilizers **Compazine** (prochlorperazine), **Haldol** (haloperidol), **Loxitane** (loxapine), **Mellaril** (thioridazine), **Moban** (molindone), **Navane** (thiothixene), **Permitil** and **Prolixin** (fluphenazine), **Proketazine** (carphenazine), **Quide** (piperacetazine), **Serentil** (mesoridazine), **Sparine** (promazine), **Stelazine** (trifluoperazine), **Taractan** (chlorprothixene), **Thorazine** (chlorpromazine), **Tindal** (acetophenazine), **Trilafon** (perphenazine), **Vesprin** (triflupromazine)

| Also Uses | This Could Result |
|---|---|
| Aluminum-containing Antacids and Diarrhea Medicine<br><br>  **AlternaGel, Aludrox, Basaljel, Diar-Aid, Di-Gel, Gaviscon, Gelusil, Kaopectate, Maalox, Mylanta, Phosphajel, Rheaban, Riopan, Robalate, Rolaids,** etc. | These compounds containing aluminum can glom on to antipsychotic medication while in the stomach and prevent proper absorption into the bloodstream. The answer to this drug interaction is simple. Don't take the antacids or diarrhea drugs within several hours of swallowing the head medicine. |

*Any dosage alterations *must* be supervised by a physician!

## Major Tranquilizers *cont.**

**If a person who is consuming** tranquilizers **Compazine** (prochlorperazine), **Haldol** (haloperidol), **Loxitane** (loxapine), **Mellaril** (thioridazine), **Moban** (molindone), **Navane** (thiothixene), **Permitil** and **Prolixin** (fluphenazine), **Proketazine** (carphenazine), **Quide** (piperacetazine), **Serentil** (mesoridazine), **Sparine** (promazine), **Stelazine** (trifluoperazine), **Taractan** (chlorprothixene), **Thorazine** (chlorpromazine), **Tindal** (acetophenazine), **Trilafon** (perphenazine), **Vesprin** (triflupromazine)

### Also Uses

Anticholinergic Medications

**Akineton, Anaspaz, Artane,** Atropine, Belladonna, **Bellafoline, Bentyl, Cogentin, Disipal, Donnatal, Kemadrin, Lomotil, Pagitane, Phenoxene,** Scopolamine, **Trest, Trocinate,** etc.

### This Could Result

These "anticholinergic" drugs are used for many purposes—treating ulcers and many other gastrointestinal disorders, diarrhea, parkinsonism, motion sickness, asthma, and several other diseases. Anticholinergic medications interact with many of the antipsychotic drugs in at least two different ways. The anticholinergics may block the positive antipsychotic effects of the major tranquilizers.

These two types of medicines also share the same types of adverse reactions. When you combine two drugs that have the same kinds of side effects you can

*Any dosage alterations *must* be supervised by a physician!

**Major Tranquilizers** *cont.\**

**If a person who is consuming** tranquilizers **Compazine** (prochlorperazine), **Haldol** (haloperidol), **Loxitane** (loxapine), **Mellaril** (thioridazine), **Moban** (molindone), **Navane** (thiothixene), **Permitil** and **Prolixin** (fluphenazine), **Proketazine** (carphenazine), **Quide** (piperacetazine), **Serentil** (mesoridazine), **Sparine** (promazine), **Stelazine** (trifluoperazine), **Taractan** (chlorprothixene), **Thorazine** (chlorpromazine), **Tindal** (acetophenazine), **Trilafon** (perphenazine), **Vesprin** (triflupromazine)

**This Could Result** *cont.*

expect adverse reactions. In this case, dry mouth, dilated pupils, rapid pulse, constipation, and difficulty in urination may become common. But some of the medications like **Artane** may reduce side effects, such as muscle twitches, from antipsychotic drugs. There is no simple solution to the problem except to be aware of it and request careful dosage adjustment by a physician.

\*Any dosage alterations *must* be supervised by a physician!

## Major Tranquilizers *cont.*

**If a person who is consuming** tranquilizers **Compazine** (prochlorperazine), **Haldol** (haloperidol), **Loxitane** (loxapine), **Mellaril** (thioridazine), **Moban** (molindone), **Navane** (thiothixene), **Permitil** and **Prolixin** (fluphenazine), **Proketazine** (carphenazine), **Quide** (piperacetazine), **Serentil** (mesoridazine), **Sparine** (promazine), **Stelazine** (trifluoperazine), **Taractan** (chlorprothixene), **Thorazine** (chlorpromazine), **Tindal** (acetophenazine), **Trilafon** (perphenazine), **Vesprin** (triflupromazine)

| Also Uses | This Could Result |
|---|---|
| Blood-Pressure Medication<br>**Hylorel, Ismelin** | If you are taking **Ismelin** (guanethidine) to control your blood pressure, don't take major tranquilizers as well. The antipsychotic medications can blunt the effectiveness of **Ismelin,** causing your blood pressure to rise. The recently released antihypertensive drug **Hylorel** (guanadrel) probably interacts in the same manner, although this is still unproven.<br><br>If you must take a major tranquilizer and blood-pressure medicine at the same time, it will be necessary to talk to a physician about an antihypertensive drug that does not interact. |

*Any dosage alterations *must* be supervised by a physician!

## Major Tranquilizers *cont.**

**If a person who is consuming** tranquilizers **Compazine** (prochlorperazine), **Haldol** (haloperidol), **Loxitane** (loxapine), **Mellaril** (thioridazine), **Moban** (molindone), **Navane** (thiothixene), **Permitil** and **Prolixin** (fluphenazine), **Proketazine** (carphenazine), **Quide** (piperacetazine), **Serentil** (mesoridazine), **Sparine** (promazine), **Stelazine** (trifluoperazine), **Taractan** (chlorprothixene), **Thorazine** (chlorpromazine), **Tindal** (acetophenazine), **Trilafon** (perphenazine), **Vesprin** (triflupromazine)

| Also Uses | This Could Result |
|---|---|
| Drugs That Cause Sedation<br><br>Alcohol, Antidepressants (tricyclic), Antihistamines, **Atarax, Ativan,** Barbiturates: **Alurate, Amytal, Butisol, Fiorinal, Gemonil, Lotusate, Luminal, Mebaral, Mysoline, Nembutal,** phenobarbital, **Seconal, Tuinal; Centrax,** Codeine, **Dalmane, Demerol, Dicodid, Dilaudid, Doriden, Equanil, Halcion, Librax, Librium, Miltown,** Morphine, **Noctec, Noludar, Paxipam, Percocet, Percodan, Placidyl, Restoril,** | So you think a tranquilizer is a tranquilizer. Wrong! "Major tranquilizers" are completely different animals from "minor tranquilizers." They are much more potent and are generally prescribed only for severe psychological disturbances or psychosis. The more correct term for this class of drugs is "antipsychotic" medications. They are not all as sedating as their common name implies, but some can knock you for quite a loop, especially **Mellaril** and **Thorazine.**<br><br>When a sedative or any of the listed drugs is taken in the presence of one of these major tranquilizers, hazard- |

*Any dosage alterations *must* be supervised by a physician!

## Major Tranquilizers *cont.* *

**If a person who is consuming** tranquilizers **Compazine** (prochlorperazine), **Haldol** (haloperidol), **Loxitane** (loxapine), **Mellaril** (thioridazine), **Moban** (molindone), **Navane** (thiothixene), **Permitil** and **Prolixin** (fluphenazine), **Proketazine** (carphenazine), **Quide** (piperacetazine), **Serentil** (mesoridazine), **Sparine** (promazine), **Stelazine** (trifluoperazine), **Taractan** (chlorprothixene), **Thorazine** (chlorpromazine), **Tindal** (acetophenazine), **Trilafon** (perphenazine), **Vesprin** (triflupromazine)

| Also Uses *cont.* | This Could Result *cont.* |
|---|---|
| Serax, Talwin, Tranxene, Valium, Vistaril, Xanax, etc. | ous intensification of central nervous system depression may occur—drowsiness, unsteadiness, confusion, fatigue, etc. A serious fall in blood pressure is also possible. |

Any dosage alterations *must* be supervised by a physician!

## MAO INHIBITORS*

This class of drugs is used to treat both psychological depression and high blood pressure. One antibiotic has even been shown to have MAO-inhibiting properties. Because they suppress the action of a crucial enzyme in the body, *mono*amine *o*xidase (MAO), they are incompatible with a variety of substances requiring this enzyme. Such interactions can be extremely dangerous.

*Note:* It usually takes at least two weeks for the enzyme blocking effects of the MAO inhibitors to wear off. During this "washout" period, you will still be susceptible to most of the drug interactions listed below. Consider this time-lag before taking any additional drugs or eating the foods listed below.

---

**If a person who is consuming** MAO inhibitors **Marplan** (isocarboxazid), **Nardil** (phenelzine), **Parnate** (tranylcypromine) (antidepressants)

*or*

**Eutonyl** (pargyline), **Eutron** (pargyline plus methyclothiazide) (blood-pressure medication)

*or*

**Furoxone** (furazolidone) (antibiotic)

| Also Uses | This Could Result |
|---|---|
| Antidepressants (Tricyclic) | See table listing *Antidepressants*. |

---

*Any dosage alterations *must* be supervised by a physician!

## Mao Inhibitors *cont.**

This class of drugs is used to treat both psychological depression and high blood pressure. One antibiotic has even been shown to have MAO-inhibiting properties. Because they suppress the action of a crucial enzyme in the body, *m*onoamine *o*xidase (MAO), they are incompatible with a variety of substances requiring this enzyme. Such interactions can be extremely dangerous.

*Note:* It usually takes at least two weeks for the enzyme-blocking effects of the MAO inhibitors to wear off. During this "washout" period, you will still be susceptible to most of the drug interactions listed below. Consider this time-lag before taking any additional drugs or eating the foods listed below.

---

**If a person who is consuming** MAO inhibitors **Marplan** (isocarboxazid), **Nardil** (phenelzine), **Parnate** (tranylcypromine) (antidepressants)

*or*

**Eutonyl** (pargyline), **Eutron** (pargyline plus methyclothiazide) (blood-pressure medication)

*or*

**Furoxone** (furazolidone) (antibiotic)

| Also Uses | This Could Result |
|---|---|
| Antiparkinsonism Drugs<br><br>**Dopar, Larodopa, L-Dopa** | The MAO inhibitors seem to rev up the activity of these drugs for parkinsonism. The potential for side effects increases as well, and very high blood pressure and a racing heart rate may result. |

---

*Any dosage alterations *must* be supervised by a physician!

## Mao Inhibitors *cont.**

This class of drugs is used to treat both psychological depression and high blood pressure. One antibiotic has even been shown to have MAO-inhibiting properties. Because they suppress the action of a crucial enzyme in the body, *monoamine oxidase* (MAO), they are incompatible with a variety of substances requiring this enzyme. Such interactions can be extremely dangerous.

*Note:* It usually takes at least two weeks for the enzyme-blocking effects of the MAO inhibitors to wear off. During this "washout" period, you will still be susceptible to most of the drug interactions listed below. Consider this time-lag before taking any additional drugs or eating the foods listed below.

**If a person who is consuming** MAO inhibitors **Marplan** (isocarboxazid), **Nardil** (phenelzine), **Parnate** (tranylcypromine) (antidepressants)

*or*

**Eutonyl** (pargyline), **Eutron** (pargyline plus methyclothiazide) (blood-pressure medication)

*or*

**Furoxone** (furazolidone) (antibiotic)

| Also Uses | This Could Result |
|---|---|
| Blood-Pressure Medicine<br><br>  **Esimil, Ismelin** | MAO inhibitors can counteract the blood-pressure-lowering effects of **Ismelin** and **Esimil** (guanethidine). Either switch to another drug regimen or have the doctor reevaluate the dose of this antihypertension medication. |

*Any dosage alterations *must* be supervised by a physician!

## Mao Inhibitors *cont.**

This class of drugs is used to treat both psychological depression and high blood pressure. One antibiotic has even been shown to have MAO-inhibiting properties. Because they suppress the action of a crucial enzyme in the body, *mono*amine *o*xidase (MAO), they are incompatible with a variety of substances requiring this enzyme. Such interactions can be extremely dangerous.

*Note:* It usually takes at least two weeks for the enzyme-blocking effects of the MAO inhibitors to wear off. During this "washout" period, you will still be susceptible to most of the drug interactions listed below. Consider this time-lag before taking any additional drugs or eating the foods listed below.

---

**If a person who is consuming** MAO inhibitors **Marplan** (isocarboxazid), **Nardil** (phenelzine), **Parnate** (tranylcypromine) (antidepressants)

*or*

**Eutonyl** (pargyline), **Eutron** (pargyline plus methyclothiazide) (blood-pressure medication)

*or*

**Furoxone** (furazolidone) (antibiotic)

| Also Uses | This Could Result |
|---|---|
| Decongestants, Cold Remedies, Asthma Medications<br><br>**Actifed, Afrinol, Alka-Seltzer Plus Cold Tablets, Allerest, A.R.M., Bronitin, Comtrex, Contac, Coricidin D, Dainite-KL, Dimetapp, Dristan,** | This drug interaction can be fatal. NEVER take a cold or allergy remedy when taking an MAO inhibitor unless you are absolutely sure it does not contain a decongestant or related compound. The reaction caused by mixing these two medicines can cause huge increases in |

---

*Any dosage alterations *must* be supervised by a physician!

## Mao Inhibitors *cont.**

This class of drugs is used to treat both psychological depression and high blood pressure. One antibiotic has even been shown to have MAO-inhibiting properties. Because they suppress the action of a crucial enzyme in the body, *monoamine oxidase* (MAO), they are incompatible with a variety of substances requiring this enzyme. Such interactions can be extremely dangerous.

*Note:* It usually takes at least two weeks for the enzyme-blocking effects of the MAO inhibitors to wear off. During this "washout" period, you will still be susceptible to most of the drug interactions listed below. Consider this time-lag before taking any additional drugs or eating the foods listed below.

---

**If a person who is consuming** MAO inhibitors **Marplan** (isocarboxazid), **Nardil** (phenelzine), **Parnate** (tranylcypromine) (antidepressants)

*or*

**Eutonyl** (pargyline), **Eutron** (pargyline plus methyclothiazide) (blood-pressure medication)

*or*

**Furoxone** (furazolidone) (antibiotic)

| Also Uses *cont.* | This Could Result *cont.* |
|---|---|
| **Drixoral, Fedrazil, Marax, Novafed, Ornade, Primatene, Propadrine, Sine-Aid, Sinutab, Sudafed, Tedral, Triaminic,** and just about all cold remedies that have *"decongestant"* on the label. | blood pressure, perhaps leading to a stroke. As with tyramine-containing foods (see below), severe headache, vomiting, and fever are manifestations of this drug interaction. |

---

*Any dosage alterations *must* be supervised by a physician!

## Mao Inhibitors *cont.**

This class of drugs is used to treat both psychological depression and high blood pressure. One antibiotic has even been shown to have MAO-inhibiting properties. Because they suppress the action of a crucial enzyme in the body, *monoamine oxidase* (MAO), they are incompatible with a variety of substances requiring this enzyme. Such interactions can be extremely dangerous.

*Note:* It usually takes at least two weeks for the enzyme-blocking effects of the MAO inhibitors to wear off. During this "washout" period, you will still be susceptible to most of the drug interactions listed below. Consider this time-lag before taking any additional drugs or eating the foods listed below.

---

**If a person who is consuming** MAO inhibitors **Marplan** (isocarboxazid), **Nardil** (phenelzine), **Parnate** (tranylcypromine) (antidepressants)

*or*

**Eutonyl** (pargyline), **Eutron** (pargyline plus methyclothiazide) (blood-pressure medication)

*or*

**Furoxone** (furazolidone) (antibiotic)

| Also Uses | This Could Result |
|---|---|
| Diabetes Medicine, Insulin | See table listing *Diabetes Medication (Oral)*. |

| Also Uses | This Could Result |
|---|---|
| Diet Pills<br><br>  **Ayd's Extra Strength,**<br>  **Benzedrine,**<br>  **Biphetamine, Control,** | The drug interaction here is the same as for cold remedies (above) and the tyramine-containing foods |

---

*Any dosage alterations *must* be supervised by a physician!

## Mao Inhibitors *cont.**

This class of drugs is used to treat both psychological depression and high blood pressure. One antibiotic has even been shown to have MAO-inhibiting properties. Because they suppress the action of a crucial enzyme in the body, *monoamine oxidase* (MAO), they are incompatible with a variety of substances requiring this enzyme. Such interactions can be extremely dangerous.

*Note:* It usually takes at least two weeks for the enzyme-blocking effects of the MAO inhibitors to wear off. During this "washout" period, you will still be susceptible to most of the drug interactions listed below. Consider this time-lag before taking any additional drugs or eating the foods listed below.

**If a person who is consuming** MAO inhibitors **Marplan** (isocarboxazid), **Nardil** (phenelzine), **Parnate** (tranylcypromine) (antidepressants)

*or*

**Eutonyl** (pargyline), **Eutron** (pargyline plus methyclothiazide) (blood-pressure medication)

*or*

**Furoxone** (furazolidone) (antibiotic)

| Also Uses *cont.* | This Could Result *cont.* |
|---|---|
| **Desoxyn, Dexatrim, Dexedrine, Didrex, Dietac, Grapefruit Diet Plan with Diadax, Ionamin, Preludin, Pondimin, Prolamine, Sanorex, Tenuate, Voranil,** etc. | (below). It too can prove fatal. |

*Any dosage alterations *must* be supervised by a physician!

## Mao Inhibitors *cont.\**

This class of drugs is used to treat both psychological depression and high blood pressure. One antibiotic has even been shown to have MAO-inhibiting properties. Because they suppress the action of a crucial enzyme in the body, *monoamine oxidase* (MAO), they are incompatible with a variety of substances requiring this enzyme. Such interactions can be extremely dangerous.

*Note:* It usually takes at least two weeks for the enzyme-blocking effects of the MAO inhibitors to wear off. During this "washout" period, you will still be susceptible to most of the drug interactions listed below. Consider this time-lag before taking any additional drugs or eating the foods listed below.

---

**If a person who is consuming** MAO inhibitors **Marplan** (isocarboxazid), **Nardil** (phenelzine), **Parnate** (tranylcypromine) (antidepressants)

*or*

**Eutonyl** (pargyline), **Eutron** (pargyline plus methyclothiazide) (blood-pressure medication)

*or*

**Furoxone** (furazolidone) (antibiotic)

| Also Uses | This Could Result |
|---|---|
| Narcotic Analgesic (Pain Medication)<br><br>**Demerol, Mepergan** | Heavy-drug pain medicine like **Demerol** and **Mepergan** (both meperidine), when mixed with an MAO inhibitor, can have very unpredictable effects, ranging from nervous system excitement and high blood pressure to nervous system depression and |

---

*\*Any dosage alterations *must* be supervised by a physician!

## Mao Inhibitors *cont.**

This class of drugs is used to treat both psychological depression and high blood pressure. One antibiotic has even been shown to have MAO-inhibiting properties. Because they suppress the action of a crucial enzyme in the body, *mono*amine *o*xidase (MAO), they are incompatible with a variety of substances requiring this enzyme. Such interactions can be extremely dangerous.

*Note:* It usually takes at least two weeks for the enzyme-blocking effects of the MAO inhibitors to wear off. During this "washout" period, you will still be susceptible to most of the drug interactions listed below. Consider this time-lag before taking any additional drugs or eating the foods listed below.

---

**If a person who is consuming** MAO inhibitors **Marplan** (isocarboxazid), **Nardil** (phenelzine), **Parnate** (tranylcypromine) (antidepressants)

*or*

**Eutonyl** (pargyline), **Eutron** (pargyline plus methyclothiazide) (blood-pressure medication)

*or*

**Furoxone** (furazolidone) (antibiotic)

|  | **This Could Result** *cont.* |
|---|---|
|  | low blood pressure. The result has led to coma followed by death. Avoid this combination at all costs. |

---

*Any dosage alterations *must* be supervised by a physician!

## Mao Inhibitors *cont.*\*

This class of drugs is used to treat both psychological depression and high blood pressure. One antibiotic has even been shown to have MAO-inhibiting properties. Because they suppress the action of a crucial enzyme in the body, *mono*amine *o*xidase (MAO), they are incompatible with a variety of substances requiring this enzyme. Such interactions can be extremely dangerous.

*Note:* It usually takes at least two weeks for the enzyme-blocking effects of the MAO inhibitors to wear off. During this "washout" period, you will still be susceptible to most of the drug interactions listed below. Consider this time-lag before taking any additional drugs or eating the foods listed below.

---

**If a person who is consuming** MAO inhibitors **Marplan** (isocarboxazid), **Nardil** (phenelzine), **Parnate** (tranylcypromine) (antidepressants)

*or*

**Eutonyl** (pargyline), **Eutron** (pargyline plus methyclothiazide) (blood-pressure medication)

*or*

**Furoxone** (furazolidone) (antibiotic)

| **Also Uses** | **This Could Result** |
|---|---|
| Tyramine-containing Foods<br><br>  Avocados, Bananas (ripe), Beer, Caffeine, Cheese (aged), Chicken Liver, Chocolate (lots of it), Fava Beans, Fermented Sausages (Salami, Pepperoni, Bologna, etcetera), Figs | Look out! This interaction could be lethal. All these foods contain tyramine or other related chemicals, which, in the presence of MAO inhibitors, could increase your blood pressure so much that you might blow a blood vessel in the brain. |

---

\*Any dosage alterations *must* be supervised by a physician!

## Mao Inhibitors *cont.**

This class of drugs is used to treat both psychological depression and high blood pressure. One antibiotic has even been shown to have MAO-inhibiting properties. Because they suppress the action of a crucial enzyme in the body, *monoamine oxidase* (MAO), they are incompatible with a variety of substances requiring this enzyme. Such interactions can be extremely dangerous.

*Note:* It usually takes at least two weeks for the enzyme-blocking effects of the MAO inhibitors to wear off. During this "washout" period, you will still be susceptible to most of the drug interactions listed below. Consider this time-lag before taking any additional drugs or eating the foods listed below.

---

**If a person who is consuming** MAO inhibitors **Marplan** (isocarboxazid), **Nardil** (phenelzine), **Parnate** (tranylcypromine) (antidepressants)

*or*

**Eutonyl** (pargyline), **Eutron** (pargyline plus methyclothiazide) (blood-pressure medication)

*or*

**Furoxone** (furazolidone) (antibiotic)

| Also Uses *cont.* | This Could Result *cont.* |
|---|---|
| (canned), Pickled Herring, Pineapple, Raisins, Red Wine, Sauerkraut, Yeast Extract, Yogurt | Terrible headache, vomiting, fever, and high blood pressure are some warning signals. |

---

*Any dosage alterations *must* be supervised by a physician!

## ANTIANXIETY AGENTS, SEDATIVES, SLEEPING PILLS, MINOR TRANQUILIZERS*

If a person is consuming *the barbiturates:* **Alurate** (aprobarbital), **Amytal** (amobarbital), **Butisol** (butabarbital), **Fiorinal** (containing butalbital), **Gemonil** (metharbital), **Lotusate** (talbutal), **Luminal** (phenobarbital), **Mebaral** (mephobarbital), **Nembutal** (pentobarbital), **Seconal** (secobarbital), **Tuinal** (amobarbital plus secobarbital)

*or*

*The benzodiazepines:* **Ativan** (lorazepam), **Centrax** (prazepam), **Dalmane** (flurazepam), **Halcion** (triazolam), **Librium** (chlordiazepoxide), **Paxipam** (halazepam), **Restoril** (temazepam), **Serax** (oxazepam), **Tranxene** (clorazepate), **Valium** (diazepam), **Xanax** (alprazolam)

*or*

*Others:* **Atarax** and **Vistaril** (hydroxyzine), **Doriden** (glutethimide), **Equanil** and **Miltown** (meprobamate), **Noctec** (chloral hydrate), **Noludar** (methyprylon), **Paral** (paraldehyde), **Placidyl** (ethchlorvynol), **Sedamyl** (acetylcarbromal), **Triclos** (triclofos), **Trancopal** (chlormezanone), **Tybatran** (tybamate), **Valmid** (ethinimate), etc.

| Also Uses | This Could Result |
|---|---|
| Alcohol<br><br>　Beer, Hard Stuff, Wine | No good! Sure, you have done it and nothing happened. Don't press your luck. Booze and tranquilizers or sleeping pills *do not mix.* This combination is an unfortunate and common reason for visits to emergency rooms. There is an additive effect, which produces deep |

*Any dosage alterations *must* be supervised by a physician!

## Antianxiety Agents, Sedatives, Sleeping Pills, Minor Tranquilizers *cont.**

**If a person is consuming** *the barbiturates:* **Alurate** (aprobarbital), **Amytal** (amobarbital), **Butisol** (butabarbital), **Fiorinal** (containing butalbital), **Gemonil** (metharbital), **Lotusate** (talbutal), **Luminal** (phenobarbital), **Mebaral** (mephobarbital), **Nembutal** (pentobarbital), **Seconal** (secobarbital), **Tuinal** (amobarbital plus secobarbital)

*or*

*The benzodiazepines:* **Ativan** (lorazepam), **Centrax** (prazepam), **Dalmane** (flurazepam), **Halcion** (triazolam), **Librium** (chlordiazepoxide), **Paxipam** (halazepam), **Restoril** (temazepam), **Serax** (oxazepam), **Tranxene** (clorazepate), **Valium** (diazepam), **Xanax** (alprazolam)

*or*

*Others:* **Atarax** and **Vistaril** (hydroxyzine), **Doriden** (glutethimide), **Equanil** and **Miltown** (meprobamate), **Noctec** (chloral hydrate), **Noludar** (methyprylon), **Paral** (paraldehyde), **Placidyl** (ethchlorvynol), **Sedamyl** (acetylcarbromal), **Triclos** (triclofos), **Trancopal** (chlormezanone), **Tybatran** (tybamate), **Valmid** (ethinimate), etc.

### This Could Result *cont.*

sedation leading to a pronounced deterioration in coordination. Any task that requires attention, especially driving, must be ruled out. This drug interaction may lead to a big fall in blood pressure as well as breathing failure. If you want to live, don't mix 'em!

*Any dosage alterations *must* be supervised by a physician!

## Antianxiety Agents, Sedatives, Sleeping Pills, Minor Tranquilizers *cont.**

**If a person is consuming** *the barbiturates:* **Alurate** (aprobarbital), **Amytal** (amobarbital), **Butisol** (butabarbital), **Fiorinal** (containing butalbital), **Gemonil** (metharbital), **Lotusate** (talbutal), **Luminal** (phenobarbital), **Mebaral** (mephobarbital), **Nembutal** (pentobarbital), **Seconal** (secobarbital), **Tuinal** (amobarbital plus secobarbital)

*or*

*The benzodiazepines:* **Ativan** (lorazepam), **Centrax** (prazepam), **Dalmane** (flurazepam), **Halcion** (triazolam), **Librium** (chlordiazepoxide), **Paxipam** (halazepam), **Restoril** (temazepam), **Serax** (oxazepam), **Tranxene** (clorazepate), **Valium** (diazepam), **Xanax** (alprazolam)

*or*

*Others:* **Atarax** and **Vistaril** (hydroxyzine), **Doriden** (glutethimide), **Equanil** and **Miltown** (meprobamate), **Noctec** (chloral hydrate), **Noludar** (methyprylon), **Paral** (paraldehyde), **Placidyl** (ethchlorvynol), **Sedamyl** (acetylcarbromal), **Triclos** (triclofos), **Trancopal** (chlormezanone), **Tybatran** (tybamate), **Valmid** (ethinimate), etc.

| Also Uses | This Could Result |
|---|---|
| Oral Anticoagulants | See table listing *Oral Anticoagulants (Blood-thinning Drugs).* |

*Any dosage alterations *must* be supervised by a physician!

## Antianxiety Agents, Sedatives, Sleeping Pills, Minor Tranquilizers *cont.**

---

**If a person is consuming** *the barbiturates:* **Alurate** (aprobarbital), **Amytal** (amobarbital), **Butisol** (butabarbital), **Fiorinal** (containing butalbital), **Gemonil** (metharbital), **Lotusate** (talbutal), **Luminal** (phenobarbital), **Mebaral** (mephobarbital), **Nembutal** (pentobarbital), **Seconal** (secobarbital), **Tuinal** (amobarbital plus secobarbital)

*or*

*The benzodiazepines:* **Ativan** (lorazepam), **Centrax** (prazepam), **Dalmane** (flurazepam), **Halcion** (triazolam), **Librium** (chlordiazepoxide), **Paxipam** (halazepam), **Restoril** (temazepam), **Serax** (oxazepam), **Tranxene** (clorazepate), **Valium** (diazepam), **Xanax** (alprazolam)

*or*

*Others:* **Atarax** and **Vistaril** (hydroxyzine), **Doriden** (glutethimide), **Equanil** and **Miltown** (meprobamate), **Noctec** (chloral hydrate), **Noludar** (methyprylon), **Paral** (paraldehyde), **Placidyl** (ethchlorvynol), **Sedamyl** (acetylcarbromal), **Triclos** (triclofos), **Trancopal** (chlormezanone), **Tybatran** (tybamate), **Valmid** (ethinimate), etc.

---

| Also Uses | This Could Result |
|---|---|
| Antidepressant Medication<br><br>    **Adapin, Asendin, Aventyl, Desyrel, Elavil, Endep, Janimine, Ludiomil, Norpramin, Pamelor, Pertofrane, Sinequan, Surmontil, Tofranil, Triavil, Vivactil** | This one is pretty common. Too many doctors prescribe antianxiety agents for depression and then add a potent antidepressant on top of it. Although probably not as dangerous as alcohol, antidepressants also exaggerate the sedative effects of minor tranquilizers and |

---

*Any dosage alterations *must* be supervised by a physician!

## Antianxiety Agents, Sedatives, Sleeping Pills, Minor Tranquilizers *cont.*\*

**If a person is consuming** *the barbiturates:* **Alurate** (aprobarbital), **Amytal** (amobarbital), **Butisol** (butabarbital), **Fiorinal** (containing butalbital), **Gemonil** (metharbital), **Lotusate** (talbutal), **Luminal** (phenobarbital), **Mebaral** (mephobarbital), **Nembutal** (pentobarbital), **Seconal** (secobarbital), **Tuinal** (amobarbital plus secobarbital)

*or*

*The benzodiazepines:* **Ativan** (lorazepam), **Centrax** (prazepam), **Dalmane** (flurazepam), **Halcion** (triazolam), **Librium** (chlordiazepoxide), **Paxipam** (halazepam), **Restoril** (temazepam), **Serax** (oxazepam), **Tranxene** (clorazepate), **Valium** (diazepam), **Xanax** (alprazolam)

*or*

*Others:* **Atarax** and **Vistaril** (hydroxyzine), **Doriden** (glutethimide), **Equanil** and **Miltown** (meprobamate), **Noctec** (chloral hydrate), **Noludar** (methyprylon), **Paral** (paraldehyde), **Placidyl** (ethchlorvynol), **Sedamyl** (acetylcarbromal), **Triclos** (triclofos), **Trancopal** (chlormezanone), **Tybatran** (tybamate), **Valmid** (ethinimate), etc.

### This Could Result *cont.*

sleeping pills. The most sedating antidepressants are **Adapin** and **Sinequan** (doxepin), **Desyrel** (trazodone), **Elavil** (amitriptyline), **Ludiomil** (maprotiline), and **Surmontil** (trimipramine), so watch out especially for these. Be damn careful if you mix these two kinds of drugs together.

\*Any dosage alterations *must* be supervised by a physician!

**Antianxiety Agents, Sedatives, Sleeping Pills, Minor Tranquilizers** *cont.**

**If a person is consuming** *the barbiturates:* **Alurate** (aprobarbital), **Amytal** (amobarbital), **Butisol** (butabarbital), **Fiorinal** (containing butalbital), **Gemonil** (metharbital), **Lotusate** (talbutal), **Luminal** (phenobarbital), **Mebaral** (mephobarbital), **Nembutal** (pentobarbital), **Seconal** (secobarbital), **Tuinal** (amobarbital plus secobarbital)

*or*

*The benzodiazepines:* **Ativan** (lorazepam), **Centrax** (prazepam), **Dalmane** (flurazepam), **Halcion** (triazolam), **Librium** (chlordiazepoxide), **Paxipam** (halazepam), **Restoril** (temazepam), **Serax** (oxazepam), **Tranxene** (clorazepate), **Valium** (diazepam), **Xanax** (alprazolam)

*or*

*Others:* **Atarax** and **Vistaril** (hydroxyzine), **Doriden** (glutethimide), **Equanil** and **Miltown** (meprobamate), **Noctec** (chloral hydrate), **Noludar** (methyprylon), **Paral** (paraldehyde), **Placidyl** (ethchlorvynol), **Sedamyl** (acetylcarbromal), **Triclos** (triclofos), **Trancopal** (chlormezanone), **Tybatran** (tybamate), **Valmid** (ethinimate), etc.

| Also Uses | This Could Result |
|---|---|
| Birth-control Pills | See table listing *Birth-control Pills (Oral Contraceptives).* |

| Also Uses | This Could Result |
|---|---|
| **Vibramycin** (doxycycline) | See tables listing *Tetracycline Antibiotics* and *Anticonvulsant Medications (for Epilepsy).* |

*Any dosage alterations *must* be supervised by a physician!

## Antianxiety Agents, Sedatives, Sleeping Pills, Minor Tranquilizers *cont.***

**If a person is consuming** *the barbiturates:* **Alurate** (aprobarbital), **Amytal** (amobarbital), **Butisol** (butabarbital), **Fiorinal** (containing butalbital), **Gemonil** (metharbital), **Lotusate** (talbutal), **Luminal** (phenobarbital), **Mebaral** (mephobarbital), **Nembutal** (pentobarbital), **Seconal** (secobarbital), **Tuinal** (amobarbital plus secobarbital)

*or*

*The benzodiazepines:* **Ativan** (lorazepam), **Centrax** (prazepam), **Dalmane** (flurazepam), **Halcion** (triazolam), **Librium** (chlordiazepoxide), **Paxipam** (halazepam), **Restoril** (temazepam), **Serax** (oxazepam), **Tranxene** (clorazepate), **Valium** (diazepam), **Xanax** (alprazolam)

*or*

*Others:* **Atarax** and **Vistaril** (hydroxyzine), **Doriden** (glutethimide), **Equanil** and **Miltown** (meprobamate), **Noctec** (chloral hydrate), **Noludar** (methyprylon), **Paral** (paraldehyde), **Placidyl** (ethchlorvynol), **Sedamyl** (acetylcarbromal), **Triclos** (triclofos), **Trancopal** (chlormezanone), **Tybatran** (tybamate), **Valmid** (ethinimate), etc.

| Also Uses | This Could Result |
|---|---|
| Steroids | See table listing *Cortisone-type Anti-Inflammatory Medication.* |

| Also Uses | This Could Result |
|---|---|
| Ulcer Medication | See table listing **Tagamet** (cimetidine). |

*Any dosage alterations *must* be supervised by a physician!

## TAGAMET (CIMETIDINE)*

**Tagamet** is a potent and very popular ulcer medication. It is one of the most frequently prescribed drugs in this country and has made its manufacturer, Smith, Kline & French, a small mint. Although a very useful drug, it is connected to a whole host of drug interactions. A newer, similar drug, **Zantac** (ranitidine) is just as effective and seems less likely to produce nasty interactions.

If a person who is consuming **Tagamet**

| Also Uses | This Could Result |
|---|---|
| Anticoagulants (Oral)<br><br>**Athrombin-K, Coumadin, Coufarin, Dicumarol, Hedulin, Miradon, Panwarfin** | Warning! This can be a very serious drug interaction. **Tagamet** decreases the body's ability to metabolize and get rid of the oral anticoagulant, effectively causing a buildup of the blood thinner in the body. A serious bleeding episode (read that hemorrhage) might result. As of this writing it appears that **Zantac** does not interact adversely with oral anticoagulants and seems to be a safer alternative. |

*Any dosage alterations *must* be supervised by a physician!

## Tagamet *cont.*\*

If a person who is consuming **Tagamet**

| Also Uses | This Could Result |
|---|---|
| Anticonvulsant Medication<br><br>**Dilantin, Mesantoin, Peganone** | The dose of these epilepsy medications should probably be decreased if it's necessary to take **Tagamet** at the same time. **Tagamet** causes a buildup of the anticonvulsant in the body which may result in toxicity from this unintentional overdose. Again, a switch to **Zantac** may be the easiest answer. Otherwise, have the doctor run some blood tests and modify dosage. |

\*Any dosage alterations *must* be supervised by a physician!

**Tagamet** *cont.*\*

If a person who is consuming **Tagamet**

| Also Uses | This Could Result |
|---|---|
| Asthma Medication<br><br>  Aminophylline, **Bronkodyl, Choledyl,** Oxtriphylline, **Respbid, Slo-Phyllin, Somophyllin, Sustaire, Synophylate, Theobid, Theo-Dur,** Theophylline, etc. | These asthma medications are all different forms of theophylline. Unfortunately, theophylline can be quite dangerous in overdose, and when **Tagamet** is combined with this asthma drug, a very serious interaction can result leading to theophylline toxicity. See the *Asthma* chapter for a detailed account of this frightening drug interaction. |

\*Any dosage alterations *must* be supervised by a physician!

## Tagamet *cont.*\*

If a person who is consuming **Tagamet**

| Also Uses | This Could Result |
|---|---|
| Beta Blockers<br><br>**Inderal, Lopressor** | This is probably a very common interaction given that both **Tagamet** and **Inderal** are two of the most frequently prescribed drugs in the country. But, as you have learned earlier in this chapter, **Tagamet** inhibits the liver's ability to metabolize many other drugs. When this interaction occurs with either of these two beta blockers, excessively slow heart rate and blood pressure may result. Using another noninteracting beta blocker is an option if **Tagamet** treatment is a must. **Zantac** may be less likely to interact and presumably could be used safely in place of the **Tagamet** if your doctor doesn't want to switch beta blockers. |

\*Any dosage alterations *must* be supervised by a physician!

## Tagamet *cont.*\*

If a person who is consuming **Tagamet**

| Also Uses | This Could Result |
|---|---|
| Minor Tranquilizers, Antianxiety Agents, Anticonvulsants, Sleep Medications (All Benzodiazepines)<br><br>**Centrax, Clonopin, Dalmane, Halcion, Librium, Librax, Paxipam, Tranxene, Valium, Valrelease, Xanax** | **Tagamet** messes up the liver's ability to metabolize and deactivate these commonly prescribed sedatives. Since more tranquilizer is left in your bloodstream, excessive sedation may result. **Tagamet** may cause mental confusion on its own, especially in older people, so this combination can produce a real double whammy. **Ativan, Restoril,** and **Serax** don't interact in this manner because the liver isn't in charge of their metabolism. They are safer alternatives if a sedative or sleeping pill is really needed. |

\*Any dosage alterations *must* be supervised by a physician!

## TETRACYCLINE ANTIBIOTICS*

**If a person who is consuming** tetracycline **Achromycin V, Cyclopar, Robitet, Sumycin,** and **Tetrex** (tetracycline), **Achrostatin V** (tetracycline plus nystatin), **Declomycin** (demeclocycline), **Minocin** (minocycline), **Mysteclin-F** (tetracycline plus amphotericin B), **Rondomycin** (methacycline), **Terramycin** (oxytetracycline), **Vibramycin** (doxycycline), etc.

| Also Uses | This Could Result |
|---|---|
| Anticonvulsants (applies to **Vibramycin** only) | See table listing *Anticonvulsant Medications (for Epilepsy).* |

| Also Uses | This Could Result |
|---|---|
| Barbiturates (applies to **Vibramycin** only) | The antibiotic benefits of **Vibramycin** could be diminished. |

*Any dosage alterations *must* be supervised by a physician!

## Tetracycline Antibiotics *cont.**

**If a person who is consuming** tetracycline **Achromycin V, Cyclopar, Robitet, Sumycin,** and **Tetrex** (tetracycline), **Achrostatin V** (tetracycline plus nystatin), **Declomycin** (demeclocycline), **Minocin** (minocycline), **Mysteclin-F** (tetracycline plus amphotericin B), **Rondomycin** (methacycline), **Terramycin** (oxytetracycline), **Vibramycin** (doxycycline), etc.

### Also Uses

Foods Containing High Concentrations of Calcium

Almonds, Buttermilk, Cheese, Cottage Cheese, Cream, Custard, Ice Cream, Milk (whole or nonfat), Pizza with Cheese, Pudding, Vegetables (green), Yogurt, etc.

### This Could Result

Damn! Here is a paradox that really hurts. The tetracycline antibiotics can screw up our stomachs. Look out for indigestion, heartburn, and diarrhea. It also kills off lots of good bacteria in our intestines. Milk products tend to diminish the stomach upset and replace some of the good guys that have been killed. Unfortunately, these foods contain high calcium levels and will drastically cut down on the effectiveness of the tetracyclines. Avoid eating these foods close to the time you take your antibiotic. In fact, never swallow tetracycline one hour prior to, during, or two hours following a meal if you want it to work. The exceptions here are **Vi-**

*Any dosage alterations *must* be supervised by a physician!

## Tetracycline Antibiotics *cont.*\*

If a person who is consuming tetracycline **Achromycin V, Cyclopar, Robitet, Sumycin,** and **Tetrex** (tetracycline), **Achrostatin V** (tetracycline plus nystatin), **Declomycin** (demeclocycline), **Minocin** (minocycline), **Mysteclin-F** (tetracycline plus amphotericin B), **Rondomycin** (methacycline), **Terramycin** (oxytetracycline), **Vibramycin** (doxycycline), etc.

| | **This Could Result *cont.*** |
|---|---|
| | bramycin and (probably) **Minocin,** which can be taken with any type of food. |

| **Also Uses** | **This Could Result** |
|---|---|
| Indigestion Aids and Antacids<br><br>**Alka-Seltzer, Amphojel, Bromo-Seltzer, Di-Gel, Eno, Gelusil, Maalox, Mylanta, Pepto-Bismol, Phillips' Milk of Magnesia, Rolaids,** Sodium Bicarbonate, **Tums,** etc. | Oh no! The same crummy problem here. After a few days of tetracycline therapy, the one thing you do need is an antacid. It is the last thing you should take. The ingredients in antacids have a great affinity for the tetracyclines (again, the exceptions are **Vibramycin** and **Minocin**). The resulting interaction can block proper absorption of these antibiotics and inhibit effectiveness. So, much as you may be tempted, avoid antacids if you want your tetracycline to work completely. |

\*Any dosage alterations *must* be supervised by a physician!

## Tetracycline Antibiotics *cont.*\*

**If a person who is consuming** tetracycline **Achromycin V, Cyclopar, Robitet, Sumycin,** and **Tetrex** (tetracycline), **Achrostatin V** (tetracycline plus nystatin), **Declomycin** (demeclocycline), **Minocin** (minocycline), **Mysteclin-F** (tetracycline plus amphotericin B), **Rondomycin** (methacycline), **Terramycin** (oxytetracycline), **Vibramycin** (doxycycline), etc.

| Also Uses | This Could Result |
|---|---|
| Iron Products, Vitamins with Iron<br><br>**Berroca Plus, Centrum, Feosol, Feostat, Fergon, Fer-In-Sol,** Ferrous Sulfate, **Ferusal, Geritol, Hematinic, Mol-Iron, Niferex, One-a-Day Plus Iron, Stuartinic, Super Plenamins, Theragran M,** etc. | This interaction is the same as that with dairy products or antacids. Do not take any iron-containing preparation with a tetracycline. Since many of these products are available over the counter, read the labels of multivitamin and mineral formulas very carefully to see if they contain iron. |

\*Any dosage alterations *must* be supervised by a physician!

## Tetracycline Antibiotics *cont.**

**If a person who is consuming** tetracycline **Achromycin V, Cyclopar, Robitet, Sumycin,** and **Tetrex** (tetracycline), **Achrostatin V** (tetracycline plus nystatin), **Declomycin** (demeclocycline), **Minocin** (minocycline), **Mysteclin-F** (tetracycline plus amphotericin B), **Rondomycin** (methacycline), **Terramycin** (oxytetracycline), **Vibramycin** (doxycycline), etc.

| Also Uses | This Could Result |
|---|---|
| Heart Medication<br><br>   **Lanoxin,** Digoxin | This interaction occurs in less than 10 percent of patients receiving the combination, but it can be very serious. Tetracycline raises the blood levels of **Lanoxin** (digoxin) in susceptible individuals, and the chances of a toxic buildup are increased.<br><br>   Beware: This interaction can occur months after you have taken the antibiotic. If this combination is absolutely necessary, your doctor should monitor your digoxin blood levels carefully. |

*Any dosage alterations *must* be supervised by a physician!

## Tetracycline Antibiotics *cont.**

**If a person who is consuming** tetracycline **Achromycin V, Cyclopar, Robitet, Sumycin,** and **Tetrex** (tetracycline), **Achrostatin V** (tetracycline plus nystatin), **Declomycin** (demeclocycline), **Minocin** (minocycline), **Mysteclin-F** (tetracycline plus amphotericin B), **Rondomycin** (methacycline), **Terramycin** (oxytetracycline), **Vibramycin** (doxycycline), etc.

| Also Uses | This Could Result |
|---|---|
| Penicillin Antibiotics<br><br>**Amcill, Ampicillin, Amoxil, Bicillin, Cyclapen-W, Dynapen, Geocillin, Larotid, Omnipen, Pentids, Pen-Vee K, Pfizerpen, Polycillin, Prostaphlin, Spectrobid, Tegopen, Unipen, V-Cillin K, Versapen, Wycillin,** etc. | If your doctor prescribes a penicillin antibiotic at the same time as one of the tetracyclines, he or she should be sent back to medical school. We're talking basic incompetence here, folks. Because these two classes of antibiotics work in a completely different manner, combining them markedly reduces therapeutic efficiency. |

*Any dosage alterations *must* be supervised by a physician!

Although the drug interactions that have been listed and discussed are among the most frequent and important, they do not represent even a fraction of the vast numbers of deleterious and sometimes fatal reactions that occur each year. With the help of your doctor and pharmacist, you should be able to avoid such dangerous complications.

Use the table frequently. In fact, every time you must take a drug, consult this chapter (or the ones in *People's Pharmacy-2* and *The New People's Pharmacy*) in order to make sure there are not special foods, over-the-counter products, or other drugs that might be incompatible with it.

But do not be lulled into a false sense of confidence if it appears that your drug does not interact with anything. These tables hardly even scratch the surface. Always consult your doctor if you are not sure about something. And do not let your physician beat around the bush about side effects.

If your doctor doesn't know whether two drugs will be safe together, try consulting a pharmacist. Many pharmacists know more about drugs and drug interactions than your family doctor. Unfortunately, they too often fall into the rut of taking pills from one bottle and putting them into another (the "count, pour, lick, and stick" syndrome). Take the time to find a pharmacist who will help you with all of your drug-related questions.

Ultimately, the only way you are going to improve the odds against an adverse drug interaction is to become extremely conscious of what prescription drugs, nonprescription drugs, and other chemicals you put into your body. Try to avoid taking more than one drug at a time. When you must take multiple medications, monitor your own system's reactivity and sensitivity. At the first sign of trouble, head for your doctor's office. Better yet, use the phone.

# References

1. Jick, Hershel. "Drugs—Remarkably Nontoxic." *N. Eng. J. Med.* 291(16):824–828, 1974.

2. Ibid.

3. Kotulak, Ronald, and Van, Jon. "Many Doctors Suffer 'Rx Fever.'" *Chicago Tribune,* Oct. 9, 1980, p. 1.

4. Long, Glenda. "The Effect of Medication Distribution Systems on Medication Errors." *Nursing Research* 31(3):182–191, 1982.

5. Friedman, Marion. "Iatrogenic Disease: Addressing a Growing Epidemic." *Postgraduate Medicine* 71(6):123–129, 1982.

6. Ibid.

7. Hoffman, Robert S. "Diagnostic Errors in the Evaluation of Behavioral Disorders." *JAMA* 248:964–967, 1982.

8. Friedman, op. cit.

9. Feely, John, and Wood, J. J. Alastair. "Effects of Cimetidine on the Elimination and Actions of Ethanol." *JAMA* 247:2819–2821, 1982.

10. Seitz, Helmut K., et al. "Increased Blood Ethanol Levels following Cimetidine But Not Ranitidine." *Lancet* 1:760, 1983.

11. "Ethanol and Cimetidine." *Drug Interaction Newsletter* 4(2):7–8, 1984.

12. Mangini, Richard J., ed. *Drug Interaction Facts.* St. Louis: Lippincott, 1984, p. 425.

13. Ibid.

14. Kramer, P., et al. "Effect of Influenza Vaccine on Warfarin Anticoagulation." *Clin. Pharmacol. Ther.* 35:416–418, 1984.

15. Huff, Barbara B., ed. *Physicians' Desk Reference,* 38th ed. Oradell, N.J.: Medical Economics, 1984, p. 1666.

16. Ames, Bruce N. "Dietary Carcinogens and Anticarcinogens." *Science* 221:1256–1264, 1983.

## Table References

1. Mangini, Richard J., ed. *Drug Interaction Facts.* St. Louis: J. B. Lippincott Co., 1984.

2. American Pharmaceutical Society. *Evaluations of Drug Interactions,* 2d ed. Washington, D.C.: American Pharmaceutical Society, 1978.

3. American Pharmaceutical Society. *Evaluations of Drug Interactions.* 2d ed. *Supplement.* Washington, D.C.: American Pharmaceutical Society, 1980.

4. Kastrup, Erwin K.; Boyd, James R.; and Olin, Bernie R., eds. *Facts and Comparisons.* St. Louis: J. B. Lippincott Co., 1983.

# 7

---

# Allergy: Oh, My Aching Nose

---

*What's it all about?* • *How to spot an
allergy at twenty paces* • *Salad-bar suicide: Watch out for sulfites* • *Finding
the culprit* • *Skin testing: Is it worth the
effort and expense?* • *Playing allergy
detective on your own* • *Doing something about allergy* • *Allergy treatment:
A shot in the dark?* • *Antiallergy alternatives* • *The pharmacological solution:
Antihistamine advances and steroid
sprays* • *Anaphylaxis: A matter of life
and death* • *Helping yourself.*

---

If every executive in the pharmaceutical industry were told tomorrow that all illnesses would be eradicated overnight, many
of them might faint or, worse yet, suffer massive coronaries.
After all, they'd be out of a job. If they were allowed to choose
a few problems to keep, I'll bet one they would be loath to lose
would be allergy. There's a potful of money being made by scores
of companies selling hundreds of different pills, shots, and lotions for a widespread ailment that's miserable to have and keeps
coming back relentlessly year after year.

Americans spend over $600 million annually trying to soothe
their stuffy, swollen sinuses, stifle sneezes, and relieve runny
noses. Nobody really has a clue as to how many allergy victims

there are. I have read estimates that range from twenty-two million to thirty-five million—even all the way up to sixty million (one out of every four people in the United States).[1-3] There are at least fifteen million hay fever sufferers alone.[4]

They say that misery loves company. Well, if you've got allergies, you certainly have plenty of company. Yup, me too. I've got hay fever, and I assure you that it takes a fellow victim to really appreciate the problem.

I often wonder how many allergy or ENT (ear, nose, and throat) specialists know what it's like to walk around with stopped-up sinuses. You can't smell or taste worth beans. Once-enjoyable sports activities turn into torture, and when it comes to thinking, forget it. Basically you just walk around in a daze trying not to moan and groan so often that you alienate everyone around you. This maddening malady has the power to reduce even the strongest among us to a quaking mass of swollen nasal tissue, teary eyes, and general misery.

Many folks first try to help themselves. But most people who take over-the-counter antihistamines in their effort to seek some relief know that means Space City. I can only liken the experience to walking under water. You feel weak and wiped out. There's a very good reason why virtually all allergy remedies carry some kind of caution along the lines of "Do not drive or operate heavy machinery, as this product may cause drowsiness."[5] People who attempt to do something that requires coordination or concentration could be a menace to themselves as well as everyone around them.

Nasal sprays may bring temporary improvement, but if you use such decongestants for longer than three days you court disaster in the form of addiction. Cold-turkey withdrawal brings on rebound nasal congestion. When you stop spritzing your nose, the little blood vessels that were constricted by medicine go wild and begin to dilate. That leads to super stuffiness, which can be worse than the original allergy. It can also last a good while after the nasal spray is stopped.

When people become frustrated with self-treatment, they often seek out specialists. Many allergists have become rich off

our misery as they turn us into pincushions with their desensitization shots. But now it's time to rattle their cages—the bottoms haven't been cleaned in quite a while. In addition, we will
astound you with some exciting new advances in the treatment
of allergy. The day is rapidly approaching when you may be
able to experience impressive relief without suffering side
effects that make you wonder whether the cure is worse than
the disease.

## What's It All About?

Allergy used to be a big black hole—a mystery ailment that left
researchers almost as puzzled as the patients who were plagued
with symptoms. There are still far more questions than answers,
but at long last immunologists are beginning to unlock some of
the secrets.

Let's get one thing straight right off the bat. Allergy is really
a garbage-bag term—a catchall word for the body's inappropriate responses to substances it believes are foreign. The immune
system is charged with the responsibility of defending our bodies
from microscopic invaders, like bacteria and viruses, and of
conducting search-and-destroy missions for cancerous cells. The
allergic response appears to be an overreaction: immunity run
amok. Symptoms can range from a stuffy nose caused by pollen,
dust, or animal dander to hives, eczema, stomach upset, asthma,
or life-threatening anaphylactic shock.

No one knows why one person reacts like crazy to that damn
old ragweed pollen, while someone else may be oblivious to the
pollen count and respond instead to peanuts. House dust, animal
fur, seafood, a drug, or even cold weather or strenuous exercise
can trigger an allergic reaction. The list of potential "allergens"
keeps growing as the list of chemicals in our environment ex-
pands.

Some people are so hypersensitive they may react to perfume,
cosmetics, detergents, pesticides, tooth powders, food additives,
or hundreds of other synthetic substances. There are even cases

of women who are allergic to semen. Intercourse can bring on hives, wheezing, and in the most extreme situation, shock.

While we don't know why some people respond so bizarrely, we are slowly beginning to get a handle on how the reaction is triggered. Let's take a slow-motion look at the chain of events leading to allergy symptoms.

In comes a pollen particle, or a bit of protein from certain types of seafood, or some dust. The body says, "Ah ha, foreign substance" and starts to churn out *antibodies*. These custom-tailored antibodies are a perfect chemical fit with that one particular invading substance (called an *antigen* or *allergen*).

The antigen and antibody latch on to one another, forming a chemical "key" that fits perfectly into the "lock" on a particular kind of cell known as a mast cell. Mast cells are found all over the body, but they are especially prevalent in the nose, skin, lungs, and digestive tract. Locked up inside the mast cell are lots of little packets of a substance you've heard referred to in hay fever and allergy commercials—histamine. In goes the key, click goes the lock, and out spills the histamine.

Once upon a time, we thought that histamine was the major culprit in allergic reactions. This theory had it that once freed from mast cells, histamine made its way to target cells located in the nose, eyes, and breathing passages. These target cells had special receptors just waiting for histamine to arrive. When it did, the receptors were thought to act like tiny switches that set in motion the swelling, tearing, itching, sneezing, and wheezing.

Antihistamines found in many popular allergy remedies supposedly blocked histamine from reaching the target, thereby preventing symptoms. But there was a problem with this grand theory. As any allergy victim knows, antihistamines are only partially effective. That's because they don't do such a hot job blocking the *other* unpleasant chemicals released by mast cells.

We have just recently learned that these other chemicals—*leukotrienes*—are turned loose when your nose is exposed to ragweed.[6] And it turns out that leukotrienes are much worse than histamine when it comes to causing inflammation and irritation. That's the bad news. The good news is that at least now we know what the enemy is. Presumably, we will someday have antileukotrienes much as we have antihistamines today, and together they will truly help relieve allergy symptoms.

## How to Spot an Allergy at Twenty Paces

Now that you know what an allergic reaction is, how do you recognize it? If ragweed pollen is the trigger, identifying it is hardly a problem. Runny, itchy, stuffy nose and watery eyes, sneezing, occasional headaches, and a general case of the blahs that doesn't go away until the first good frost—these enable most people to recognize seasonal hay fever.

On the other hand, some of the symptoms can look a lot like those of a cold, so it may not strike you that allergies are the offender until you note that the problem surfaces year after year, appearing and disappearing at about the same times.

Nonseasonal allergies such as animal-dander and house-dust allergies may be harder to recognize. Just as "hay fever" has nothing to do with either hay or fever, house-dust allergies are in fact a reaction to a microscopic mite whose home is the dust in your home, or the cotton bedding and furniture stuffing. Mixed together, these substances form a veritable allergy cocktail, but it's one that will leave you feeling low, not high.

Some people are allergic to food. Not all food, thank goodness, but specific foods, very often those with certain protein structures. Food allergies can be tough to identify, since the reaction can come quite a while after the food's been eaten, and it may be hard to single out the guilty party from an entire meal. Food allergy really isn't as common as many people believe. In children the accepted incidence is from 0.3 percent to about 7.5 percent.[7] Fortunately, children often outgrow many of their food allergies as the body's immune system matures.

Some babies fed on formula show signs of food allergy very early in life. A switch to a different formula, or to breast-feeding if that is possible, usually brings relief. Human milk seems to be less likely than formula to cause this kind of problem for babies, but occasionally a breast-feeding mother will notice that a food she herself eats (including cow's milk) may produce a colicky, allergic response in her infant.[8]

The symptoms of food allergy are many, and a person may experience abdominal discomfort, cramps, nausea, skin rashes, swelling, and even asthma. Indeed, some rashes of undetermined nature could be due to unrecognized food allergies. In one study, 92 percent of the children with atopic dermatitis (described as "the itch that rashes") were allergic to one or more foods. When they ate the offending food, more than half the children got worse rashes.[9]

Very occasionally food allergies can provoke anaphylactic shock. This life-threatening allergic reaction should be regarded as a medical emergency. The more common foods that cause allergic reactions are eggs, dairy products, wheat, peanuts and other nuts, soybeans, chicken, and seafood.[10]

Sometimes it's not the food itself that causes problems but rather an unsuspected chemical that has been added either as a coloring agent or a preservative. Here is a letter we received from one of our newspaper column readers describing a severe allergic reaction to sulfite:

A year ago last August we went out to dinner, and after only three bites of salad I had to go straight to the hospital.

My face and lips had swelled to five times their regular size. I was extremely red, my blood pressure and pulse were very high, and I was wheezing and having trouble breathing. I also had a rash all over my body.

Since then, I've had to have emergency treatment half a dozen times. After hearing news reports, we suspected it might be an allergic reaction to sulfite. I called the restaurants I had reacted in, and sure enough, they were washing their lettuce and some produce in this chemical.

I now carry Adrenalin with me at all times, and try to be

extremely cautious about what I eat. These reactions are frightening, and being rushed to the emergency room is very traumatic. I am 34, married, and have two children. My family has been wonderful and supportive, but these allergic episodes put a strain on all of us.

Once again we are reminded how inadequate the Food and Drug Administration's regulation of food additives can be. Sulfite preservatives serve only one purpose—to keep old food looking fresh instead of stale and soggy. The fruit and vegetables that sit and wait a long time at the salad bar may turn brown and mushy before you get there, cutting down on their customer appeal. Many restaurants dip lettuce and other salad ingredients in sulfite so that their premade salad bars will look great for long periods of time.

Who'd ever suspect that the wine served with dinner also contained sulfite, or that the lovely shrimp cocktail, the avocado dip, or tempting fruit compote was dripping with a drug that might make certain people violently ill? The menu rarely lists the chemical content of foods.

Artificial colors such as tartrazine (FD&C Yellow No. 5) which is found in a wide variety of prepared foods on supermarket shelves can also bring on allergic symptoms such as hives and wheezing. People with asthma are especially vulnerable. They have a hard enough time coping with their ailment without having to worry about the food they eat. But until the FDA decides to do something about the hidden additives in food, people with asthma and those sensitive to sulfite and tartrazine will have to be extracautious anytime they eat out or buy packaged food.

Egg allergies pose another problem. Many vaccines are grown in eggs, and the purified vaccines may still contain minute traces of egg. The medical community is still somewhat undecided whether it is safe to give certain vaccinations to children who are allergic to eggs.

The vaccines in questions are rubella (German measles),

rubeola (the other measles variety), influenza, typhus, mumps, yellow fever, and rabies.[11] The consensus is that vaccination may still be safe for most people allergic to eggs except those who have experienced especially severe reactions after eating eggs or who have markedly positive skin tests.[12] Before being vaccinated, however, be sure to inform your doctor if you have any egg or chicken allergies.

## Finding the Culprit

It should be apparent by this point that there are literally hundreds of substances to which you can become allergic. Even drugs can produce serious allergic reactions. Dermatologists have estimated that as many as 10 percent of the patients in American hospitals suffer drug-related skin reactions. Penicillin, sulfa, codeine, aspirin, antiinflammatory agents (like **Butazolidin, Clinoril, Feldene, Indocin, Motrin, Nalfon, Naprosyn, Rufen,** and **Tolectin**) or water pills (diuretics) are just some of the medications that can cause eruptions resembling acne or hives—or even a rash resembling measles.

One newspaper column reader reported to us that she was "ready to peel off my skin. The itching was unbearable and I couldn't get any sleep. At first I thought it was allergies, but I was following my usual routine, with no strange foods, soaps, or anything else." It took several weeks to figure out that the rash was a consequence of a blood-pressure drug she had been taking for years.

With so many allergens around you, how can you ever hope to isolate the particular ones responsible for your individual misfortune? Allergists have managed to convince millions of Americans that something called a skin test is a fine diagnostic tool for identifying the culprit.

Skin testing is an impressive-looking procedure, to say the least. The test is done by a placing a large number of extracts of the likely suspects on small areas of exposed skin—usually the back or forearm. The skin is then pricked with a needle, allowing the extracts to get into the skin. The test is "positive" when the skin that has been pricked with the extract turns red and itchy. If you respond like this to several substances, you may end up feeling as though you'd been attacked by a horde of very hungry and virulent mosquitoes.

Unfortunately, an extensive (and expensive) series of skin tests may only fool the patient into believing that he or she has a whole bunch of weird allergies. How is the poor allergy sufferer to know that the doctor's solemn pronouncement that feathers, Alternaria (a fungus), house dust, milk, strawberries, potatoes, dog dander, and dandelion are the sources of the problem could have little more basis in fact than a fairy tale?

You see, the skin test is a notoriously unreliable technique. If the doctor forgets to mention this, it could be a diagnostic rip-off. It's not so much the result as it is proper interpretation of the results that is essential to a sound diagnosis.

Two of the more famous experts in the field of allergy and immunology, Drs. P. S. Norman and L. M. Lichtenstein, have observed, "Positive skin tests to an allergen may be found in individuals who disclaim symptoms to that allergen."[13] In other words, lots of people who have never experienced any symptom of allergy to a particular agent may react to it in a skin test.

Dr. David S. Pearlman, in a chapter in a major pediatrics textbook, further amplifies this statement: "A positive skin test suggests only that . . . antibody is present in the skin. It may reflect a past, present, or potential clinical hypersensitivity, . . . *but it is not necessarily clinically significant.*[14]

Dr. Emmett Holt, Jr., a pediatrician who has studied allergy shots in children, says that a person who exhibits a positive skin reaction to a test

**can be classified as allergic, and often is. But does this mean that the allergen in question is responsible for allergic symptoms from which he may suffer? Originally—in the early days of allergy—this was thought to be so, and heroic**

efforts were made to avoid all allergens to which the skin
reacted. Some patients were given lists of over four hundred
things to avoid. Fortunately, it soon became apparent that
this extreme point of view could not be upheld. Positive skin
reactions were found in many persons with no history of
allergy.[15]

Other factors complicate this already muddied picture. Drs.
Robert Zeilger and Michael Schatz point out that "Appropriate
concentrations of allergens . . . must always be employed in skin
testing. All too frequently, excessive concentrations of allergens
are used for skin testing which elicit nonspecific irritating reactions which are therefore nondiscriminating."[16] In other words,
by using a sledgehammer instead of a flyswatter to squash that
pesky insect, the doctor may hit more than he reckoned on.

Even if you react positively to an appropriate dose of skin-test
allergen, are you truly allergic to that substance? Perhaps not.
The National Institute of Allergy and Infectious Diseases concluded in a government report, "Present skin tests often fail to
indicate which of a variety of agents is actually responsible for
the disease because of the complex nature of the antigen (allergen) being used. A patient sensitive to elm pollen, for example,
will often cross-react with many other pollens as well, and only
by prolonged observation is the culprit allergen identified."[17]

Skin tests are not without possible side effects. There is always
the chance, albeit slight, that you may react violently to the
substance being administered—the reaction we've referred to as
anaphylactic shock. To add insult to injury, it's possible for the
test to make you sensitive to the material you're being tested
with, even if you weren't allergic to it before!

Dr. Holt sums it up: "Allergic patients . . . frequently gave skin
reactions that could not be blamed for their symptoms. Cases
were also encountered of marked sensitivity with a negative skin
test." He also states, "It has seemed to me somewhat illogical to
regard the skin test as significant when it confirms the history,
and to disregard it when it fails to do so. By doing so one is really
relying only on the history."[18]

## Playing Allergy Detective on Your Own

What all this says is that any "allergy" proclaimed solely on the basis of a skin test may be a work of fiction. It can be awfully expensive as well, since the next step the doctor may propose could be a multiyear program of "desensitization shots."

Before doing that, try playing detective yourself. If you start to sneeze and itch when a cat enters the room, you don't have to pay a hundred bucks to find out you've got a cat allergy. If you have been sleeping comfortably on a feather pillow for years with no nasal stuffiness when you awake, it's unlikely you suffer from a feather allergy, despite what the allergist may tell you. An accurate diagnosis can only be made by careful observation and a detailed clinical history, confirmed by a skin test that is cautiously interpreted.

I don't want to throw the baby out with the bathwater, but I wouldn't mind changing the water. Skin testing can be useful when it is done by a physician who is completely aware of all of its inherent problems. A well-done and properly interpreted skin test may be a valuable diagnostic tool, but only for allergies to pollens, drugs, some foods, and some animals. The *Harvard Medical School Health Letter* says, "There is little or no support for the notion that other substances can be tested in this way."[19]

Some doctors feel that "challenge" testing is a good, cheap technique for determining specific sensitivity. It involves exposure to the suspected irritant. If there is a reaction that slowly decreases once the irritant is removed, there's a good chance the offender has been found. Many research studies use this method as an indicator that a specific allergy exists. If the response can be repeated on separate occasions, you are halfway home.

Of course, few things in life are perfect, and that holds true for challenge testing too. Even momentary exposure and withdrawal of an allergen may cause a prolonged allergic reaction. As with skin testing, the test itself may produce a profound, occasionally dangerous, reaction.

In addition, one allergen's effect may be to make you more susceptible to another. For example, during hay-fever season the family cat could make your symptoms worse, although during the rest of the year your sensitivity to cats alone is minimal. Or you might find it impossible to sleep in your down sleeping bag at the end of summer (during the pollen plague), even though there was absolutely no problem during June or July.

This "priming" effect also explains why you are still suffering hay-fever symptoms in late October, well after the pollen disappears. By increasing your sensitivity to other allergens, the ragweed makes you more susceptible to house dust kicked up by the furnace. That's why it may take a month or two before your reactivity diminishes and life returns to normal.

All this is to say that challenge testing is successful only if you can isolate individual suspects. Trying to determine whether or not a feather pillow is partly responsible for your stuffy nose would be ridiculous in the middle of hay-fever season if you are already so stopped up you can't breathe.

You might assume that there must be some better way to test for allergies than to turn yourself into a human pincushion or to expose yourself to something that will make you feel miserable. You're right, at least partially. There is a relatively new and simple blood test called the RAST (for *r*adio*a*llergo *s*orbent *t*est). Its advantages are that it is no more dangerous or uncomfortable than drawing a blood sample. It can be performed on persons in whom skin testing would be impossible, such as patients with skin disorders like eczema.

Unfortunately, the RAST may not be as accurate as a well-done skin test. False-negative results (the test says you're not allergic when you really are) occur in up to 16 percent of those tested, and false-positive findings (results that show that you're allergic when you really aren't) appear in about the same percentage.[20] Although this is one diagnostic tool that will undoubtedly improve with time, it is now only partially useful in testing for allergies and in standardizing the potency of allergen extracts.

## Doing Something About Allergy

Okay, now you know what you're allergic to, or at least what your allergist thinks you're allergic to. But what to do? It doesn't take a lot of smarts, if you're allergic to shrimp or chocolate, to figure out that you should skip the shrimp Newburg and chocolate mousse. But sometimes avoiding the allergen is tricky. In that case, the allergist may recommend a course of "desensitization" shots, commonly known as allergy or hay-fever shots. The big question is, are these shots worth the financial investment and the trauma of being poked with needles for years to come, not to mention the risk of experiencing a severe reaction to the treatment itself?

Desensitization, hyposensitization, immunotherapy, or allergy shots by any other name all involve injecting small quantities of an extract of the allergen to which the patient is presumably sensitive. By gradually increasing the concentration of the extract, the doctor hopes to build up the patient's tolerance for the evil substance. The usual procedure is to start the injections at a very low dose and to then increase the dose with each subsequent injection until an "optimum" dose is reached without discomfort.

The initial shots are usually given at weekly or semiweekly intervals. Once the upper limit is reached, the injections are continued at this maintenance dose at intervals of anywhere from every other week to every six weeks. Although beneficial results may appear within the first six months or so, the maximum benefits often are not achieved for three years or more. After four years of good results, the doctor may consider trying to discontinue treatment and see if the symptoms return. That, my friends, is a lot of shots. Along the way, your wallet will be thoroughly shot through, as well.

So much for the principle. What makes it work (when it does)? Nobody knows for sure, but lots of people have ideas. One guess is that by injecting, say, ragweed-pollen extract throughout the year, the doctor gets your body to slow down its manufacture of antibody. There is evidence that highly allergic individuals make too many "bad guy" antibodies (dubbed IgE), and that the shots slowly reestablish a more proper balance.

Another possibility is that the shots actually stimulate manufacture of a different type of antibody, termed a *blocking antibody* (IgG). This "good guy" antibody presumably interferes with the ability of the antigen-antibody duo to get to the mast cell and unlock the histamine that's hiding there. Keep the histamine locked up, and you shouldn't have to suffer with sniffles and sneezes.

Over the past several years, immunologists and allergists have gone nuts trying to measure and correlate blocking antibody levels with clinical improvement. They assumed that if allergy shots could increase the amount of "good" blocking antibody circulating in the body, they could prove that their whole approach to desensitization was a success.

The theory looks good on paper, but levels of blocking antibody clearly don't tell the whole story. In many patients, blocking antibodies are found after a course of allergy shots, but there is no firm correlation between the levels of these antibodies and symptom relief. The exceptions are patients given desensitization shots for bee-sting allergies. In this relatively small group the blocking antibody levels correlate better with actual improvement.

At the time of this writing the only certainty is that we still don't know completely how desensitization shots work. But the really important question for the allergy sufferer is not so much *how* they work, but *if* they work.

The answer is an unqualified maybe. The caveats should be stated up front—desensitization works for some people some of the time. Successful treatment depends on what allergy you're being treated for, the potency of the extracts being used, a proper dose being given, and how the individual responds to therapy. Even when desensitization works, there is no cure, just a decrease in symptoms.

Let's start with the success stories. Desensitization shots for children and adults who are allergic to bee stings can be remarkably effective. This is particularly good news since bee-sting eactions can be quite severe, even deadly. (See pages 316–319 or a more complete discussion.)

The older method of desensitization required grinding up the entire body of the offending insect and injecting an extract. This was the shotgun approach. Whole-bee extracts only conferred about a 40-percent protection rate. But if a pure venom extract is used, the success rate zooms towards the 90 percent to 95 percent range.

Many physicians who'd faithfully administered the whole-body extracts for years stuck to their guns for a while, but mounting evidence has produced clear proof that venom extracts are the superior protectors. There are now licensed preparations for five venoms: honey bee, yellow jacket, yellow hornet, white-faced hornet, and wasp.

But if the results of venom therapy are encouraging, the results of pollen desensitization are less so.

Desensitization by means of pollen-extract injection has been around for more than seventy years. However, the evidence supporting the success of immunotherapy is still controversial. In the last several years, studies have begun to show that allergy shots with ragweed, grass, and some tree pollens can be moderately successful. But the debate is far from over, and desensitization for other allergies remains pretty much unproven. Dr. Philip Norman at Johns Hopkins University, in a paper on the future of desensitization therapy, had this to say:

**Placebo-controlled studies with other pollens, molds, and animal danders are completely lacking. Indeed, the variety of allergenic substances in the environment that may at times cause symptoms is so great as to make it improbable that studies which require so much labor will be performed even for the more important allergens.[21]**

Even though desensitization shots have only been proven effective for a few kinds of allergy, their use is far more widespread. A *JAMA (Journal of the American Medical Association)* article states benignly, "In practice, the method is used with

other inhalent antigens *besides those* in which clinical efficac
has been satisfactorily demonstrated, although further studie
with these antigens are needed [my emphasis]."[22] In other words
if your allergist wants to desensitize you with some esoteri
mold, food, pollen, or animal-dander extract, he may be usin
an unproven and potentially dubious treatment.

Why would a doctor treat someone with an unproven remedy
The answer is probably not greed or insensitivity, but an over
zealous reliance on historical precedence and personal observa
tion.

Dr. Emmett Holt, Jr., has offered this observation on the "i
it's lasted this long it must be good" theory:

**The value of specific diagnosis and therapy is not to be
determined by the fact that these procedures have survived
for half a century. Bloodletting in medicine lasted for a
much longer time. Nor should one be convinced by the fact
that considerable numbers of patients are certain of benefit
received. When blind studies of any doubtful therapy are
carried out, there are always substantial numbers of patients who have received placebos who are altogether certain of the benefit they have received. Psychological factors
have an extraordinary way of coloring results.**[23]

When Dr. Holt refers to "blind studies," he does not mea
that the researchers go around wearing blindfolds. He mean
that the study is designed so that personal prejudice canno
influence the results of the investigation.

Allergists who may subconsciously find it difficult to forget th
economic factors involved in injection therapy must go out o
their way to plan experiments that remove psychological influ
ence. One such approach is to organize a study in which neithe
the doctor nor the subject will know what is being administered
One set of patients receives true extract; the other group receive
a placebo in the form of saltwater injections or a "nonactive"
mimic of the true extract. In this manner, the study will b

scientifically valid and is called "double-blind" because no one knows who got what until the probe ends.

It is shocking how few good double-blind tests have been carried out over the years. A recent analysis by Dr. R. C. Godfrey provides the following gloomy overview:

> **Results of the better trials lead to a mixed picture, ranging from improvement in 60–80% of patients with pollen-induced hay fever to negative results in some trials of desensitization against house dust mite and other allergens. On one point nearly all trials are agreed, namely the strong placebo effect. Around 40% improve with saline (salt water) injections only. This argues, not unexpectedly, that there is a strong psychological element in "the needle."[24]**

Small though the advantage seems to be, some will choose to pursue allergy shots. Those who do should be aware, however, that they may be about to become part of a medical experiment.

## Allergy Treatment: A Shot in the Dark?

Even if your doctor decides to try desensitization with one of the hay-fever pollens that do work for some people, there are lots of pitfalls. One of them is that when the doctor gives you an allergy shot, he or she may not really know how much of a dose you're getting!

Sound incredible? You perhaps think of medicine as a science of great precision, with sterile fluids measured out in the most precise of quantities. Indeed, that's often true. But not when it comes to allergy shots.

Investigators have described many pollen preparations as nothing more than extremely crude extracts.[25] Commercial and experimental pollen extracts vary incredibly in their potency. Drs. Bloch and Salvaggio report, "Analyses of short ragweed pollen, grass pollen, and Alternaria [a type of mold spore] extracts disclosed a thousandfold difference in potency among materials claimed by manufacturers to have approximately the same potency."[26] That means that your doctor may not have the faintest idea of how much active ingredient you're getting.

The way around this dilemma is to experiment on each patient until the "right" dose is found. The way this works is that the doctor starts with a dose so small he's certain (well, pretty certain) it won't cause an adverse reaction. The amount is then cranked up progressively until it does you some good, stopping somewhere below the amount that will definitely do harm.

This "poke-and-pray" method of dosing people is hardly ideal, but it seems the best that allergists can do at the moment. You probably can't get away without some adverse reactions if you expect the treatment to work.

This dosing method dates back to 1911, when allergy shots first appeared on the scene. It is not, however, the only method in current use. Another one is the Rinkel Method, named for the doctor who invented it, and it is based on using very carefully calibrated low doses of pollen extract. The only wrinkle with Rinkel is that it doesn't appear to work very well.

Dr. Thomas Van Metre and a host of colleagues at Johns Hopkins did a definitive double-blind study, stating,

> **The Rinkel method of immunotherapy is widely used in the United States at the present time. Proponents claim that it provides very satisfactory relief from symptoms of hay fever. However, it has not been proved effective for this purpose by suitable controlled double-blind studies.**[27]

They did such a study and concluded, "Rinkel-method immunotherapy with ragweed pollen extract was no more effective than placebo given in imitation of the Rinkel method."[28] Not surprisingly, there were also no side effects noted with this low-dose method. Now that, my friend, is *dynamite!* If you do decide to go in for hay-fever shots, you might want to make sure your allergist is *not* following the Rinkel method.

All right, already. By now you are either bored to tears with all this nonsense, or you have a vested interest in some sort of conclusion. In a nutshell, what all this means is that the value of allergy shots is still controversial. While they may help some folks with hay fever, there is real doubt about other forms of therapy, and no good evidence that they will prevent or improve asthma. Summing up, Dr. Godfrey offers the following bombshell:

> It is hard to find any clear reason why the present practice of desensitization should continue. The treatment is expensive, relatively ineffective, and not without serious side effects. Its indication for diseases which are on the whole trivial are hard to see. It would be a different matter if desensitization were the only treatment available for a life-threatening condition. In the future we may see an improvement in the theory and practice of immunotherapy, but at the moment such an improvement seems distant. I see no reason to continue desensitization in its present form.[29]

As you can see, allergy injections are quite an opportunity for you, the patient. They're an opportunity to pay for an expensive course of treatment during which you may get an imprecisely measured quantity of a material that may provide little or no beneficial effect. If you go for that, I've got a bridge to sell you. And it will cost less than a course of allergy shots.

## Antiallergy Alternatives

If allergy shots don't appear tremendously appealing, does that mean learning to suffer and enjoy it? NO. Definitely not. There are many other ways to tame your raging allergy beast.

The first is the most obvious, and thus probably the most overlooked. It's cheap, simple, highly effective, has absolutely no side effects, and can be done without even taking a trip to the doctor's office. This magic solution consists of avoiding or getting rid of whatever it is that irritates you (we're talking about allergies, now, not coworkers and neighbors—that's a separate problem).

This approach may be a little painful, though, since it may involve getting rid of a favorite feather pillow or a comfortable armchair. It might be a faithful pet or a special brand of cosmetics that has to go. If dust is the culprit, most cotton or kapok stuffing material should be eliminated and frequent vacuuming instituted. Cotton mattresses may have to be encased in plastic or replaced with a water bed.

For some, the synthetic substances that have become so much a part of our modern way of life may have to go. Formaldehyde in carpets, permanent-press clothing, or house insulation may be the enemy. For others the problem may be plastic, foam rubber, polyester, or vinyl.

Locating and eliminating the allergens in your life can be a real nuisance. Lots of folks would rather suffer than kick their favorite cat out of the house. And dusting is a real chore. Nevertheless, if you can keep away from the things that cause your allergies, you will no longer have to suffer.

It's a lot more difficult to avoid the seasonal pollens. You can't stop breathing for the summer, and it's rarely practical to move to the Antarctic for the duration. There are, however, a few helpful hints that can make the hay-fever season more bearable. If you live in the country, mow down the ragweed growing around your property before it has a chance to pollinate. Encourage children to play indoors, or as far away as possible from ripe ragweed fields.

Air-conditioning can be a real help. While it doesn't actually filter the air, it allows you to shut your windows during the summer months. Even window-box type units can substantially decrease the amount of pollen drifting into your house.[30] Dehumidifiers and electronic air filters may also help pull dust and pollen out of the air. Pollen masks, available at most pharmacies, make you look as if you're about to perform surgery, but they do cut down the pollen you breathe in.

There is one other simple, nonhazardous technique for relieving the stuffy nose associated with allergy. Have you ever noticed that when you sit or lie down, your allergy symptoms tend to get worse? And that when you get up or are more active, your nose seems to open up a little bit?

There is a very good scientific explanation for this phenomenon. The extra stuffiness associated with resting is related to a general decrease in nervous-system activity. When the nervous system is more at rest, blood vessels tend to relax. Doctors call this *diminished vascular tone,* and it's a factor in causing nasal congestion.

According to a renowned allergy specialist, Dr. Paul M. Seebohm, "Another way to reverse the congestive effect of rhinitis [stuffy nose] is with exercise. [We've] demonstrated complete reversal of obstructive congestion to be associated with a vigorous 3-minute step-type exercise."[31] This simple exercise effort produced better results than a potent medication, and you can bet it cost a heck of a lot less. Next time you're fed up with swollen sinuses, why not try a little exercise? The price is right.

There could come the day when, having given away the cat, the mattress, and your best down jacket, you thoroughly dust the house, turn on the air-conditioner, place a dust mask over your nose, jog in place but still suffer the allergy miseries. Your best efforts to go it alone have failed. You can't afford long, luxurious ocean cruises away from all the irritants, and you simply refuse to stop breathing. It's time to explore some other alternatives for tackling the allergy problem.

## The Pharmacological Solution

The first stop will be antihistamines. There's strong agreement among medical people (a rarity in itself) that antihistamines are the drugs of choice, particularly in preference to those controversial allergy shots. The highly respected *Medical Letter* says: "Desensitization for pollen allergy appears to be justified only in patients in whom oral antihistamines or topical intranasal corticosteroids have failed."[32]

The *Harvard Medical School Health Letter* says it another way: "The cost, inconvenience, and (modest) risk of immunotherapy make it appropriate only for patients who are disabled by their symptoms but cannot take antihistamines without drowsiness or other adverse effects."[33]

The way antihistamines work is quite fascinating. Earlier in this chapter I discussed how the irritating antigen and antibody produced by the body's immune system cling together and act as a key to fit in the lock on a mast cell and release histamine, which then goes to target cells and causes those all-too-familiar allergy symptoms. As its name implies, an *anti*histamine works against histamine, blocking it from reaching the target cell and thus blocking all those unpleasant consequences.

But which antihistamine should you use? There are at least eighteen different antihistamines on the market, marketed under at least four hundred different brand names.[34] Clearly, your doctor or allergist can't be an expert on each one. Additionally, no two people react quite the same way to a given product. Antihistamines are notorious for their tremendous variability in both effectiveness and side effects. No one, including your doctor, can predict with assurance a person's response to a particular brand.

As mentioned early in this chapter, the most common side effect encountered with antihistamine therapy is drowsiness, and the elderly may be particularly affected. Fortunately, some people are more resistant to this lethargic, unpleasant, space-cadet feeling. But for those of us who are susceptible, it becomes necessary to experiment until we discover the product that produces the least amount of drowsiness.

In many cases, the drowsy feeling will become much less noticeable after you take the medication for a week or so. For best results, antihistamines should be taken all day, not just when you feel stuffy. Even though people vary in the degree of drowsiness they feel with the different antihistamines, certain of these compounds are notorious for their sleepmaking ability—so much so that they're now used as ingredients in over-the-counter sleeping pills such as **Compoz, Sominex Formula 2, Nytol with DPH, Sleep-Eze 3** (diphenhydramine), **Somnicaps** (pyrilamine), and **Unisom** (doxylamine).

One antihistamine that is considered to have a relatively low drowsiness potential is chlorpheniramine, found in such popular products as **Allerest, Chlor-Trimeton, Contac, Coricidin, Dristan, Sinarest,** and **Sine-Off.** Brompheniramine is also supposed to be reasonably well tolerated. It is contained in **Dimetane** and **Dimetapp.** Triprolidine (**Actidil** and **Actifed**) is another antihistamine that may be a little less likely to slow you down. Clemastine (**Tavist**) and cyproheptadine (**Periactin**) are intermediate on the drowsiness scale, while diphenhydramine (**Benadryl** and **Benylin**) and promethazine (**Phenergan**) can knock you for a loop.

Another important consideration is cost. Almost inevitably these preparations cost less when prescribed by their generic rather than brand names. And they're cheaper still when bought as nonprescription medications. In the last several years a surprising number of prescription-only antihistamines have been approved for over-the-counter sale. You no longer need your doctor's approval to purchase **Actifed, Benadryl, Benylin, Chlor-Trimeton, Dimetane,** or **Drixoral.**

No matter which antihistamine you select, remember that one person's antihistamine is another person's sleeping potion. Selecting an antihistamine is a trial-and-error proposition for which I offer the following general suggestions:

- **Start with an OTC product containing a single antihistamine ingredient. Combination products often provide a witches' brew of decongestants, pain relievers, caffeine, and lots of other garbage you don't need. Those suffering from high blood pressure must avoid decongestants, which can aggravate hypertension.**
- **Select an antihistamine with the lowest tendency to cause unpleasant side effects such as sedation.**
- **Take the minimum possible dose on a constant, around-the-clock basis rather than waiting until symptoms set in and then gobbling down a huge dose.**
- **Be alert to the onset of side effects, and either reduce the dose or switch to another drug.**
- **Take very seriously the warning you will find on ALL antihistamines about not driving, operating dangerous machinery, or doing anything else that requires maximum mental alertness.**

One final word of encouragement about antihistamines. New-generation compounds appear to offer allergy relief without producing drowsiness or impairing driving ability. One medication called terfenadine has recently been approved by the FDA for sale under the brand name **Seldane.** Preliminary tests have researchers excited. One investigator, Dr. Charles E. Buckley III, an allergy specialist at Duke University, reports that it "causes an incidence of sedation and dryness no greater than that observed with placebo."[35]

Besides a greatly reduced tendency to produce the sleepies, terfenadine also seems less likely to interact unpleasantly with drugs such as alcohol and **Valium.** Other antihistamines often increase their sedative effect. As an added bonus, **Seldane** is effective when taken only twice daily, while most other antihistamines need to be taken three or four times a day to be effective.

Another allergy fighter in the pipeline is called astemizole. It's of much more recent vintage, just from the early 1980s. Though it hasn't been widely tested yet, the first results look quite positive. Somewhere between two thirds and three fourths of those taking the drug experienced relief from drippy noses and sneezing, while complaints about drowsiness were reported to be "practically nil." With a half-life of over one hundred hours, astemizole hangs around the system longer than any other antihistamine, so it's possible to get effective relief by taking it no more than once a day.

So for allergy sufferers there's definitely help and hope within sight. No longer will sneezers and weepers be faced with a choice of suffering along with their symptoms or being too doped up and drowsy to function at work or safely drive a car.

## The Future Is Now

Hold on to your hat. That's not all the good news. You won't have to wait for the FDA to approve these exciting antihistamines to get some relief. A quiet revolution in allergy treatment is making life a lot more bearable during the sneezin' season. One of the latest advances in allergy treatment is steroid nasal sprays, and they are available right now.

Steroids (cortisonelike drugs) are extremely strong substances that have a wide range of effects on body systems. They're particularly good at reducing swelling, and for many years it's been no secret to doctors that steroids were effective against allergy symptoms.

The problem is that the steroids are powerful drugs with an imposing list of very severe side effects, including susceptibility to infection, cataracts, stomach ulcers, weakness, glaucoma, water retention, weight gain, and psychological disturbances. That hardly makes them candidates for treating a runny nose that's annoying but far from life-threatening. You don't shoot at ants with an elephant gun, even if they are pesky little critters.

Enter the nasal spray version. Researchers discovered that applying steroids directly to the source of the problem allowed the drugs to do their good work without spreading extensively through the body and wreaking the havoc caused by more traditional oral steroids.

**Vancenase** and **Beconase** (beclomethasone diproprionate), and **Nasalide** (flunisolide) are all available as nasal sprays, and the evidence is strong that they offer symptomatic relief from seasonal allergy symptoms. **Decadron Turbinaire** (dexamethasone) is another, somewhat older, steroid nasal spray. However, it is not as active topically and may have more side effects associated with its use. For this reason, I'd stick to the newer models.

Up to 85 percent of hay-fever sufferers get excellent relief using these prescription nose sprays.[36] Most people tolerate the medicine well, though some of them experience an occasional nosebleed, sneezing, and temporary itching and burning. The sprays do not seem to be absorbed readily into general circulation, so the body doesn't alter its other functions in response to this outside source of steroid. The potential for trouble is there, however, if you overuse the sprays. There have been several reports of cases in which a hole has developed in the septum, the cartilage between the two nostrils. Check with your doctor periodically to make sure you aren't getting into trouble.

If none of the above works, don't despair—at least not yet—because there remains at least one more rabbit in the hat. **Nasalcrom** (cromolyn sodium) nasal spray is yet another alternative, and a good one. Whereas antihistamines block the effects of histamine after it has been released into the circulation, cromolyn actually keeps the mast cells from releasing the histamine in the first place.

Although there may be some temporary stinging, sneezing, burning, or irritation, many good studies show that **Nasalcrom** works to lessen "mouth breathing, stuffy nose, runny nose, postnasal drip and sneezing."[37] The evidence is usually based on diaries kept by the patients, recording how many times they blew their nose or sneezed, how much antihistamine they had to take to get relief, and so forth.

Dr. R. K. Chandra and colleagues took it one simple step further. They did what so many physicians forget to do; they asked their patients how they liked it. Some 78 percent of their patients rated cromolyn either "excellent" or "good," and only 4 percent thought that it had no effect. When patients were given a placebo without knowing it, only 6 percent of the people rated the placebo anything more than "fair" and 78 percent could detect no measurable improvement.[38] Enough said.

## Anaphylaxis: A Matter of Life and Death

So far we've just been talking about "simple" allergies. Because the problem has become so common these days, people are complacent and casual about their allergic disorders. There's one kind of allergic reaction about which one can afford to be neither casual nor complacent, because it can easily be a matter of life and death. Believe it or not, this threat to life comes from something as mundane as an insect sting.

It may be hard to grasp the threat posed by anaphylactic shock after thinking in terms of hay fever or poison ivy, but believe me, this is a whole different ball game.

*Anaphylaxis* is a big word which denotes the total collapse of the system in allergic reaction to such diverse substances as penicillin, the cephalosporin antibiotics, insulin, local anesthetics, chymopapain, and even strenuous exercise, as well as insect stings. It may begin with a marked local reaction (a bee sting that really swells up and lasts) or a generalized itching. This may be followed by agitation, red and itching eyes with a runny nose, nausea and vomiting, diarrhea, coughing and wheezing, a rapid pulse, and heart palpitations.

Some or all of these symptoms can appear within a few minutes to a half hour after the offending substance gets into the body. Occasionally, the delay will be longer. The symptoms can rapidly go from bad to worse—respiratory-tract spasms can make breathing very difficult, and accumulation of fluids in the throat may also seriously interfere with respiration. Shock sets in, followed by loss of consciousness. At this point death becomes a possibility, due to the severe strain placed on the heart.

Obviously, this kind of serious reaction demands quick recognition and medical response. Even if you haven't had a serious response to an insect sting or a drug before, it is not impossible for a new one to develop.

There are thirty kinds of insects that produce allergic symptoms, with the worst and most frequent offenders being yellow jackets, wasps, hornets, bees, and fire ants. In the United States, about one hundred deaths each year are attributed to stings from these insects, with more people dying every year from insect stings than snakebites.[39]

Any insect sting that produces excessive and prolonged swelling or a sense of uneasiness should be a warning flag. You could be developing an allergy that will later be life-threatening. Very often that first sting gets your immune system to producing antibodies that lie in wait until a second or third episode, each of greater severity, until anaphylactic shock results.

If a sting brings on a feeling of impending doom, palpitations, generalized itching, tingling sensations, shortness of breath, or wheezing, move quickly. You could have less than thirty minutes to live once the toxic venoms are injected into your skin.

Fast action will save your life. If you are close to a doctor's office or a hospital, go there immediately as an emergency patient. Unfortunately, help isn't always at hand, which means you must be prepared to take care of yourself. In the summertime you *must* carry a kit containing an injection of epinephrine (adrenalin). Any doctor or nurse can show you how to properly deliver what could literally be a lifesaving injection.

Two excellent emergency kits are available, but both require a prescription. The **Ana-kit** contains a syringe preloaded with two doses of epinephrine, two sterilizing swabs, chewable antihistamine tablets, and a tourniquet, all in a box smaller than a pack of cigarettes. The directions are very clear, but make sure you go over them with your doctor and know them thoroughly BEFORE an emergency arises. Once trouble starts, every minute counts, and that's no time to be reading directions.

If you're squeamish about injecting yourself with even a small needle, consider the **EpiPen Auto-Injector.** It's about the size and shape of a medium-sized cigar and remarkably easy to use. All you do is remove the cap and press the cartridge against your thigh or shoulder. The mechanism contains a spring-loaded syringe, with which you inject a premeasured dose of epinephrine almost painlessly. Having two or three of the kits allows you to distribute them in several locations to make certain that one is always handy when trouble strikes.

Do *not* store such kits in the car's glove compartment, since heat destroys epinephrine. In fact, epinephrine, like all drugs, will eventually decompose and have to be replaced. Look at the expiration date on the package and make sure you keep yours up-to-date.

Remember, this self-treatment is only a stopgap emergency measure. Have someone rush you to a doctor or call an ambulance. Children who suffer from insect-sting allergy can probably use the **EpiPen** more easily than the **Ana-kit** and should be trained thoroughly in its use. Physicians can order a special training device from the company.

**EpiPen** is available in most pharmacies, and it also comes in a pediatric dose. If you need more information, you can write to Center Labs, Channel Drive, Port Washington, NY 11050. But remember, all epinephrine kits require a doctor's supervision and prescription.

People who are allergic to insect stings often receive desensitization shots in the hopes of preventing a fatal accident. This is probably a good precaution, but it does involve some risk. For one thing, there is always the possibility that a skin test or the allergy shot itself will provoke anaphylactic shock. For another thing, desensitization shots are reported to provide up to 95 percent protection, but such shots shouldn't be allowed to cover you in a false cloak of security. Although less likely today because of much more effective venom extracts, there are reports of people who had desensitization shots from whole-body extract and later died of insect stings.

One patient died from a sting, even though he had received a desensitization shot five days before being stung.[40] Tragically, this person died in the doctor's waiting room. This case serves as a reminder that anaphylactic shock is a major emergency and should be treated as such.

Another patient died within fifteen minutes of being stung. He, too, had received his last desensitization shot within the week. These cases are presented not to scare anyone unnecessarily but merely to illustrate the point that immunotherapy is not foolproof and must be backed up with immediate emergency procedures when the risk of anaphylaxis presents itself.

## Allergy: Helping Yourself

Allergy, then, is still very much a medical mystery, although the veil is slowly being lifted to reveal the mechanisms by which everything from fur to feathers to pollen sets the alarm bells ringing for the body's immune system.

Until a lot more becomes known, however, allergy treatment is still a pretty hit-and-miss proposition to which you, the patient, can often contribute as much as the physician.

Think before running off to the doctor and assuming the cure must come from the medical establishment. For all the great advances of recent years, we're still left with more questions than answers. We know, in broad outlines, what sets the allergic reaction in motion, but the details of its actions remain to be settled. What we don't know can (and does) fill a textbook, and a futile search for relief can only aid in filling the doctors' pockets.

A reasonable approach starts with knowing what can and can't be expected from each test or medication. Skin testing is a crude, incomplete, and often inaccurate means of determining what's irritating you. It will very often provide a false positive answer, typing you as "allergic" to things that aren't really the problem any longer.

Desensitization, long the mainstay of allergy "treatment," works to some extent for a limited number of people and probably only for a few types of allergy, like ragweed-induced hay fever. It's imprecise, time consuming, expensive, and extremely uncertain in its result.

There's a lot you can do for yourself before spending money on dubious cures. First, try and remove what's bothering you from the vicinity. Toss out the pillows or the cat. Allergic patients are often sensitive to animals, cotton or kapok stuffing material, and feathers.

Then consider a trial of an over-the-counter antihistamine. If one type doesn't work or makes you drowsy, try another.

If none of those efforts does the trick, approach the doctor about trying the new non-sedating antihistamine called **Seldane** or a steroid nasal spray. The spray could provide safe and effective relief. Cromolyn (**Nasalcrom**) is another good alternative.

Allergy is one of those things for which medical science just simply doesn't have a magic bullet. Not only is there no cure, but the pursuit of relief can be a long, arduous, and sometimes futile effort. It's an effort in which the patient can and should play a major role. When it comes to treating allergy, ask a lot of questions before taking the doctor's word or treatment, and try the easy, inexpensive solutions first.

And if you need one last consolation prize to help you grin and bear it, try this one on for size. There are some very preliminary, but nevertheless tantalizing reports in the medical literature that allergy may be associated with less risk of cancer.[41] Perhaps the misery of suffering the symptoms of an overactive immune system will be rewarded by diminished risk of malignant disease.

# References

1. Rust, Tommy. "Respiratory Allergies: How to Avoid 'Em, How to Live with 'Em." Press Release from the American Association for Respiratory Therapy, Oct. 1982.

2. Mathews, Kenneth, P. "Respiratory Atopic Disease." *JAMA* 248:2587–2610, 1982.

3. Hochman, Gloria. "A Frightening Diagnosis: Allergic to 20th Century." *Philadelphia Inquirer Magazine,* printed in the *Raleigh News and Observer,* Mar. 25, 1984, p. 3C.

4. Mathews, op. cit.

5. Contac Product Information.

6. Creticos, Peter, S., et al. "Peptide Leukotriene Release after Antigen Challenge in Patients Sensitive to Ragweed." *N. Engl. J. Med.* 310:1626–1630, 1984.

7. Buckley, Rebecca H., and Metcalfe, Dean. "Food Allergy." *JAMA* 248:2627–2631, 1982.

8. Anon. "Colicky Babies and Breast Milk." *Tufts University Diet & Nutrition Letter.* 1(9):1, 1983.

9. Sampson, Hugh A. "Role of Immediate Food Hypersensitivity in the Pathogenesis of Atopic Dermatitis." *J. Allergy Clin. Immunol.* 71:-473–480, 1983.

10. Buckley, op. cit.

11. Miller, J. Randall; Orgel, Alice H.; and Meltzer, Eli O. "The Safety of Egg-containing Vaccines for Egg-allergic Patients." *J. Allergy Clin. Immunol.* 71:568–573, 1983.

12. Ibid.

13. Norman, P. S.; Lichtenstein, L. M.; and Ishizaka, K. "Diagnostic Tests in Ragweed Hay Fever." *J. Allergy Clin. Immunol.* 52:210–224, 1973.

14. Kempe, C., et al. *Current Pediatric Diagnosis and Treatment.* 7th ed. Los Altos: Lange Medical Publications, 1982, p. 917.

15. Holt, Emmett Jr., "A Nonallergist Looks at Allergy." *N. Engl. J. Med.* 276:1449–1454, 1967.

16. Zeigler, Robert S., and Schatz, Michael. "Immunotherapy of Atopic Disorders." *Med. Clin. North Am.* 65(5):987–1012, 1981.

17. U.S. Department of Health, Education, and Welfare. *Immunology—Its Role in Disease and Health.* Bethesda, Md.: National Institute of Allergy and Infectious Disease, 1976. (DHEW publication No. (NIH) 77–940), p. 87.

18. Holt, op. cit.

19. *The Harvard Medical Health Letter.,* "Allergies, pt. 1" VI(8):1–2, Jun. 1981.

20. Bloch, Kurt J. and Salvaggio, John E. "Use and Interpretation of Diagnostic Immunologic Laboratory Tests." *JAMA* 248:2734–2758, 1982.

21. Norman, Philip S. "An Overview of Immunotherapy: Implications for the Future." *J. Allergy Clin. Immunol.* 65(2):87–96, 1980.

22. Patterson, Roy, and Norman, Phillip. "Immunotherapy-Immunomodulation." *JAMA* 248:2759–2772, 1982.

23. Holt, op. cit.

24. Godfrey, R. C. "Desensitization to Allergy: Why Do It?" *Med. Trib.* 25(18):35, Jun. 27, 1984.

25. Ibid.

26. Bloch, op. cit.

27. Van Metre, Thomas E., et al. "A Controlled Study of the Effectiveness of the Rinkel Method of Immunotherapy for Ragweed Pollen Hay Fever." *J. Allergy Clin. Immunol.* 65:288–297, 1980.

28. Ibid.

29. Godfrey, op. cit.

30. Solomon, William R.; Burge, Harriet A.; and Boise, Jean R. "Exclusion of Particulate Allergens by Window Air-conditioners." *J. Allergy Clin. Immunol.* 65:305–308, 1980.

31. Seebohm, Paul M. "Allergy." *Family Practice,* ed. H. F. Conn. Saunders, 1973, pp. 898, 902.

32. *Medical Letter* 15:55–56, 1973.

33. *The Harvard Medical School Health Letter* "Allergies—Part II." VI(9):1–2, 5, 1981.

34. Kastrup, Erwin K., and Boyd, James R., eds. *Facts and Comparisons.* St. Louis: J. B. Lippincott, Oct. 1983, p. 188.

35. "Antihistamines Relieve Symptoms of Hay Fever without Drowsiness." *Medical World News* 25(5):111–112, 1984.

36. Webb, Robert D. "Steroids in Allergic Disease." *Med. Clin. North Am.* 65:1073–1081, 1981.

37. "Cromolyn Sodium Nasal Spray for Hay Fever." *Medical Letter* 25:89–90, 1983.

38. Chandra, R. K.; Heresi, Gloria; and Woodford, G. "Double-Blind Controlled Crossover Trial of 4% Intranasal Sodium Cromoglycate Solution in Patients with Seasonal Allergic Rhinitis." *Ann. Allergy* 49:131–134, 1982.

39. Patterson, Roy, and Valentine, Martin. "Anaphylaxis and Related Allergic Emergencies including Reactions Due to Insect Stings." *JAMA* 248:2632–2636, 1982.

40. Torsney, Philip J. "Treatment Failure: Insect Desensitization." *J. Allergy Clin. Immunol.* 52:303–306, 1973.

41. Motoki, Tatsuya, et al. "Low Serum Histamine in Malignant Disease." *N. Engl. J. Med.* 310:391–392, 1984.

# 8

## Asthma: From a Medical Quagmire to a Quiet Revolution

*The ins and out of asthma • Old-fashioned remedies hold hidden hazards • New inhalers offer better relief: Albuterol, metaproterenol, and terbutaline • Theophylline: The big step • Coffee: First aid for asthma • Watch out for drug interactions • Intal: An attractive alternative • Cortisone: The last resort • Steroid sprays: Safer, yes, but not risk-free • Hope for the future.*

Asthma is awful. There is nothing more frightening than not being able to catch your breath. I should know. When I was a child, I would wake up in the middle of the night wheezing and gasping for air. Those were terrifying times for my mother as well as for me.

Luckily, I grew out of my asthma. Lots of people aren't so fortunate. Nine million Americans (half of them children) suffer periodic bouts of breathlessness. The attacks may be nothing worse than a temporary wheeze after exercise, or they may range all the way up to a life-and-death fight for air that sends the victim rushing to an emergency room for oxygen and a shot of adrenalin.

Although doctors are still a long way from curing asthma, there have been some extraordinary breakthroughs in the understanding of this devastating disease. More importantly, since I wrote the first edition of *The People's Pharmacy,* the treatment of asthma has changed enormously. A quiet therapeutic revolution has occurred, and today most people can control their symptoms without trading that relief for severe adverse drug reactions. And researchers are on the brink of some even more important discoveries that eventually may lead to the virtual elimination of asthma.

Now before you get the idea that old Joe has become a starry-eyed dreamer, let me hasten to add that the therapeutic trail still has plenty of thorns, and if people aren't careful they can get pricked pretty badly. There are a surprising number of asthma products on pharmacy shelves, many of which appear to be the remnants of a bygone era. Some of the potions still being given to asthmatics are either useless or dangerous, and there's nothing to protect these sufferers except their own wits.

But despite the pharmaceutical pitfalls that still persist, this chapter is really more about success than failure. So sit back, take a deep breath, and relax. You are going to learn how a series of small drug developments has led to dramatic advances in asthma treatment.

## The Ins and Outs of Asthma

Asthma is a molecular mistake on the part of the body's defense system. For reasons we don't yet understand, an asthmatic's lungs react to an irritant—smoke, dust, aerosol sprays, perfume, temperature changes, even emotional stress—by releasing chemical substances that cause the small, smooth muscles surrounding the lung's air passages to constrict. The result can only be described as terrifying.

The partial closing off of these small paths or tunnels creates difficulty in breathing, and the characteristic asthmatic wheeze becomes audible. Think about your vacuum cleaner for a minute.

Have you ever caught something in the nozzle and listened to the motor start to strain and whine as it tried to suck in air past the obstruction? It may not be a perfect analogy, but at least you get some idea of what happens in the lungs when airflow is restricted. To the asthmatic having such an attack, the sensation is one of slow suffocation.

We used to think that asthma had its roots stuck in the allergy quagmire, and that here was a place where desensitization shots (see Chapter 7) might well be justified. We now know, however, that immunotherapy is not very helpful.[1] It is also clear that antihistamines aren't much good either. That's probably because histamine isn't the primary culprit causing the chest tightness.

Instead, researchers have discovered that chemicals produced in the body called *prostaglandins* and *leukotrienes* (the same nasties that can cause a stuffy nose from ragweed pollen) can produce bronchoconstriction.[2, 3] The release of these chemicals may be triggered by all sorts of things that have nothing to do with allergy, including infection (colds, for example), emotional stress, or exercise.

The ultimate solution to the asthma nightmare will probably come when compounds are created that can interrupt the chemical cascade that leads to the production of pesky prostaglandins and troublesome leukotrienes. But asthmatics need not wait until the last piece to the puzzle is found. There are drugs available today that go a long way toward relaxing runaway lung muscles and relieving symptoms.

## The First Rung on the Ladder

Most doctors recognize the value of a "stepped care" approach, in which they first try the smallest amounts of the least potent drugs, escalating to more powerful agents only when the lighter artillery has proved ineffective. When I wrote the first edition of *The People's Pharmacy,* ephedrine was considered a good first choice for most asthma victims. After all, few drugs have such an impressive track record. It has been used for at least five thousand years. Records show that physicians of ancient Greece and China made use of the medicinal properties of the ephedra plant.

Ephedrine acts to relax the muscle spasms which constrict the airways and restrict airflow. For folks with mild breathing problems, this medication works reasonably well. And since ephedrine is available generically as well as over-the-counter, it can be quite inexpensive.

But despite its long history and relative safety, there are problems with ephedrine, and today there is little reason to rely on this old-fashioned remedy. For one thing, it is not very helpful for patients who have a chronic daily breathing problem. When it is taken continuously (more than three times a day, every day) its effectiveness is reduced considerably.

Another problem with ephedrine is a lack of specificity. What I mean is that it affects more than just the lungs. This drug can stimulate the heart, leading to increased force of contractions and raised blood pressure. Obviously, anyone with hypertension, heart disease, or other health problems, such as thyroid disease or prostate trouble, should steer clear. In addition, ephedrine may activate the nervous system and cause nervousness, irritability, trembling, and trouble sleeping.

Because of this tendency to make people nervous and jumpy, drug companies often create combination products containing sedatives such as phenobarbital. Including a barbiturate along with ephedrine theoretically is supposed to offset the stimulant action—a little like driving with your foot on the gas pedal and the brake simultaneously. A few brand names that include phenobartibal include **Amodrine, Bronkotabs, Primatene P, Quadrinal, Tedral, Thalfed,** and **Verquad.**

Some combinations lack only the eye of a toad or the ear of a bat to resemble alchemists' concoctions. The combo rarely solves the problem it sets out to handle, but what it may manage to do is make the primary problem worse. Asthmatics are often drug-sensitive. They are the last people who should be dosed with extra, unnecessary chemicals, yet there they are receiving prescriptions for sedative-containing drugs which actually depress the functioning of their already overextended respiratory systems.

Although there are many inappropriate combination products on the market, one that makes me especially nervous is **Dainite-KI** made by Wallace Laboratories. It contains no fewer than six active ingredients. Along with ephedrine there's aminophylline (a powerful drug we'll discuss in a moment), phenobarbital (the sedative), benzocaine (a local anesthetic), potassium iodide (an expectorant), calcium carbonate (an antacid), and tartrazine (a food coloring).

The addition of tartrazine is one of the most incomprehensible aspects of this conglomeration. Tens of thousands of asthmatics have an allergylike sensitivity to tartrazine (FD&C Yellow No. 5). This dye can produce wheezing, difficulty breathing, a runny nose, and hives. Aspirin-sensitive patients are particularly vulnerable to tartrazine. Since anywhere from 10 percent to 39 percent of all asthmatics may develop breathing problems from aspirin, you can see that this is a humongous problem.[4]

As for the other ingredients of **Dainite-KI,** they're not much more sensible. Pulmonary specialists have called for the elimination of potassium iodide (the expectorant) from asthma products on the grounds that it is of questionable benefit and can produce toxicity (rash, goiter, acne).[5]

Asthmatic patients are a highly variable lot. According to Dr. Irwin Ziment, professor of medicine at UCLA,

> **Asthmatic patients vary even more than the drug products that they use. One patient may be completely relieved by a particular agent taken in small dosage every few hours, whereas another ostensibly similar patient may fail to obtain adequate benefit when using the same agent in even larger dosage on a much more frequent basis.[6]**

That means it's an incredibly difficult task to adjust an asthma patient to the proper dose of *one* drug. Add several together and the situation rapidly goes from difficult to absurd, and along the way it becomes a true health hazard.

Editors of the respected journal *The Medical Letter on Drugs and Therapeutics* complain that products which "combine theophylline [aminophylline is a form of theophylline] with ephedrine and a small dose of barbiturate or other sedatives make it impossible to increase the theophylline dose to achieve an appropriate blood level without increasing the doses of the other components. Therefore these preparations may be less effective than single-entity theophylline . . ."[7] If there is a moral to this tale it is that people should try to start with single-ingredient asthma drugs. If additional medicines are needed, they can be added one at a time and in the proper dosage.

## Next Stop: The Inhalers

The next rung on the asthma-treatment ladder is often an inhaler which provides droplets of a drug directly to the afflicted lung muscles, rather than releasing a drug into the body's general circulation. The goal here is to obtain relief that's both quicker and less likely to provoke unwanted side effects, and for the most part that promise has been fulfilled when inhalers are used properly.

The most popular drugs used in inhalers these days are albuterol (**Ventolin** and **Proventil**), metaproterenol (**Alupent** and **Metaprel**) and terbutaline (**Brethine** and **Bricanyl**). All three are quite effective, longer acting, and less likely than old-fashioned aerosols to stimulate the heart. Epinephrine (**Adrenalin, Asthmahaler, Bronitin Mist, Bronkaid Mist, Primatene Mist, Medihaler-EPI, Vaponefrin**) and isoproterenol (**Isuprel, Medihaler-ISO, Norisodrine**) have been around for ages. But they are short-acting and in high doses can produce angina or irregular heart rhythms for some people.

Another advantage to albuterol, metaproterenol, and terbutaline is flexibility. They come as pills or as aerosols. The oral form provides a more gradual and longer lasting effect, whereas the

aerosols provide faster onset and, as we've said, may have somewhat fewer side effects. Pills tend to produce tremor (which may
disappear after several days) and in larger doses can cause nervousness, headache, palpitations, nausea, and sweating. Nevertheless, these newer drugs are less likely to affect the heart and
overall represent an important therapeutic advance.

There is a hitch, however, and it has to do with how people
actually use their asthma aerosols. It turns out that swallowing
pills can be a whole lot easier than trying to breathe in medicine
through the lungs. One study showed that up to 77 percent of
the patients using these inhalers did so improperly and thus
defeated the purpose of the drug.[8] Wrong placement of the aerosol in the mouth, failure to time inhaling with actuation of the
device, and incorrect breathing and breath-holding were all complicating factors. Even after further detailed instruction, about
15 percent of the patients—primarily the very young and very
old—still won't be doing it right.[9, 10] Clearly what is required is
good communication with a doctor or respiratory therapist and
plenty of supervised practice.

Another problem associated with bronchodilator sprays, as
they're called, is overuse. A person who suffers from asthma gets
highly anxious during an attack and will do anything to open
those vital breathing passages. This often means taking puff after
puff from the inhaler. Soon a person's nebulizer may become a
crutch, producing physiological as well as psychological habitua-
tion.

Some physicians feel that constant overuse of inhalers (especially the older-fashioned epinephrine and isoproterenol types)
actually makes an asthmatic's problem worse by causing the
system to overreact with constriction after a brief period of relief.
One team of doctors found many of their long-term asthmatic
patients "were returned to relatively good health by only one
change in their management—the discontinuation of aerosolized
adrenergic drugs."[11]

Inhalers may also tend to dry the lung secretions, which ag-
gravates things for the asthmatic who may be faced with a thick

mucous plug that can't be expelled and which can provoke a prolonged, difficult-to-treat attack.

An even more serious situation is the possibility that these drugs could react with another asthma medicine to cause potentially fatal heartbeat irregularities. Animal research has shown that isoproterenol (**Isuprel**, etc.) may interact with drugs of the cortisone class (**Decadron**, prednisone, etc.) to produce serious heart-rhythm disturbances.[12, 13]

## Theophylline: The Big Step

The next step is a big one, because it means calling in a drug whose increased effectiveness is bought at the price of an increased risk of side effects. Theophylline (and the closely related aminophylline) is a first cousin to the caffeine found in coffee and cola. By the way, if you're caught without your asthma medication at hand when an attack strikes, a few cups of strong coffee wouldn't be a bad bet as first aid.

What's that, you say? Joe has finally flipped his lid with this one? Coffee therapy for an asthma attack sounds like an old wives' tale, not something a doctor would ever recommend. Well, physicians have been recommending it for over a hundred years, and a recent article in the *New England Journal of Medicine* titled "The Bronchodilator Effects and Pharmacokinetics of Caffeine in Asthma" tells it all:

> In 1859 Dr. Hyde Salter stated, "One of the commonest and best reputed remedies of asthma, one that is almost sure to have been tried in any case that may come under our observation, and one that in many cases is more efficacious than any other, is strong coffee . . ."
>
> We have shown that caffeine is as effective a bronchodilator as theophylline in young patients with asthma. . . . We do not recommend caffeine for regular use as a bronchodilator. However, caffeine, in any of its commonly available

forms, may have value for temporary use as a bronchodilator when prescribed antiasthma medications are not readily
available.[14]

A different group of researchers confirmed these findings in
adults. Reporting to their colleagues at the American College of
Chest Physicians, the UCLA team found that "three cups of
coffee (averaging a total of 433 mg of caffeine) produced a 20
percent peak increase in forced expiratory volume—equivalent
to that produced by 200 mg of aminophylline, a commonly
prescribed bronchodilator."[15]

Clearly, coffee is strong medicine. But it's not something that
fits easily into a pillbox, and getting the dose right is not so easy
either. That's why doctors usually recommend the pharmaceutical equivalent—theophylline or aminophylline.

These medications have had a checkered career. Over the last
several decades they have experienced peaks and valleys in popularity. Things are on the upswing again with the addition of
newer, slow-releasing theophylline formulas such as **Theo-Dur,
Theobid, Slo-phyllin Gyrocaps, Somophyllin-CRT**, and many
more. These sustained-release forms mean a patient who formerly had to figure out a way to get his or her medication down
four to six times a day can now make do with twice-daily doses.
This is especially helpful for people who used to have to wake
up in the middle of the night to take their medicine.

Another valuable new formulation is something called **Theo-
Dur Sprinkle**, a twelve-hour theophylline designed for children
or adults who have a hard time swallowing tablets. These capsules are designed to be opened up so the "minipellets" can
literally be sprinkled on food such as apple sauce, Jell-O, or what
have you. I really have to take my hat off to Key Pharmaceuticals for spending the money to develop and market **Theo-Dur
Sprinkle**, a perfect answer for people who hate the thought of
downing horse-sized capsules.

While much has been done to make theophylline more convenient, it still remains a difficult drug to handle. The problem is
that the gap between getting enough and getting too much is

pretty narrow; and as noted above, asthmatics are notorious for the wide differences in how their bodies process drugs. The same dose put into two asthmatics of the same age, height, and weight can produce very different blood levels, and thus very different therapeutic results. It's all quite unpredictable, despite years of effort and lots of fancy computer models. The most common side effects include stomach upset, heartburn, nausea, skin rash, and nervousness.

Theophylline metabolism can be affected by age (children use it up more quickly than adults), smoking (smokers metabolize it at a much greater rate), and the use of other drugs, particularly the ulcer medicine **Tagamet** (cimetidine) and the antibiotic erythromycin (**E-Mycin, Ilosone**, and others), which slow the rate at which the body breaks down and eliminates theophylline.

Consider the case of an eighty-year-old man who was taking theophylline and **Tagamet** simultaneously. When his theophylline dose was boosted from 300 mg to 400 mg daily, it took him only four days to develop stomach pain, which the doctors took to be a sign of his ulcer getting worse. They quadrupled his **Tagamet** intake, and three days later he died with four times the accepted maximum level of theophylline in his blood.[16]

The stomach pain was not his ulcer, but a warning sign of theophylline toxicity. When the doctors upped the **Tagamet** they lowered his ability to get rid of theophylline, which accumulated until it apparently helped to kill him.

Now please don't get me wrong. I think theophylline is good medicine. This was obviously an extreme case, but it does point out that the drug is potent and potentially dangerous. A useful practice is to measure blood levels on a routine basis, especially after starting treatment or after changing the dose. This enables the doctor to tailor the dose so as to keep the level in the "therapeutic" range, and to tell when the concentration is climbing so high as to become hazardous.

Unfortunately, this practice isn't yet widespread, and most theophylline therapy is still an exercise in guesstimation. If you are taking theophylline, make sure that your progress is monitored by your doctor, and that you never increase the dose or

take extra medication without her advice. By the way, it
wouldn't be a bad idea to keep a record of your blood levels. Ask
the doctor for the lab results. The ideal range is between ten and
twenty micrograms per milliliter of plasma.

Most important, remember the warning signs of theophylline
toxicity: stomach pain, headache, nausea, and vomiting. These
signs usually (but unfortunately not always) are the early warnings of more severe toxicity. To prevent any adverse drug interactions, make sure that your doctor knows all the medicines
you are taking.

## Intal: An Attractive Alternative

For many asthmatics, another option is **Intal** (cromolyn). I can't
quite understand why **Intal** isn't more popular in the United
States. Despite wide acceptance in Great Britain and other European countries where it has been used since 1968, physicians in
the United States seem reluctant to embrace **Intal** for what it is
—a very effective drug with very few side effects.

It is particularly attractive because it can be safely used in
conjunction with the inhalers mentioned earlier, such as **Alupent**, **Metaprel**, **Brethine**, **Bricanyl**, **Proventil**, or **Ventolin**.
Theophylline, on the other hand, could be a problem in combination with these aerosols, as the interaction may increase toxicity,
especially to the heart.[17]

**Intal** doesn't work for all asthmatics (estimates range from 52
percent to 89 percent[18]), especially those seriously debilitated,
but in most cases it probably deserves a try before taking a
chance with the riskier, harder-to-control drugs such as theo-
hylline or the steroids.

Much research has been devoted to understanding how **Intal**
works, and it now seems clear that its primary activity is to
prevent the group of cells known as mast cells from releasing
their symptom-producing substances. In essence, **Intal** acts to
block the first step in the sequence of physiological events that
lead to an asthma attack.

**Intal** is especially useful for children, and other drugs like theophylline or steroids can often be eliminated or reduced following a good response to **Intal**. Some doctors are reevaluating their criticisms of **Intal** and their praise of theophylline.

Dr. Jay Selcow is one such physician. He and his colleagues had tested **Intal** in 1973 in a group of very ill asthmatic children who had required around-the-clock theophylline plus steroid therapy. At that time, the researchers decided that **Intal** wasn't as effective as the other two drugs (this was probably due to the seriousness of their patients' conditions). However, several more years of experience with theophylline and steroids convinced them of a need to reconsider this judgment.

> **We constantly encountered a significant number of children with pronounced theophylline side effects despite careful monitoring of serum theophylline blood levels, the use of controlled-release theophylline products, and the use of lower doses initially. Not only were there obvious gastrointestinal side effects, but many parents after careful questioning admitted that their children "just were not the same" when taking theophylline. Many children became disagreeable, rude, and argumentative, seemed to develop poor attention spans with decreased school performance, and sometimes hyperactivity interfered with normal sleep.[19]**

The doctors undertook a second study, this time using children with mild to moderate asthma. "Our attitude at the commencement of the . . . study was that **Intal** was ineffective but safe, whereas theophylline was effective but we were seriously questioning its safety."[20]

The results of the new study were a surprise to the docs. Their initial reluctance about **Intal** was replaced by real enthusiasm. The new data clearly showed that **Intal** was as effective if not better than theophylline, and had many fewer side effects.

They concluded, "Our results confirm . . . that **Intal** is a very effective and safe agent. It was significant to us that in the **Intal** group we were generally able to reduce either the **Intal** dosage or the concomitant bronchodilator dosages or both."[21]

While Dr. Selcow is now a convert, many of his fellow physicians remain unswayed by the mounting evidence in favor of using **Intal** as a first-line agent rather than a drug of last resort. Why? One reason may be that many of the earlier studies panning **Intal** were seriously flawed because they didn't continue the tests long enough to see the full results.[22]

Other reasons for reluctance, cited by Dr. Bernard Berman of Tufts University,[23] boil down to three major areas. First, **Intal** was introduced into the United States in 1973, just when theophylline was riding a crest of newfound popularity because of improved blood-level monitoring tests and computer-derived dosing regimens. Theophylline was a "high-tech" drug and doctors tended to prescribe it in preference to **Intal**.

Second, many doctors don't understand **Intal**. It doesn't work like the other more familiar asthma medications, and even today there are some questions about how it works. We think that by protecting or stabilizing the cells which contain histamine, the drug keeps the lungs from overreacting to stress or allergic irritations.

Third, since the doctors weren't familiar with this new drug, their patients didn't get the education they needed to properly use the **Intal** inhaler. **Intal** comes as a dry powder in a small gelatin capsule which gets inserted into the whirling inhaler ("Spinhaler"). A needle inside the inhaler pierces the capsule and the powder is released. When you start inhaling, the powder is propelled by a blower out the opening and into your lungs.[24]

Proper use of the Spinhaler is essential for the **Intal** to be at all effective, but getting the hang of it can be a little tricky. About the only common side effect with **Intal** is bronchial irritation from using the Spinhaler, and some people find inhaling this dry powder rather unpleasant.

Other less common side effects include skin problems and leg weakness or pain. A "nebulized" liquid form of **Intal** is also available, but its use requires wearing a facemask, a feature not likely to meet with overwhelming consumer acceptance. This form of **Intal** administration is probably most useful for young children and others unable to tolerate or properly use the Spinhaler.

For the inhaled **Intal** powder to reach the lungs, the airways must be as clear as possible. For this reason, the doctor may recommend you take a puff of a bronchodilator inhaler first, then wait five or ten minutes before using **Intal**.

It's important to understand what **Intal** is and isn't good for. **Intal** is very useful in preventing attacks of asthma, but it won't help you out once an attack starts. In fact, inhaling the powder in the middle of an attack may make the asthma worse. For those who've identified their particular attack "triggers," a spray of **Intal** about a half hour before playing with the cat, mowing the lawn, strenuously exercising, or whatever incites their lungs to riot, will usually prevent the attack.

There's a tendency on the part of both doctors and patients to give up on **Intal** too soon. The drug takes *at least* four weeks, and usually longer, to have maximum effect. During that time it must be taken correctly and at the prescribed frequency (usually four times daily).

**Intal** is certainly no miracle cure, but it can provide an enormous amount of relief for many of the asthmatics who use it. And the drug is remarkably safe, at least in comparison with other asthma medications. If you have asthma and have not yet given **Intal** a good shot, you might consider asking your doctor about it.

## At the End of the Line

In any stepped-care scheme, there's always something at the end of the line—the court of last resort. Or, in this case, the cortisone of last resort. For the asthma patient who is still having trouble after theophylline or one of the aerosol inhalers like albuterol, metaproterenol, or terbutaline, and cromolyn has failed to solve the problem, it's time to roll out the heavy artillery in the form of cortisone derivatives.

Now, it used to be that doctors would prescribe oral medications like **Cortef** (hydrocortisone or cortisol), **Delta-Cortef** (prednisolone), **Meticorten** (prednisone), **Cortone** (cortisone), **Aristocort** (triamcinolone), **Medrol** (methylprednisolone), **Decadron** (dexamethasone), and **Celestone** (betamethasone).

Even though the list of cortisone-type drugs is long, they're pretty much the same, being synthetic modifications of cortisol, a natural hormone. Such steroids are used for an incredible number of diseases and conditions. They are injected into the bruised and battered knees of football players and the elbows of tennis bums in order to relieve the inflammation associated with abused joints. They are taken orally by patients with rheumatoid arthritis to decrease the pain and swelling. They are even used as cancer chemotherapy for children and adults with leukemias and lymphomas. They are also used for a variety of allergic conditions, for preventing tissue rejection in some organ-transplant operations, and, of course, for bronchial asthma.

Despite their many uses, steroids cannot cure anything. At best they may relieve symptoms, and that can sometimes be lifesaving. In most instances, however, they afford the promise of relief but at the cost of physical and psychological addiction.

Continued use of these medications can produce some very serious adverse reactions such as increased susceptibility to infections. Steroids may even mask the signs of infection by suppressing the body's normal defense mechanisms. Other adverse reactions include increased blood pressure from fluid retention, thinning of the bones, menstrual irregularities, psychological disturbances, complications in diabetes management, growth suppression in children, impaired wound healing, and skin problems. These drugs seem to help cause ulcers or make them worse. They may also bring on cataracts, produce muscle cramps and weakness, and make people depressed or nervous.

Anyone who has taken high-dose steroids for any length of time is truly addicted and can't just stop cold turkey. If you do suddenly stop taking your medication, your body is left defenseless, since your system can no longer manufacture its own supply of this essential hormone. Slow withdrawal under a doctor's care is imperative. Very gradual tapering over a period of many weeks to months is necessary for your body to recover its normal hormonal function.

The really big question is, are the benefits of cortisone-like drugs worth the risk for asthma patients? According to Drs. Vincent Fontana and Angelo Ferrara of the Department of Pediatric Allergy at St. Vincent's Hospital and Medical Center of New York:

> **The insidious side effects that follow long-term steroid therapy are what concern us, and they should be considered by all physicians. It has been our experience, and certainly the experience of others who have been left with the responsibility of "weaning" children from steroid therapy, that the most disastrous effects of cortisone treatments are not metabolic. The more important iatrogenic effects [illness caused by doctors] are: addiction, the postponement of proper allergic investigations and management, emotional changes, and, last but not least, unresponsiveness of the child to all other anti-asthmatic medications after he has been on steroid therapy for a long period of time . . . a grave responsibility rests with the physician who starts a child on steroids except in life-threatening situations. After years of steroid therapy, these children become both pulmonary and emotional cripples who ultimately become the responsibility of the convalescent homes.[25]**

In a report prepared by the Drug Committee of the Research Council of the American Academy of Allergy, some startling facts came to light. Of 122 patients, 76 were "steroid dependent." That is, they could have given up the drugs only with great difficulty, if at all. The side-effect rate was 2.44 per patient.

This heavy-duty committee concluded, "The Committee does not condone the use of any of the corticosteroids, unless a life-threatening situation is involved. Before corticosteroid therapy is undertaken, every other means of controlling the patient should be attempted."[26]

Okay, you've got the picture. We have pounded the message into your head until you're scared to death of steroids. Prepare for an about-face. There's something new on the market, and it truly offers a much safer alternative to oral cortisone. In recent years, drug companies have come up with an aerosol form or, in other words, a steroid spray.

Beclomethasone diproprionate (**Beclovent** and **Vanceril**) is inhaled much the same way the bronchodilators are. This way, the medicine gets right to the lungs where it is needed rather than first circulating from the stomach to the bloodstream to the whole body, and eventually to the constricted breathing passages. Far less drug is absorbed, and side effects are minimal. Sometimes yeast infections (Candida) can occur in the mouth, but if people rinse the throat with water after using the drug the likelihood of such infections may be diminished.

As with **Intal**, inhaled steroids aren't any good at taking care of an attack once it gets going. They are never for use "as needed," but should instead be used on a regular basis.

The point is that steroid sprays like **Beclovent** and **Vanceril** are far less dangerous than oral cortisone. Safer, yes . . . risk free, no! They can be lifesaving in case of severe asthma, and no one hesitates using them in such instances. But the message is still that steroids are always potentially dangerous and should be saved for the very last rung on the ladder.

Because of the complex nature of asthma, there are times when no one drug will do the trick. For many asthmatics, relief comes only from a careful combination of medications. The key here is *careful.* As I noted earlier, the asthmatic already starts out with two strikes against him when it comes to dealing with drugs, and willy-nilly combinations are more likely to aggravate than eliminate the problem.

Combination therapy should be reserved for those persons who have not been able to achieve adequate relief by using optimal doses of a single drug. Adding another drug increases the risk of adverse reactions and makes the drug treatment more complicated. On the other hand, the occasional use of an inhaled bronchodilator can complement pretty much any drug regimen for asthma, and is frequently used with persons already on cromolyn or inhaled steroids. The possible combinations are endless, and getting the right one requires patience, persistence, and excellent communication between the patient, his family, and the physician or respiratory therapist.

## Hope for the Future

Experimental research, as always, proceeds along several paths at once. At this point it is impossible to predict which path will lead to some new breakthrough in asthma treatment, but several avenues look promising.

Vitamin C, which has been proposed to be the cure or preventive for just about every disease afflicting mankind, has been touted for asthma relief as well, and there's a modest amount of research to support that belief. Experimentally, Vitamin C has shown some activity in both animal[27] and human[28] tests.

If Vitamin C does work, however, it works moderately well at best. It can prevent some of the bronchoconstriction seen in mildly asthmatic patients under test conditions, but its practical value for most asthmatics is uncertain. Taking several hundred milligrams three or four times a day probably won't hurt anything.

There's a lot more hope for relief with the use of two drugs whose major application is the treatment of heart problems. Verapamil (**Isoptin** and **Calan**) and nifedipine (**Procardia**) are two in a category of drugs referred to as calcium channel blockers. Doctors found that patients taking these drugs for their heart conditions had a coincidental improvement in their asthmatic symptoms.[29] Experiments showed that these drugs can prevent exercise-induced asthma as well,[30] though the use of calcium channel blockers expressly for treatment of asthmatics awaits further testing.

One drug almost certain to find use in treating asthma will be ipratropium bromide, a close cousin of atropine. It's long been known that atropine is effective in treating asthmatics, especially when all else fails. However, atropine has many unpleasant side effects. In addition, researchers thought that atropine would dry up the secretions in the lungs, an adverse reaction that could be disastrous to a person with asthma.

This fear severely limited the use of atropine in asthmatics. A 1975 study showed that this theoretical concern just wasn't borne out by what was observed clinically, and that atropine had little effect on bronchial secretions.[31] The other side effects of atropine were still a problem, though, so the chemical wizards went to work modifying the drug's structure. The result was ipratropium, which isn't spread around throughout the entire body system when it's inhaled.

When used as an inhaler, ipratropium has very few side effects and can be very effective. For some patients, ipratropium is as effective as albuterol in relieving acute attacks, but the combination is better than either alone.[32] Exactly which patients will benefit most from ipratropium is still unknown, but the drug is a welcome addition to the arsenal in the asthma wars.

While predicting the future is always a risky business, I'm very optimistic about the continuing improvements in asthma treatment. Since the last edition of this book was published, the number of options available to the asthmatic has increased enormously, and people are now living much more comfortably with their condition. Researchers are slowly teasing out the causes of asthma and when they are known, more rational treatments should emerge.

As I already mentioned, a chemical class of biological compounds known as the leukotrienes is looking more and more like the principal villain in this story,[33] and drug manufacturers are working on leukotriene compounds in an attempt to find a molecule that will block their harmful effects and prevent asthma attacks in the first place.

No matter what medical science manages to come up with, though, it's the asthma patient who will be on the front lines in the fight against the disease. Anyone suffering from asthma must be constantly vigilant to identify and steer clear of things that aggravate the condition. Pollutants, aerosol sprays, noxious odors, tobacco smoke, and chemicals must be avoided at all costs. And remember, asthmatics are also more likely to be allergic to aspirin and related drugs.

Managing asthma requires a close, cooperative working relationship between doctor and patient. This relationship is the key to successful treatment, and it will be worth any asthmatic's while to look long and hard for a doctor who has the patience and knowledge to deal carefully and properly with the disease, who undertakes drug therapy conservatively, and who communicates frankly.

Asthma is a serious lung disease. It shouldn't be underestimated, nor should it be overtreated. Therein lies the dilemma. Less is more is definitely the answer here. Don't use anything that isn't absolutely necessary, and don't use anything that's necessary more often than you must or in any way other than as instructed.

The new therapeutic drugs, combined with old standbys, offer a lot of options and a lot of hope for relieving the fear and discomfort that comes with being asthmatic. Knowing what's available and when it should be used puts you on the inside track to get the best available treatment, which is what every asthmatic is entitled to.

# References

1. Foreman, John C., and Lichtenstein, Lawrence M. "Clinical Pharmacology of Acute Allergic Disorders." *Ann. Rev. Med.* 31:181–190, 1980.

2. Hardy, Christopher Charles, et al. "The Bronchoconstrictor Effect of Inhaled Prostaglandin D2 in Normal and Asthmatic Men." *N. Engl. J. Med.* 311:209–213, 1984.

3. Goetzl, Edward J. "Asthma: New Mediators and Old Problems." *N. Engl. J. Med.* 311:252–253, 1984.

4. "Proceedings of the Symposium on Current Clues to the Understanding of Aspirin-sensitive Asthma." *J. of Asthma* 20 (Suppl. 1):1–3, 1983.

5. Hendles, Leslie, and Weinberger, Miles. "A Time to Abandon the

Use of Iodides in the Management of Pulmonary Diseases." *J. Allergy Clin. Immunol.* 66(3):177–178, 1980.

6. Ziment, I. "Bronchodilator Therapy." Boehringer Ingelheim, 1982.

7. "Drugs for Asthma." *Medical Letter on Drugs and Therapeutics* 24:83–86, 1982.

8. Appel, D. "Faulty Use of Canister Nebulizers for Asthma." *J. Family Pract.* 14:1135–39, 1982.

9. Kirillof, L. H., and Tibbals, S. C. "Drugs for Asthma." *Am. J. Nursing.* 83:55–61, 1983.

10. Settipane, G. A., et. al. "Adverse Reactions to Cromolyn." *JAMA* 241:811, 1979.

11. Caplin, Irvin, and Haynes, J. T. "Complications of Aerosol Therapy in Asthma." *Annals of Aller.* 27:659, 1969.

12. Guideri, G., et al. "Extraordinary Potentiation of Isoproterenol Cardiotoxicity by Corticoid Pretreatment." *Cardiovasc. Res.* 8:775–786, 1974.

13. Green, M., et al. "Role of Alpha and Beta-adrenergic Activation in Ventricular Fibrillation Death of Corticoid-Pretreated Rats." *J. Pharm. Sci.* 69:441–444, 1980.

14. Becker, Allan B., et al. "The Bronchodilator Effects and Pharmacokinetics of Caffeine in Asthma." *N. Engl. J. Med.* 310:743–746, 1984.

15. Simmons, Kathryn. "Caffeine Opens Airways for Asthmatics." *JAMA* 251:441, 1984.

16. Anderson, J. R., et al. "A Fatal Case of Theophylline Intoxication." *Arch. Int. Med.* 143:559–560, 1983.

17. Lehr, David and Guideri, Giancarlo. "More on Combined Beta-Agonists and Methylxanthines in Asthma." *N. Engl. J. Med.* 309:1581–1582, 1983.

18. Penna, P. M. "Asthma." In Herfindal, E. T., and J. L. Hirschman, eds. *Clinical Pharmacy and Therapeutics,* 2d ed. Baltimore: Williams and Wilkins Co., 1979, p. 398.

19. Selcow, J. E., Mendelson, L., and Rosen, J. P. "A Comparison of Cromolyn and Bronchodilators in Patients with Mild to Moderately Severe Asthma in an Office Practice." *Ann. Allergy* 50:13–18, 1983.

20. Ibid.

21. Ibid.

22. Berman, B. A., and Ross, R. N. "Cromolyn." *Clin. Rev. Allergy* 1:105–121, 1983.

23. Ibid.

24. Kirillof, op cit.

25. Fontana, Vincent J. "Statistics, Mortality, and Asthma." *J. of Allergy.* 41:58–59, 1968.

26. Brown, Earl B. "Reply to Corticosteroid Therapy in Asthma." *J. of Allergy* 41:60, 1968.

27. Dawson, W., and West, G. B. "The Nature of Antagonism of Bronchospasm in the Guinea Pig by Ascorbic Acid." *J. Pharm. Pharmacol.* 17:595–596, 1965.

28. Mohsenin, V., et. al. "Effect of Ascorbic Acid on Response to Methacholine Challenge in Asthmatic Subjects." *Am. Rev. Respir. Dis.* 127:143–147, 1983.

29. Midtbo, K. "Possible Antiallergic Effect of the Calcium Entry Blocker Verapamil." *Curr. Ther. Res.* 33:724–725, 1983.

30. Patel, K. R., and Kerr, J. W. "Calcium Antagonists in Experimental Asthma." *Clin. Allergy* 12 (supp.):15–20, 1982.

31. Lopez-Vidriero, M. T., et. al. "Effect of Atropine on Sputum Production." *Thorax* 30:543–547, 1975.

32. Leahy, B. C., et. al. "Comparison of Nebulized Salbutamol with Nebulized Ipratropium Bromide in Acute Asthma." *Br. J. Dis. Chest* 77:159–163, 1983.

33. Griffin, M., et. al. "Effects of Leukotriene D on the Airways in Asthma." *N. Engl. J. Med.* 308:436–439, 1983.

# 9

# Contraception: Birth of a Controversy

---

*Effectiveness of various contraceptive techniques • The Pill: Risks and benefits • Interactions: How the Pill gets along with other drugs • How the Pill is changing • The Intrauterine Device (IUD): Copper 7, Dalkon Shield, Lippes Loop, Saf-T-Coil • Vasectomy: The men's turn at bat • New advances in birth control • How terrific is **Today?**: The contraceptive sponge • LHRH.*

---

So you don't want to make a baby. What you *do* want is a simple, safe, and effective means of contraception. Good luck! Despite the advances of the past quarter century, no one has yet discovered anything that resembles an ideal method of birth control.

Contraception has everything needed to make a perfect controversy. It involves a highly complex physiological system, and as if that weren't enough, any decision carries strong social, moral, religious, and cultural overtones. No wonder there have been pitched battles around this issue. In recent years, the biggest fights have been in the medical community itself, primarily about safety.

You may have heard a lot about the side effects of birth-control pills, but which are mostly mythical and which are real hazards? What's the real story on the **Dalkon Shield**, and are all IUDs alike? Will there ever be a safe, effective birth-control pill for men? What people want is an uncomplicated, sure way of preventing pregnancy, without risk. Unfortunately, there are some drawbacks to almost any contraceptive technique available today, and before you choose one, it only makes sense to know as much as possible about it.

How do you select your contraceptive? First off, it's got to work. Let's take a look at how well the major methods protect against pregnancy over a period of one year:

## Effectiveness of Various Contraceptive Techniques

| | |
|---|---|
| Vasectomy | almost 100% |
| Female sterilization | almost 100% |
| Combination Pill (oral contraceptive) | above 99% |
| MiniPill (oral contraceptive) | 97% to 98% |
| IUD (intrauterine device) | 92% to 99% |
| Condom *and* foam | 95% to above 99% |
| Condom alone | 64% to 97% |
| Contraceptive sponge | 85% to 90% |
| Diaphragm | 80% to 98% |
| Foam spermicides | 71% to 98% |
| Jelly and cream spermicides | 64% to 96% |
| Rhythm method | 53% to 99% |

As you can see, some of these methods have a pretty wide range of effectiveness. While condoms, diaphragms, and the rhythm method *can* be almost as effective as the Pill, they have to be used properly, consistently, and conscientiously to rack up that kind of record. Used casually or haphazardly, they may end up being only a bit better than taking your chances with nothing at all!

While we can tell you the numbers and what's involved medically in each method, nobody but the people involved can say what the varying risks of pregnancy mean to them. Some might prefer to postpone pregnancy for a while but would not be unhappy should they conceive; others would have their lives devastated by an unwanted pregnancy.

All these factors interact and make it impossible to point at any one method of birth control and say, "Use that, it's the best thing." Lots of options are available, so let's take a look at what there is to work with, and the pluses and minuses of each approach.

## The Pill

The first big revolution in contraception came with the discovery of oral contraceptives—the Pill. This new concept seemed to be the answer to everyone's prayers. It was unobtrusive, easy to use, didn't interfere with anyone's pleasure or spontaneity, *and,* best of all, it worked remarkably well. If a woman just remembered to take the thing each day, she had contraceptive protection that was anywhere from five to five hundred times more reliable than other options.

At first, men and women, freed of the fear of an unwanted pregnancy, didn't pay much attention to side effects. But after a time—and once the nervous nellies who feared the Pill would turn American youth into degenerate sex maniacs began to quiet down—medical worries began to arise. By now the Pill has been revealed, reviled, studied, restudied, blessed, cursed, and condemned—sometimes all at the same time.

A series of studies in the late 1960s and early 1970s linked the oral contraceptives (OCs) to all sorts of maladies, including thrombophlebitis (a painful irritation of a vein caused by formation of a blood clot), pulmonary embolism (a clot that breaks loose and lodges in the lungs), gallbladder disease, noncancerous liver tumors, visual problems, a higher risk of some types of cancer, and an increased risk of heart attack and stroke.

For years, proponents of the Pill dealt with these issues by pointing out that the excess risk for any given healthy woman is quite small. (But let's not forget that even a small risk multiplied by 8.5 million women taking oral contraceptives could add up to a considerable toll.) Anyway, the Pill people used to counter, it was far safer to use OCs than to get pregnant.

Statistics from the Centers for Disease Control (CDC) indicate that by the late 1970s that was no longer true. With lower rates of death during pregnancy and childbirth, a woman runs almost as much of a risk of dying while on the Pill as she would if she got pregnant. And if she is over thirty-five, her risks with oral contraceptives are significantly higher.

On the other hand, the Pill appears to offer considerable protection against several major health problems of women, such as iron-deficiency anemia, benign breast disease, and ovarian cysts.[1] All of these protective benefits have shown up in multiple studies of large numbers of Pill users. Evidence from smaller studies also suggests that the Pill may help protect against endometrial (uterine lining) and ovarian cancer.[2] This is particularly significant, since neither of these forms of cancer is very readily detected by any available screening techniques.

The trouble is, so many of these studies seem to point in different directions because they are very complicated. Not long ago, Dr. Malcolm Pike and his colleagues at the University of Southern California reported an increased risk of breast cancer among women under twenty-five who had used the Pill for five years or more,[3] in apparent contradiction to a major study less than a year before.[4] At that time, the CDC and its more than one hundred cooperating researchers found no increased risk of breast cancer due to oral contraceptives. Perhaps because of this, the conclusions of Pike's study have been publicly questioned and criticized.[5-7]

How can both studies be right? Don't jump to the conclusion that the scientists don't know what they're doing. Look more closely: Pike and his coworkers didn't assume that all Pills are created equal. They found a relationship between the progestogen (synthetic progesterone hormone) content and the risk of breast cancer. Low-progestogen pills involved little or no excess risk for any age group, and women over twenty-five on high-progestogen pills seemed to be at only slightly greater risk. But those under twenty-five who'd been on high-progestogen OCs for several years experienced "a substantial risk of breast cancer"— substantially higher, that is, than the normal low risk of women this age. If that sounds complicated and confusing, you're right.

By the time such subtleties as age-related risk and progestogen content filtered through the popular press, though, what many women heard was simply that the Pill had again been found risky. The truth, of course, was a lot more complex. Just imagine how difficult it can be to track down either beneficial or harmful effects when they don't show up for ten or twenty years—sometimes longer—after the women started using OCs. To make matters even more confusing, differences in how, where, and when studies are conducted and analyzed can sometimes lead to differing conclusions.

## Interactions: How the Pill Gets Along with Other Drugs

Even Pill–drug interactions, which don't require quite as much patience to uncover as the long-range risks of the Pill itself, are not as widely recognized as they should be. The big exception is tobacco, and rightly so, since OCs and cigarettes make a potentially disastrous combination. Smokers on the Pill multiply their chances of a stroke by about twenty-two times over that of women who neither smoke nor take oral contraceptives. In fact, any smoker in her late thirties or older really ought to pick out a different contraceptive method, unless she's just crazy about Russian roulette. The risks of cardiovascular problems due to the Pill really soar as you start adding other risk factors, such as obesity, diabetes, or hypertension.

Other drugs that can up the ante for trouble with OCs include antibiotics, an antianxiety agent, an anticonvulsant, and at least one anti-inflammatory medication. The Pill seems to slow the body's metabolism of **Valium** (diazepam) so much that this antianxiety drug stays in the bloodstream almost twice as long as usual. For some women, this could produce symptoms of overdose, such as confusion, incoordination, and drowsiness. It is not clear whether similar drugs can interact in the same way, but women taking other antianxiety medicines such as **Librium** (chlordiazepoxide), **Ativan** (lorazepam), **Tranxene** (clorazepate), or sleeping pills such as **Dalmane** (flurazepam) should probably be alert to this possibility.

OCs can also interfere with the effectiveness of some medications. Tricyclic antidepressants such as **Elavil** (amitriptyline), **Triavil** (amitriptyline and perphenazine), **Norpramin** (desipramine), or **Tofranil** (imipramine); oral anticoagulants; anticonvulsants; oral diabetes medicine such as **Orinase** (tolbutamide), **Tolinase** (tolazamide), or **Dymelor** (acetohexamide); and guanethidine, a blood-pressure drug which also goes under the aliases **Ismelin** and **Esimil** might not work as well as they should for a woman who is taking the Pill. Since birth-control pills can raise blood pressure or trigger depression or diabetes in susceptible women, some of these interactions are not as esoteric or unlikely as they might seem.

**Butazolidin** (phenylbutazone), which is a potent arthritis medicine; **Dilantin** (phenytoin), often used to treat epilepsy; and antibiotics such as ampicillin, penicillin V, rifampin, sulfonamides (including **Gantrisin**), or tetracycline pose the risk of a different interaction. So do barbiturates and antimigraine preparations such as **Fiorinal**. In combination with any of these, the Pill could lose some of its contraceptive efficacy, and a woman could be surprised by an unexpected pregnancy.

The real catch-22 here is the migraine medicine, since birth-control pills can bring on migraines or make them worse. But of course *any* of these interactions leading to an unwelcome surprise can pose a big problem. If you have to take any of these drugs, it might be smart to use some other contraceptive approach instead of or in addition to OCs, just to be safe.

## How the Pill Is Changing

How do oral contraceptives work? Basically, the Pill provides synthetic versions of the hormones the body uses to regulate its reproductive cycle. In the process, they shut down the brain circuitry that gives the ovaries the signal to release an egg. No egg, no baby. The Pill also causes changes in the lining of the uterus that make it an inhospitable place for an egg to take up residence, were one in fact to be released and fertilized.

When oral contraceptives first came along, they contained relatively large doses of estrogen and progestin or progestogen, synthetic versions of the hormone progesterone. This chemical sledgehammer seemed necessary to ensure getting enough of the hormones into circulation. But when red flags started going up about problems, researchers began looking for ways to cut the dose of hormones, particularly the estrogen component believed responsible for much of the circulatory-related problems. This was done, and done so successfully that one expert now says, "The findings of many investigations in the late 1960s and early 1970s may no longer be entirely appropriate because the oral contraceptives available then had higher dosages than today."[8]

The watershed amount of estrogen in a pill is 50 micrograms (50 one-millionths of a gram). Anything above that is a high-dose pill; anything below qualifies as a low-dose pill. The lower limit is around 20 micrograms, at which level many women experience breakthrough bleeding (bleeding at some other point in the cycle besides the regular menses).

Among the low-dose pills now in use are **Lo/Ovral, Loestrin 1/20, Brevicon, Norinyl 1+35, Ortho-Novum 1/35**, and **Ovcon-35**. Some of the mid-dose pills (50 micrograms of estrogen) include **Ovcon-50, Ovral, Norinyl-1+50, Demulen, Norlestrin 1**, and **Zorane 1/50**. Remaining high-dose pills include **Ovulen** (100 micrograms), **Enovid 5 mg** (75 micrograms), **Enovid-E** (100 micrograms), **Enovid 10 mg** (150 micrograms), **Ortho-Novum 10** (60 micrograms), and **Ortho-Novum 1/80** (80 micrograms).

The newer, low-estrogen pills appear less likely to lead to heart attacks, strokes, or blood clots in the legs or lungs. They may even be less guilty of causing such common Pill side effects as nausea and vomiting, breast tenderness, cramps, change in weight, breakthrough bleeding, depression, intolerance for contact lenses, or loss of interest in sex. But we promised drawbacks for every method, and the low-dose birth-control pills are a little less effective. When a woman takes a 50-microgram to 100-microgram Pill she can forget one occasionally and still have enough of the artifical hormone circulating in her system to skate through. Not so with the low-dose version. Miss a single little Pill and the chances of experiencing either breakthrough bleeding or fertilization do go up.

By the way, just to clear up a bit of confusion, the "mini-Pill" is *not* just a low-dose combination Pill. Mini-Pills such as **Micronor, Nor-Q.D.**, and **Ovrette** are progestin-only Pills. These Pills are somewhat less effective than combination Pills. Women on the mini-Pill are also more likely to experience breakthrough bleeding, variations in menstrual cycle length, or a lack of menstrual periods.[9] But if estrogen gives you troublesome side effects, the mini-Pill might not.

A very recent addition to the Pill patrol is the triphasic Pill, of which there are now (appropriately) three—**Triphasil, Ortho-Novum 7/7/7**, and **Tri-Norinyl**. These are the next logical step for combination Pills. Instead of supplying a fixed ratio of estrogen to progestin throughout the twenty-one days a woman takes the Pill, the triphasics vary the relationship of these two hormones every few days in an effort to mimic the natural reproductive cycle more closely. Early studies show that these OCs seem to have relatively little effect on cholesterol and other blood components; hopefully, they will eventually prove to have the least risk yet of causing blood clotting and heart attack problems.[10]

By providing the hormones on a schedule that follows the woman's natural cycle, the triphasics manage to reduce the total amount of hormone administered during the month by almost one third below that even of a low-dose pill. Since the adverse effects known for OCs to date have been dose related, any reduction in hormone content is a welcome one, though it will be many, many years before we can say with any degree of certainty whether these triphasics have now gotten the drug level down to a point where many or most women aren't at greater risk when taking the Pill.

All this leaves any woman who wants to use the Pill with a dilemma. First, is the Pill safe for her at all? And second, which Pill should she use?

If a woman, no matter what her age, smokes, has any blood-vessel disease (including high blood pressure), any evidence of heart problems, epilepsy, diabetes, liver disorders, or gallbladder problems, or if she developed toxemia during a previous pregnancy, she'd be wise to seek other forms of contraception. All of these health problems have been shown to put a woman at considerably higher risk when she's taking birth-control pills, and there's as yet no definitive evidence the lower-dose pills will reduce that risk.

"Women over the age of 30 (and certainly over the age of 40)," writes one researcher, "who smoke or have any of the risk factors mentioned should use contraceptive methods other than the Pill. . . . For the older woman who is in good health and without risk factors, the new low-dose pill may be an appropriate choice if she is willing to undertake a slightly increased risk of circulatory death (knowing that the exact risk cannot be accurately estimated at this time)."[11]

So there you have it, in black and white. If you're young *and* in good health *and* a nonsmoker, the latest Pill may provide the contraception you want at a risk you can accept. If you're older, or have any of the known risk factors, taking the Pill is a more significant gamble. If a woman *is* going to take the Pill, she should have a long talk with her doctor. Sometimes docs fall into a habit of prescribing something because it's what they've always prescribed for birth control, or because that's what the latest drug detail man had to hawk, or because they haven't had time to get up-to-date on their journal reading.

Given what we know about the dose-related effects of the hormones in birth control pills, every woman owes it to herself to get on the lowest possible dose Pill that provides effective contraception without persistent breakthrough bleeding or other unwanted side effects. While that still involves taking a chance, at least it means taking the least chance possible.

# The Intrauterine Device (IUD): Copper 7, Dalkon Shield, Lippes Loop, Saf-T-Coil

This contraceptive method has generated almost as much controversy lately as the Pill. The IUD is among the most effective birth-control techniques, and when all goes well it doesn't require much fuss and bother—not even remembering to pop a tiny tablet down the hatch every day. But despite years of experience, we don't yet know for certain how it works. And there's very disquieting evidence that when it misfires, the IUD can lead to BIG trouble.

The intrauterine device is as old as the hills. Rumor has it that Arab nomads, not wishing their female camels to be burdened with camel kiddies while crossing the deserts, would insert small stones into the animals' uteruses and thus prevent conception.

The modern, high-tech IUD isn't really all that far removed from stones in the uterus. The devices come in a bewildering variety of shapes, from loops to shields to coils. They all seem to work. The best guess (and it seems more a guess than a medical fact) is that the IUD causes a minor but persistent irritation in the uterus so that a fertilized ovum can't implant itself and start growing into a baby.

There is no doubt the IUD has its advantages. It's not a chemical, so there are none of the side effects seen with the hormonal birth-control pills. Once in place it's there to stay until removed by a doctor, and nothing need be done before having sex. Give it points for spontaneity. And it works, to the tune of about 95 percent efficiency. Its other virtues are low maintenance (no monthly charges for prescription refills) and a high success rate for restoring fertility once the thing is taken out.

Sounds great, right? Well, by now you know there has to be a catch. Here's the story:

Once there was a popular IUD named the **Dalkon Shield**. In May, 1974, the A. H. Robins Company notified the public and medical profession that its **Dalkon Shield** had been present in thirty-six women who became pregnant, developed blood poisoning, and subsequently miscarried. Four of these women died.

If only the company or the FDA had acted quickly, responsibly, and forthrightly, the matter would have been a tragic footnote in contraceptive history instead of a cause for tragic headlines. But the **Dalkon Shield** was not recalled, and within five months it had been associated with 219 infected pregnancies and 13 deaths.[12]

With such a wave of reports rolling in, you'd expect the company to respond with incredible dispatch. Instead, the A. H. Robins Company denied there was any special problem with the **Dalkon Shield**, although the company suddenly stopped distributing the device in 1974. From 1974 on, legal claims for damages started raining on the company. The claims eventually totaled more than 250,000 in number; at last count the company had paid out over $500 million.

It's hard to believe, but A. H. Robins stonewalled for almost ten years, during which time countless women unknowingly walked around with **Dalkon Shields** that might have exposed them to a far greater than normal risk of uterine infection that could cause pain, infertility, and even death.

When some of the cases finally got to federal court, documents that one judge ordered the company to preserve and produce were suddenly said to have "disappeared" when a lawyer's wife did some spring housecleaning.[13] And another batch of documents, according to the testimony of the man who had once managed the company's defense on the **Dalkon Shield** litigation, were deliberately destroyed.[14]

U.S. District Court Judge Miles Lord was so incensed by the company's conduct in his court that he summoned three top A. H. Robins officials and lectured them personally. "None of you," said the judge, "has faced up to the fact that more than nine thousand women have made claims that they gave up part of their womanhood so that your company might prosper. It is alleged that others gave their lives so you might so prosper.

"It is not enough," the judge admonished, "to say, 'I did not know,' 'It was not me,' 'Look elsewhere.' Time and time again, each of you has used this kind of argument in refusing to acknowledge your responsibility and in pretending to the world that the chief officers and directors of your gigantic multinational corporation have no responsibility for the company's acts and omissions.

". . . Confession is good for the soul, gentlemen. Face up to your misdeeds. Acknowledge the personal responsibility that you have for the activities of those who work under you. Rectify this evil situation. Warn the potential future victims and recompense those who already have been harmed."[15]

I wish I could say that Robins officials repented after hearing Judge Lord's little sermon. Instead, they resented his strong words so much that they asked the appellate court to punish him. On November 2, 1984, the judge's remarks were stricken from the court record.[16]

In late 1984 the company finally couldn't hack it anymore. A. H. Robins settled over two hundred suits that had been pending, for many millions of dollars, and then spent $4 million on an advertising campaign advising women that the company would pay for the medical examination of any woman who thought she still had a **Dalkon Shield** in place; they would pay for the removal of any IUD which did in fact prove to be a **Dalkon Shield**.

"There is substantial medical opinion," the company finally conceded in its advertisement, "that its continued use may pose a serious personal health hazard." A little slow, weren't they? Yet company president E. Claiborne Robins, Jr. claimed that this magnanimous gesture by his company was from a concern for the health of the women still using the **Dalkon Shield**, and because of what he called "unwarranted" adverse publicity and criticism.

On August 21, 1985, A. H. Robins filed for protection under chapter 11 of the Bankruptcy Code. It looked as though the $615 million the company had set aside for legal settlements on **Dalkon Shield** cases would not be enough.

The **Dalkon Shield** is *not* the only IUD to have caused infection problems. According to a study at Boston University School of Medicine, women using an IUD are almost nine times more likely to experience the serious infections called pelvic inflammatory disease (PID) than those who use other birth-control methods. Here again, though, not all IUDs are equal. These researchers discovered that the **Dalkon Shield** is the worst of the lot.[17]

The problem with PID is not just that it's produced by serious infections, though that's bad enough. It can also have nasty aftereffects, because the infection may scar the Fallopian tubes. As a result, women who have had PID sometimes have difficulty conceiving at a later time, and they may also run a risk of a dangerous ectopic (outside of the uterus) pregnancy.

Why were women developing pelvic infections, and getting pregnant, and developing blood poisoning, and having septic abortions, all with an IUD in place? Maybe, just maybe, the IUD works by causing a slight local irritation, in the form of a minor infection.

Several years ago, Dr. William J. Ledger, working in the Department of Obstetrics and Gynecology at the University of Michigan, was doing basic research on rabbits to determine how IUDs worked. Dr. Ledger discovered bacteria growing in the uteruses of rabbits implanted with a large foreign body (essentially an IUD). The organisms were sensitive to penicillin and streptomycin. Dr. Ledger and an associate concluded that "A local uterine infection can play a role in the mechanism preventing implantation when a large uterine foreign body is utilized in the rabbit."[18]

If the IUD does work by setting up an infection, does it work less well when the infection is eliminated by antibiotics? That's what Dr. Ledger found to be true for his rabbits, and another researcher confirmed the same effect in rats.[19] Bunnies and rats aren't people, of course, so who cares if they get pregnant with an IUD and an antibiotic? Well, Dr. Ledger made a startling observation on this point. During the course of his rabbit study, he encountered a number of women who'd become pregnant with an IUD in place. The conception of these pregnancies coincided with the administration of antibiotics given for unrelated medical problems.

Now, this was sort of a street-corner survey, rather than a carefully controlled medical study, so we can't say for certain that this is what's going on. But when a lot of signs point in the same direction, you're sort of inclined to think you're headed the right way.

One other interesting tidbit about pregnancy and IUDs. A study conducted at the University of Utah Medical School found that women who got pregnant while wearing IUDs were much heavier users of aspirin, downing an average of forty-one tablets a month. Those who didn't conceive averaged closer to six aspirins over the course of the month.[20] Some researchers feel that the antifertility effect of IUDs results from their stimulating in the uterine lining production of substances called prostaglandins. Good old aspirin, the painkiller more people prefer, works its magic by suppressing prostaglandin production in all parts of the body.

Another hint that it could be prostaglandins at work comes from a letter in the British medical journal *Lancet.* Two physicians report eight pregnancies in four women with IUDs who were taking anti-inflammatory drugs, either aspirin or cortisone-like drugs.[21] What makes this report particularly intriguing is the fact that these four women each became pregnant a second time while using an IUD. The doctors calculate the odds of such an event happening just due to the normal failure rate of an IUD at 1 in 10,000 woman-years. In other words, not ruddy likely.

That brings us full circle to the question of whether or not an IUD is a good method of contraception, but at this time, the question is academic. In February 1986, the G.D. Searle company voluntarily withdrew its **Cu-7** (copper seven) and **Tatum-T** IUDs, hoping to avoid future litigation. That virtually eliminates IUDs as an option for American women, with the current exception of the **Progestasert,** a hormone-containing IUD that must be replaced each year.

This is a shame because most women tolerate IUDs very well. Women with diabetes, high blood pressure or other cardiovascular problems, women over 40, and heavy smokers should stay away from oral contraceptives and might find the IUD an attractive alternative. Over two million women were using this method when Searle made its move, and most had experienced few if any problems. The most common side effects are an increased monthly flow—which is why the doctor may prescribe an iron supplement along with the IUD—and some menstrual cramping.

What about the risks of PID? Even though women using IUDs are at higher risk than those using birth-control pills or "barrier methods" of contraception such as condoms or a diaphragm, it appears that no more than 5 percent of users eventually suffer this complication. Some studies show that the percentage is much lower—around one percent.[22, 23] Women who have a variety of sexual partners are already at a higher risk of PID[24] and might want to choose a different contraceptive method.

Any woman wearing an IUD needs to know the early signs of pelvic infection so she can get medical attention promptly—and we do mean pronto, *not* next week. The warning signs include bleeding between periods, skipping a period, an exceptionally heavy period, unusual vaginal discharge, any abdominal pain aside from typical menstrual cramps, fever, or pain during intercourse. Early treatment of an infection may reduce the risk of later complications.

Other cautions we'd recommend: If any doctor starts talking about "medical diathermy," make *sure* she knows you have an IUD in place. This therapeutic use of heat often employs microwaves, and metal on an IUD, just like metal placed in a microwave oven, can attract more than its share of heat and possibly burn the uterus.

We'd also suggest that if you have to take cortisone-type medication, or any of the nonsteroidal anti-inflammatory drugs such as **Motrin, Rufen, Advil, Nuprin** (all ibuprofen), **Clinoril** (sulindac), **Tolectin** (tolmetin), **Feldene** (piroxicam), **Indocin** (indomethacin), **Naprosyn** (naproxen), or **Ponstel** (mefenamic acid), among others, large doses of aspirin or antibiotics that you add another birth-control method as a "backup" until you're no longer taking the drug. This might help you avoid becoming a contraceptive failure statistic.

So there you have them . . . advantages, disadvantages, cautions, and precautions pertaining to the IUD. By now it's surely clear why contraception is still not a simple, one-size-fits-all kind of decision.

## Vasectomy: The Men's Turn at Bat

Perhaps you've noticed something about all the birth-control methods we've talked about up to this point? Right: They're all for women.

It certainly isn't fair, but the major burden for contraception has traditionally fallen on the woman. Many feel that because most researchers and drug company executives are men, there's a bias in favor of developing contraceptive drugs and devices that work on the opposite sex.

There may be some truth to that, but it could also be that it's just plain easier to find a way to foil a single ovum once a month than it is to totally eliminate the millions of potentially impregnating sperm that go on their merry way with each ejaculation.

Which is not to say there haven't been any efforts to develop a "male Pill." There have, but each has ended in failure. Some of the birth control pills developed for men proved unsatisfactory because they simply failed to kill off enough sperm; others reduced the man's sexual desire. And a few produced female characteristics such as breast enlargement. Very few men are going to be enthusiastic about taking a contraceptive that makes them look as if they should go shopping for a training bra.

There is some exciting work being done by an international team at the University of California and in Montreal on a synthetic compound that is similar to a chemical naturally found in semen. The natural substance, called inhibin, acts as a messenger to the pituitary gland, telling it when there's sufficient FSH (follicle-stimulating hormone), a crucial link in the chain that leads to sperm production. By taking inhibin the body hasn't made, men might be able to shut down the process early and keep sperm counts—and fertility—down next to nothing.

But there is still a long way to go from synthesizing a drug in the laboratory to confirming that it can provide safe, effective, and acceptable contraception. It will require many years of testing before we will know whether inhibin will prove to be a contraceptive breakthrough or just another tantalizing dead end.

Right now the only effective male techniques of birth control remain the condom and vasectomy. Since the condom (also known as prophylactic, rubber, sheath, skin, etc.) depends to a great extent upon the motivation of the user in order to be effective, its batting average is not as good as other forms of contraception. That's not to say it can't be highly successful. It can, and it may also offer some protection against herpes and other sexually transmitted diseases. But many men don't use the device as carefully as they should, nor do many couples take advantage of the considerable extra contraceptive protection afforded by combining the condom with a sperm-killing vaginal foam.

That leaves vasectomy, a simple surgical operation in which the doctor makes a small incision to cut and tie off the tubes that carry sperm from the testes. The operation is simple and sure. It produces no change in hormones, and no alteration of a man's sex drive unless he somehow psychologically feels "castrated" by the surgery. Some men do, as evidenced by reports in the medical literature of psychological disturbances[25, 26] as well as long-term physical complaints[27] following vasectomy.

When the first edition of *The People's Pharmacy* was written, there was considerable concern about the possibility that men who'd had vasectomies would suffer a significantly higher rate of coronary heart disease. This was thought to be an outcome of their bodies producing substances to fight off the millions of sperm which were now being dumped into their systems and were being detected as a "foreign" substance by their immune systems. Some researchers feared that this immune response would end up yielding chemical substances that could damage the walls of arteries and make the men more likely to have heart or kidney trouble.

These concerns were founded on the results of animal studies in which vasectomy does seem to produce such results. We're happy to report, though, that several long-term studies in humans clearly show no increased health risk of any kind to men with vasectomies.

One study, conducted by a UCLA doctor and his colleagues, paired 10,590 vasectomized men with a like number of men identical in age, race, marital status, and other significant factors. They interviewed each to determine what health problems they experienced. "The incidence of overt cardiovascular disease found in this study," say the researchers, "was less among the vasectomized men than among the nonvasectomized men."[28] In fact, the vasectomized men came out slightly better on a number of health measures, including number of cancers and overall survival rate.

While vasectomy has now been given a clean bill of health, it continues to have one major drawback—it must be considered permanent. Men are told—or should be—that the operation is nonreversible and that restoration of fertility is practically impossible. Given the current state of the art, that must be considered true, and no man who has any question in his mind about wanting to father children should undergo a vasectomy, thinking it can be undone if his feelings change.

A lot of American couples are evidently deciding permanence is not a drawback. In 1982, sterilization became the most popular form of contraception in this country, if you lump vasectomies together with female sterilization.[29] Couples who have all the children they want and those who prefer to remain childless are opting for these permanent solutions to the contraceptive problem. But once in a while, a person changes her—or his—mind about that decision. Wouldn't it be great to have a technique that could be permanent, but could also be reversed?

One new method currently being tested might have this potential. It's called the Overblock, and it involves injecting silicone rubber into the Fallopian tubes and allowing it to harden into "plugs." With the pathway from ovary to uterus blocked, the ovum has no opportunity to meet a sperm cell and cause an unwanted pregnancy. Even if the Overblock proves irreversible, many women could be interested in it because it doesn't require surgery, dosing with hormones, or otherwise interfering with body chemistry.

The technique for placing the plugs is somewhat complex, involving a thirty- to ninety-minute procedure that can be conducted in the doctor's office under local anesthesia. Proper plug placement is confirmed by X-ray exam. So far about 20 percent of the women required a second procedure in order to get both tubes completely blocked. This percentage will presumably decline, however, as the technique is refined and perfected.

In theory, all that will be necessary to restore fertility is to literally "pull the plug," but at this time no one knows if this will really work to restore fertility. It must be considered a sterilization procedure until we have more data. If it is reversible, though, then according to one enthusiastic gynecologist, "it should become a major method of family planning."

## New Advances in Birth Control

Suppose you're not ready for a potentially permanent plug or vasectomy, and not too crazy about the Pill or the IUD? Well, take heart. First off, you've got plenty of company. And second, drug companies are scrambling hard to come up with better methods. After all, they're quite capable of counting up the numbers of people who need contraception. The market statistics are impressive, so the companies are investing in some fairly intensive research.

Perhaps the Perfect Contraceptive will emerge from this scientific effort, but more likely the number of options, methods with both pros and cons, will continue to grow. One that has already appeared on the scene is the contraceptive sponge, being sold under the brand name **Today**. The sponge (or perhaps the

Sponge) is a flat, round, polyurethane device with a dose of a spermicide in it. To use the sponge, a woman merely moistens it in water and inserts it over the cervix.

The sponge has a number of attractive features. First, it's sold over-the-counter. No doctor's visit, no prescription. Second, the device can be inserted and left in place for twenty-four hours. This answers the demand for a contraceptive device that doesn't interfere with the spontaneity many people value highly in their sexual relationships.

In clinical trials involving sixteen hundred women, the sponge was 85 percent effective. One FDA official pointed out that most of the pregnancies took place when women were still learning to use the device properly. With correct placement, the effectiveness rate appears to be roughly similar to that of the diaphragm.

The **Today** sponge was at one time supposed to be the **"2 Day"** sponge, since the original plan was that a woman would be able to keep it inserted for up to forty-eight hours. However, during the clinical trials too few women actually wore it that long for the tests to meet FDA certification rules. The company either had to change the name, or do more tests to support the forty-eight-hour feature. That's how they wound up going to market as **Today**.

The sponge is basically a combination of two old, tried-and-tested contraceptives. Placing a physical barrier over the cervix to keep sperm from getting in is the idea behind diaphragms and cervical caps. And the spermicide used in the **Today** sponge, nonoxynol-9, has been available in over-the-counter preparations for almost twenty years. By combining the two, the sponge's makers have given the device an extra measure of effectiveness. They've also created a device that's easier and more comfortable to use than a diaphragm, and which doesn't require individual fitting and thus doesn't require a doctor's intervention.

But some questions have been raised about toxic shock. While premarketing studies showed the sponge would not support growth of any of the organisms thought responsible for toxic shock, there were at least four confirmed reports of toxic shock associated with the sponge during its first year on the market. It is unclear whether the sponge was responsible, but some caution seems prudent. There is now a warning both on the outside of the **Today** package as well as in the package insert that tells women to see a doctor immediately if they have two or more symptoms of toxic shock (fever, vomiting, diarrhea, muscular pain, dizziness, or rash similar to sunburn).

An unexpected number of women using the sponge have had difficulty removing it. Because leaving the device in the body for more than twenty-four to thirty hours could increase the risk of developing toxic shock, it is important to contact the company Hotline (800) 223-2329; in California (800) 222-2329, or a physician if this problem develops. Other side effects that have been reported include vaginal irritation or infection.[30]

Lots more new contraceptives are hovering on the horizon, awaiting further research or clinical confirmation of their safety and effectiveness. For example, scientists at the University of California, San Diego, have produced a man-made version of a brain hormone which looks pretty promising as a once-a-month birth-control drug.

The natural brain hormone has the tongue-twisting name of luteinizing hormone-releasing hormone—mercifully abbreviated to LHRH by most people called upon to say it often. The lab version is 140 times as powerful as the natural stuff. In small doses, it corrects a certain infertility problem experienced by a small percentage of women. In larger doses, paradoxically, it works as a contraceptive.

Synthetic LHRH does its job by tinkering with the timing of the complex hormonal and physical apparatus of conception. Normally a woman's cycle consists of two approximately equal phases, with the midpoint being ovulation. When women are given the super-LHRH, though, they have a very long preovulation phase and a very short postovulation phase. So what? Well, the uterus continues on its old schedule, and is thus all primed and ready to receive an egg when there isn't one. About the time the ovum *does* arrive, the uterine lining is already starting to break down in preparation for a menstrual period.

One of super-LHRH's inventors, Dr. Samuel Yen, is the first to recognize the difficulties facing the substance. "The whole world is waiting for a better birth-control pill," he says, "but it is not going to come easily."

Many others are working on pills, injections, or implantable devices that would permit drugs to be taken either less often, or continuously but in much smaller doses. University of Alabama researchers have embedded a contraceptive dose of the drug norethindrone in microcapsules that can be injected, providing up to several months' protection from pregnancy as the drug is slowly released from the "tiny time pills." It's still too early to tell what side effects this may produce.

In another development, a Swiss firm is working on an anti-progesterone hormone which prevents the fertilized egg from implanting in the uterus. According to Dr. Walter Hermann at the University of Geneva, the drug has no apparent side effects and seems very promising.

For now, however, we're left with some pretty difficult choices. The methods now available all have their difficulties and downsides. Though the Pill and the IUD have hazards, they're by far the most certain forms of birth control. Simpler physical barrier methods, such as the condom and diaphragm, can be quite effective but they must (1) be used, and (2) used correctly.

As we warned you at the outset, there is no one "right" answer. In deciding on contraception, each person must weigh the risks of pregnancy against the risks of each birth control method, and then decide where the balance lies.

We feel strongly that any such choice is difficult enough without people lacking information on the true risks and benefits. In addition to the material in this chapter, anyone facing the birth control–method decision should search diligently for knowledgeable help in reviewing the choices. That help might come from a family planning center, a nurse-practitioner, or a physician.

Make certain you connect with someone who's prepared to give you all the information, rather than push their answer on you. It's a mighty serious decision, with tremendous implications for your health and happiness. There's no more important time to demand all your rights as a consumer than when deciding about birth control.

# References

1. Ory, Howard. "The Noncontraceptive Health Benefits from Oral Contraceptive Use." *Int. Fam. Planning Perspectives,* 8(3):93–95, 1982.

2. Rosenfield, Allan. "The Pill: An Evaluation of Recent Studies." *The Johns Hopkins Medical Journal* 150:177–180, 1982.

3. Pike, M. C., et al. "Breast Cancer in Young Women and the Use of Oral Contraceptives: Possible Modifying Effect of Formulation and Age at Use." *Lancet* ii:926–929, 1983.

4. The Centers for Disease Control Cancer and Hormone Study. "Long-term Oral Contraceptive Use and the Risk of Breast Cancer." *JAMA* 249:1591–1595, 1983.

5. Horwitz, Nathan. "Canadian Expert Panel Pans Pike Pill Study." *Medical Tribune,* Feb. 15, 1984, p. 7.

6. "Study Assailed for Linking Birth Control Pills, Cancer." *Raleigh News and Observer,* May 13, 1984, p. 15A.

7. "Researchers Rap Study Linking Pill to Cancer." *Durham Sun,* May 9, 1984, p. 2-C.

8. Rosenfield, Allan. op. cit., p. 177.

9. Graham, Sian, and Fraser, Ian S. "The Progestogen-only Mini-Pill." *Contraception,* 26(4):373–389, 1982.

10. "New Triphasic OC Adjusts Steroids to the Natural Menstrual Cycle." *Med. World News,* Dec. 10, 1984.

11. Speroff, Leon. "The Formulation of Oral Contraceptives: Does the Amount of Estrogen Make Any Clinical Difference?" *The Johns Hopkins Med. J.,* 150:170–176, 1982.

12. Ad Hoc Obstetric-Gynecology Advisory Committee. "Report of Safety and Efficacy of the Dalkon Shield and Other IUDs." Oct. 29–30, 1974.

13. Walsh, Mary Williams. "A. H. Robins Is Ordered to Tell Court about Missing Dalkon Shield Papers." *Wall Street Journal,* Aug. 20, 1984, p. 8.

14. Walsh, Mary Williams. "Robins Ex-Official Says He Destroyed Dalkon Shield Data." *Wall Street Journal,* Aug. 1, 1984, p. 17.

15. Lord, Judge Miles. Speech to E. C. Robins, Jr., William Forrest, and Dr. Lunsford. Minneapolis, Feb. 29, 1984.

16. Walsh, Mary Williams. "Judge's Remarks Chastising A. H. Robins in Dalkon Case Are Stricken from Record." *Wall Street Journal,* Nov. 5, 1984, p. 12.

17. Kaufman, David W., et al. "The Effect of Different Types of Intrauterine Devices on the Risk of Pelvic Inflammatory Disease." *JAMA* 250:759–762, 1983.

18. Dikshit, Suhasini, and Ledger, William J. "A Role of Antibiotics in the Contraceptive Effectiveness of an Intrauterine Foreign Body in the Rabbit." Unpublished report.

19. Wrenn, T. R., et al. *Abstracts, Society for the Study of Repro.* 3:23, 1970.

20. *News Front.* "Aspirin May Inhibit IUD Antifertility Effect." *Modern Medicine* 50(8):37–38, 1982.

21. Buhler, M., and Papiernik, E. "Successive Pregnancies in Women Fitted with Intrauterine Devices Who Take Anti-Inflammatory Drugs." *Lancet* i:483, 1983.

22. Westrom, L. "Incidence, Prevalence, and Trends of Acute Pelvic Inflammatory Disease and Its Consequences in Industrialized Countries." *Am. J. Ob. Gyn.* 138 (7, pt. 2):880–892, 1980.

23. O'Brien, F. B., et al. "Incidence of Pelvic Inflammatory Disease in Clinical Trials with Cu-7 (Intrauterine Copper Contraceptive): A Statistical Analysis." *Contraception* 27(2):111–122, 1983.

24. Burkman, R. T., and Women's Health Study. "Association between Intrauterine Device and Pelvic Inflammatory Disease." *Obstetrics and Gynecology* 57(3):269–276, 1981.

25. Johnson, M. H. *Am. J. Psychiat.,* 121:482, 1964.

26. Ziegler, F. J. "Vasectomy and Adverse Psychological Reactions. *Ann. Int. Med.* 73(5):853, 1970.

27. Wig, N. N., and Singh, S. "Psychosomatic Symptoms Following Male Sterilization." *Indian J. Med. Res.* 60:1386–1392, 1972.

28. Massey, Frank, et. al. "Vasectomy and Health." *JAMA* 252(8):-1023–1029, 1984.

29. "Study: Sterilization Now Most Popular Form of Birth Control." *Durham Sun,* Dec. 6, 1984, p. 8-A.

30. Cohen, Z., et al. "Use-Associated Problems with the Vaginal Contraceptive Sponge—A Preliminary Report." *Western J. Med.* 141:-380–381, 1984.

# 10

## Drugs and Children: Pregnancy to Puberty

---

*Most drugs NOT tested for children's use • Alcohol in cough and cold medicine can cause trouble • Drugs and pregnancy: Too much, too often, too dangerous • Alcohol, nicotine, caffeine, antibiotics, morning-sickness medicine • Drugs and the nursing mother • Cautions for kids • Common childhood problems: Diarrhea, ear infections, bedwetting, hyperactivity • Children and drug safety: Poisoning prevention • Table 1: Prescription Drugs That May Be Dangerous During Pregnancy • Table 2: Drugs and Breast Feeding.*

---

Children, it's said, should be seen and not heard. When it comes to prescription medications, children are neither seen *nor* heard because few of the medications handed out by the doctor have been properly tested on the pediatric population.

According to an American Academy of Pediatrics report to the FDA, "possibly as many as three quarters of the drugs used in hospital pediatric practice are not officially approved for the purpose for which they are commonly employed."[1] "Indeed," the report continues, "if the drugs marketed prior to 1962 are included, an even greater number of agents in current usage will be shown to lack substantial evidence of safety and efficacy."

As you've read earlier in this book, the process for testing new drugs is a long and tedious one at best, and the drug companies are not anxious to extend their financial (and legal) liabilities by going to the trouble of testing on children everything they come up with.

That's what would be required in order for the manufacturers to get labeling approval to say the drug worked on kids. It's easier, cheaper, and safer to simply say "safety and dosage have not been established for pediatric use." Such a disclaimer is colloquially called CYA (cover your a**). It is a colossal cop-out because it absolves the drug company of all blame, yet leaves the conscientious doctor hanging in limbo.

On the surface it might appear that this is a very simple matter. Any drug that has not been proved safe just should not be used. But in the real world it doesn't work that way at all.

We'll let you in on a little medical secret. When the drug companies say something like "safety and dosage have not been established for pediatric use," that does *not* necessarily mean the drug can't or shouldn't be used for children. As the American Academy of Pediatrics report so candidly states, "With few exceptions, marketed drugs find their way into widespread use and are, in fact, administered to pregnant women, infants, and children, despite disclaimer statements in the package insert."

What the drug company says, with a big wink of its corporate eye, is "Okay, doc, *you* know what this drug does, and *we* know what it does, and you know we can't say it's safe for use on children, so we're not saying anything, but . . ."

What happens then is a logical outcome of our tendency to see children as simply little big people. The doctor knows that a 150-pound person gets 15 milligrams of Drug X in order to solve Problem Y. Faced with a 50-pound child who has the same problem, simple logic tells him that 5 milligrams should do the trick.

Unfortunately, simple logic isn't always right. When it comes to drugs, children are much more (and much less) than just smaller versions of adults. Their immature organ systems often deal with drugs far differently than their grown-up version will a few years later, and the differences can lead to anything from uncomfortable reactions to deadly ones.

To take just one example, the *British Medical Journal* not long ago carried a report of three cases in which children suffered "severe and disturbing" visual hallucinations after taking small doses of Actifed, which contains the antihistamine triprolidine and the decongestant pseudoephedrine.

*Case 1*—. . . Six hours after receiving a single dose [5 ml Actifed; a three-and-one-half-year-old girl] presented screaming and unconsolable, complaining of seeing crabs, snakes, and spiders. She said that insects were biting her and that a crocodile was making a hole in her back. . . . When examined she was pushing invisible objects off herself and stamping on other invisible objects on the floor . . .

*Case 2*—A 3-year-old girl received two 5-ml doses of Actifed during the night. The following day she suddenly developed episodes of uncontrollable terror, complaining of seeing spiders and insects. On examination she was intermittently pushing and brushing away invisible objects and also hitting out and stamping . . .

*Case 3*—A 2-year-old boy with . . . frequent coughs and fevers was given Actifed and Actifed Compound in 5-ml doses at night whenever he was feverish. He was described as always being delirious when ill, seeing spiders and insects in bed and pushing them away. This was initially thought to be due to fever, but when promethazine (Phenergan) was substituted for Actifed there were no further episodes despite his fever.[2]

The doctors reporting these cases suggest that pseudoephedrine was probably the culprit, and that "it may produce visual hallucinations in children even when administered at the usual clinical dose."[3]

Pseudoephedrine, by the way, is available in a large number of cough and cold remedies such as **Actamine Liquid, Allerfrin OTC Syrup, Carbodec Syrup, Contac Severe Cold Formula Liquid, CoTylenol Cold Formula Liquid, Co-Pyronil 2, Endotussin-NN Pediatric Syrup, Fedahist Syrup, Novafed A Liquid, Novahistine DH Liquid, Nyquil Nighttime Colds Medicine Liquid, Pedi-Tot Pediatric Cough Syrup, Rhinosyn-PD Syrup, Robitussin-PE Syrup, Ryna Liquid, Sudafed Plus Syrup, Triacin Syrup,** and **Tussend Liquid.**

We have seen no reports of children experiencing visual hallucinations on such medications, but the British physicians note that:

> **Visual hallucinations are uncommon in young children, and their occurrence leads to considerable alarm if the cause is not recognised. Many parents do not regard Actifed and other decongestants as drugs when bought over the counter. . . . In addition, we have anecdotal evidence of an increased incidence of nightmares, night terrors, and behavior problems in children taking Actifed, but this is difficult to evaluate as these problems are common among children.[4]**

What all this means is that we don't have any idea how common are drug-induced psychological problems in children. Doctors are quick to blame nightmares and other unusual disturbances on the illness rather than the treatment. No adult would think to blame a nice simple OTC medicine like **Actifed, Sudafed, Nyquil,** or **Robitussin PE,** since grown-ups rarely have difficulty with these medications.

Alcohol is another problem. In most states in the United States, you have to be at least eighteen years old to buy booze. Many states won't allow beer, wine, or other alcoholic beverages to be sold to anyone under twenty-one. Yet a child can walk into almost any supermarket or drugstore in the country, plunk down a couple of bucks, and legally walk out with a bottle containing anywhere from 50- to 80-proof alcohol. In fact, many kids are given medicine with high alcohol content by their unsuspecting, well-intentioned parents.

Many of the most popular cold and cough remedies contain whopping doses of alcohol. **Nyquil, Dristan Ultra Colds Formula, Contac Severe Cold Formula,** and **Robitussin Night Relief** are 50-proof. **Comtrex, Romilar III,** and **Halls Decongestant Cough Formula** are 40-proof or more. Terpin hydrate elixir can be more than 80-proof. That's equivalent to gin, vodka, or whiskey. Even medicine designed specifically for children can contain quite a bit of alcohol. **Contac Jr.** is 20-proof.

A report by the American Academy of Pediatrics, prepared for the FDA and published in March 1984, warned that

> **even small amounts of alcohol can affect a child's central nervous system, causing decreased reaction time, muscular incoordination, and behavioral changes. Alcohol-containing medications also may affect the way other drugs behave in the child's body.**[5]

The real problem with children consuming alcohol, however, is hypoglycemia—or low blood sugar. Alcohol keeps the liver from making glucose, the simple sugar that fuels the body. This is especially a problem when children have not had much to eat, a common situation when they are ill. Because children use up glucose quickly, it doesn't take a lot of alcohol to cause hypoglycemia.

Another area where children can get into trouble is with mouthwash. No adult would ever consider drinking **Scope** or **Signal,** but according to the FDA, children may not realize the purpose or the danger of mouthwash.

> **The bright colors and pleasing flavors of these products make them particularly tempting to youngsters. The bottles, usually without child-proof caps, are easily accessible in the family bathroom. Persuasive television advertising depicts people smiling happily after using that minty green**

liquid, but they are never shown spitting it out. A young viewer might think the product is supposed to be swallowed.

Whether it is this mistaken notion or some other reason that prompts them to take a swig of mouthwash, children have been accidentally poisoned by these pretty liquids, some of which contain more alcohol than beer or wine.[6]

What is so shocking about alcohol in drugs is that in most cases it doesn't need to be there, at least not in children's medicine. The Committee on Drugs of the American Academy of Pediatrics is quite clear that the amount of alcohol in over-the-counter medication should be no more than 5 percent. These doctors go on to say that "physician supervision is suggested for children less than age 6 years using OTC preparations containing alcohol." Most important of all, they recommend that "continued efforts should be made to have alcohol removed from liquid preparations for children."[7]

So next time your child has a cold or a cough, don't just pass the **Nyquil, Comtrex,** or **Contac Jr.** In fact, why not read the label and make sure there's no alcohol, period. And while you're reading labels, you may want to think twice before giving your young person **Actifed, Sudafed,** or any other cold remedy with a decongestant. Preparations that contain ingredients such as pseudoephedrine or phenylpropanolamine (PPA) may cause insomnia or nightmares, not to mention other unpleasant psychological reactions.

If adult-tested drugs are such a problem for kids, the solution would appear obvious—any drug not proved safe just shouldn't be used. Unfortunately, things aren't quite that easy or obvious. Take away the drugs not tested for pediatric use and you'd eliminate quite a bit of the doctor's pharmacological arsenal.

To understand the dilemma, let's take a look at a hypothetical case. Jenny Jones, age nine, has suffered for five weeks with a severe ear infection, and none of the antibiotics tried so far have helped. The infection is worsening, Jenny is in intense pain and dizzy, and her mother wants *something* done—and done quickly.

The doctor knows of a drug that should kill the resistant bacteria causing Jenny's infection. The medication has been used for more than six years in adults with excellent results and few side effects. But the drug label says that "safety and dosage have not been established for pediatric use." What would you do if you had to make this decision?

Not so easy or obvious a choice, is it? Now you understand some of the problems faced by patients, doctors, and drug companies when it comes to medications for kids.

Sometimes that problem is made even worse by mundane mistakes in the directions on prescription drug labels . . . you know, "Shake well, take one teaspoon three times a day with meals." In a study of more than 2,200 prescriptions for seventy of the drugs used most frequently with children, doctors at Los Angeles County–University of Southern California Medical Center found that only 5 percent of those prescriptions "contained no errors or omissions."[8]

Now that's incredible! We're talking about a major health center here, folks. Top-notch pediatricians and residents worked in this facility. And yet most of the prescriptions they wrote were incorrect in one way or another. Although many of the mistakes were relatively minor, "more than one third of the prescriptions with dosage specified contained an error."[9] In light of this, the researchers say, "the chance of a patient's receiving sufficient medication to maintain a therapeutic blood level is about 1 in 30."[10] The kids might be better off taking their chances at the gambling tables in Las Vegas.

There *is* no one answer, no easy solution. What parents *can* do is be aware of the problems involved. This awareness must begin with pregnancy. Until children are adults in terms of their bodies' handling medication, their only protection is the vigilance of parents and the awareness of physicians.

## Drugs and Pregnancy

Everyone agrees that the process of pregnancy and birth is something of a miracle. And yet we often meddle with the delicate cellular process taking place in a mother's body by administering powerful chemicals during the nine months of gestation.

Stop and consider for a second what happens in pregnancy. Starting with just two cells, an indescribably complex series of events takes place which allows those cells to multiply and differentiate until there's a baby with trillions of cells and dozens of organs. Billions of biochemical reactions take place during those nine months. Disruption of just one may mean deformation, disability, or death for the growing fetus.

Nevertheless, some pregnant women continue taking drugs that have never been proved safe for use during pregnancy. In fact, because of the ethical considerations involved, it is unlikely there will be clinical testing of very many drugs on pregnant women. So anything a woman takes while pregnant should be considered an experiment, unless there is evidence to the contrary.

One would think that after the thalidomide tragedy, when thousands of European children were born with birth defects caused by their mothers' sleeping pills, women and doctors would have learned a painful lesson. Unfortunately, that doesn't seem to be the case. A study published in the *British Medical Journal* revealed that of 1,369 women, 97 percent took at least one medication during their pregnancy.[11]

Many other reports have come up with comparable—or worse —numbers. One found 100 percent of those surveyed used *at least* two drugs during pregnancy, and 93.4 percent took five or more.[12] A study of middle- and upper-class Houston women found they'd used an average of *ten* different drugs during pregnancy, with antibiotics and antacids heading the list. One woman took twenty-five aspirin tablets daily during her pregnancy. Asked about it, she said, "If I'd known aspirin was a drug, I wouldn't have taken it."[13]

But aspirin *is* a drug. Not only can it prolong pregnancy and labor, aspirin may increase the risk of bleeding disorders and low birth weight.

Most people overlook many of the chemicals that they commonly consume. Alcohol, nicotine, laxatives, vitamins, tranquilizers, antacids, and antinausea medications can all affect the unborn baby. Everything the doctor prescribes is a drug, but so are over-the-counter remedies.

The fetus is most susceptible to birth defects during the first few weeks of pregnancy. A woman could inadvertently expose her baby to a hazardous drug even before she realized she was pregnant. For all of these reasons, Dr. Kurt Hirschhorn of Mount Sinai Medical Center in New York emphatically told a meeting of the National Foundation–March of Dimes that no woman in her childbearing years should take any drug that is not essential to preserve her health unless she is absolutely positive she is not pregnant.[14]

Once, not so very long ago, doctors believed something called the placental barrier isolated the developing infant and prevented substances in the mother's bloodstream from reaching the fetus. But like the sound barrier, the placental barrier belongs to the past. "Until proven otherwise," experts in the field now say, "most commercially available drugs are able to pass the placenta and reach the fetus with ease."[15] Several British experts, assessing the situation, said "It is now generally considered that most (if not all) drugs present in maternal blood will reach the fetal circulation to some extent."[16]

Although an expectant mother should ideally avoid all drugs and other chemicals as much as possible, no one expects her to live on just bread and water for nine months. Obviously, a lot of women have gotten pregnant and had healthy babies while drinking, smoking, and taking both prescription and nonprescription medications. On the other hand, we would all like to improve the odds as best we can. Let's take a look at some of the chemicals that could pose potential problems.

*Alcohol*—Here's a substance that's ubiquitous in our society, and which too often is not even recognized as a drug. That little glass of white wine at lunch or a scotch-and-soda after work seem so innocuous. Yet in sufficient quantity, alcohol can cause something terrible called Fetal Alcohol Syndrome (FAS).

Babies born with FAS suffer severe birth defects. They are smaller than normal at birth and continue to be underweight; they have characteristic facial abnormalities, heart problems, and kidney complications, as well as irregularities of the fingers. Mental retardation and attention-deficit disorders are not uncommon with this syndrome.[17]

Now most of these problems are the outcome of heavy drinking, and most pregnant women aren't alcoholics. But the scary question is, how much effect does a modest alcohol intake have? Unfortunately, we don't have a good answer to that one.

Newspaper headlines variously report, on the one hand, "Liquor Linked to Pregnancy Woes,"[18] while announcing on the other that "Moderate-Drinking Pregnant Women May Not Hurt Babies."[19] With such conflicting information, what's a pregnant woman to believe?

I don't have a crystal ball or a corner on insight. But I am big on lowering risks. One group of investigators concluded that "infants exposed to alcohol in utero, even in moderate amounts, appear to suffer from a spectrum of developmental mental and motor delays. Severe problems typically present early, while the more subtle changes may become apparent only when the children enter school."[20]

That's good enough for me. Even if they're wrong and "modest" alcohol consumption doesn't cause damage, why take even the smallest risk? Swearing off the sauce for nine months seems a small price to pay to have the healthiest baby possible.

*Smoking*—It's certainly no secret that smoking isn't good for you. Everyone except the tobacco industry agrees on that. But some people don't seem to think about how maternal smoking affects the developing baby.

In late 1984, the American Cancer Society developed a hard-hitting series of television ads showing a fetus in the womb . . . smoking. "Would you give a cigarette to your unborn child?" asks the voiceover. "You do every time you smoke when you're pregnant. Pregnant mothers: Please don't smoke."

The reasons for this warning are clear. Nicotine and other byproducts of smoking enter the fetal circulation and have a wide range of effects. As far back as the 1930s, doctors reported that fetal heart rate was altered when mothers smoked.

More recently, investigators from the Maryland School of

Medicine reported the results of a study examining the effect of smoking on birth weight.[21] Birth weight is an important measure of how well an infant will do during the first months of life. Generally speaking, low-birth-weight babies have more problems, and mothers who smoke have about twice the risk of giving birth to an infant weighing less than 2,500 grams (about 5.5 pounds).

Knowing this, the Maryland researchers divided 935 pregnant smokers into two groups. One group continued smoking. The other received all kinds of support and encouragement to cut down or quit. Chemical testing shortly before birth showed that the intervention group had indeed significantly reduced their smoking habit. In fact, 43 percent had quit entirely. And the babies benefited. Infants born to the low-smoking group were on average both heavier and longer (as measured head-to-toe) than those born to women whose smoking was not reduced.[22]

In summing up the evidence on smoking and pregnancy, two reviewers conclude that "A relationship exists between maternal smoking and low birth weight, decreased length, spontaneous abortion, fetal, neonatal, and postnatal deaths, prematurity, abruptio placenta, stillbirth, placenta previa, premature rupture of the membranes, delayed crying time, decrease in fetal breathing time, impaired reading attainment, and hyperkinesis."[23]

That's quite a burden to place on a baby just so that its mother can enjoy the pleasure of smoking. We'll loudly second the American Cancer Society's plea: "Pregnant mothers, please don't smoke."

*Coffee/caffeine*—I know, I know, it's beginning to sound as though everything you like is bad. Unfortunately, very high levels of caffeine (from tea and cola drinks as well as coffee) have been linked to a higher incidence of abortion and prematurity.[24]

However, a number of studies show no deleterious effects on the outcome of pregnancy. At this time it appears there is little, if any, danger in moderate coffee consumption, moderate meaning a few cups a day. The real coffee compulsives, the ten-cup-a-day people, might be well advised to give themselves and their babies-in-waiting a break by cutting back.

*Prescription drugs*—In general, drugs are available by prescription because they are powerful chemical substances which can often cause almost as many problems as they cure. It's only logical that such medications could cause trouble for the developing fetus. Pregnant women should be the world's most reluctant consumers of prescription medication, and the last to insist that the doctor give them a prescription for every last ache and pain.

In Table 1 at the end of this chapter you'll find a partial list of prescription drugs for which there is concern about safe use in pregnant women. While many medications can cause complications when used during pregnancy, certain categories of drugs have proved particularly troublesome. Extra caution is called for when the doctor starts talking about prescribing anything in the following groups:

- *Antibiotics*—Many of the most popular types of antibiotics are either known to cause problems or are strongly suspected of doing so.

    At the top of the list is the widely used tetracycline and its chemical cousins, which appear under a bewildering array of brand names, including **Achromycin V, Aureomycin, Azotrex, Cyclopar, Deltamycin, Kesso-Tetra, Mysteclin-F, Panmycin, Robitet, Sumycin, Terramycin, Tetra-C, Tetracyn, and Tetrex.** Tetracycline can cause discoloration of baby teeth which will later emerge, and it's also responsible for impaired bone growth.

    Other antibiotics on the watch-out list include sulfas such as the sulfonamides (**Gantanol, Gantrisin, SK-Soxazole,** sulfamethoxazole, sulfisoxazole), which may cause cleft palate, anemia, and jaundice.

- *Anticonvulsants*—The epileptic woman is in a real bind. Many of the drugs commonly prescribed to prevent seizures have been linked to birth defects. **Dilantin** (phenytoin) may increase the risk of facial deformities, limb defects, and mild to moderate mental retardation. **Depakene** (valproic acid), another anticonvulsant, has been associated with a slightly increased risk of spina bifida, a condition in which the child is born with spinal-cord irregularities. Women who receive the antiepileptic drug **Tridione** (trimethadione) during their pregnancies may increase the risk of growth retardation, developmental delay, speech disturbances, and V-shaped eyebrows.[25]

Stopping medication during pregnancy, however, can also be dangerous, since the mother's uncontrolled seizures could also be harmful to both her and the fetus. If you are epileptic, you will want to discuss these issues in detail with your physician to try and minimize the risk for your baby. *Morning-Sickness Medicine*— Many pregnant women suffer from nausea, especially during the first trimester. Unfortunately, that's when the developing infant is most sensitive to drugs passing through the bloodstream.

Until recently the FDA had sanctioned only one drug for treating morning sickness—**Bendectin** (Vitamin B₆ and doxylamine). But then even **Bendectin** was removed from the market in 1984 by a manufacturer that had grown weary of a deluge of lawsuits charging that the drug caused birth deformities. As of this writing, there is no drug available which is approved for this use.

Merrell Dow, the maker of **Bendectin,** finally threw in the towel with 325 lawsuits pending. It was paying a *monthly* insurance tab of $1 million. "The burdens of continuing to market **Bendectin**," said company president David Sharrock, "have become just too heavy."[26]

There has been a long, bitter, and inconclusive debate as to whether the drug really did cause birth defects. Everyone from public-interest health groups to an FDA advisory committee has reviewed the scientific evidence, and nobody agrees on exactly what it means. In this case, as so often in medicine, the data are neither black nor white. The FDA committee felt pretty certain that **Bendectin** wasn't a strong promoter of birth defects, but at the same time it expressed "residual uncertainty" that the drug might cause problems at least once in a while.

Now here's the catchy part of the catch-22. One of the active ingredients in **Bendectin** was doxylamine, an antihistamine that is found in many OTC remedies, sometimes in higher doses than **Bendectin** contained. Products such as **NyQuil, Contac Severe Cold Formula, Nytime Cold Medicine, Decapryn, Consotuss, Vicks Formula 44 Cough Mixture, Mercodol with Decapryn,** and **Unisom** remain on the market.

That in itself isn't so shocking, but if you check the labels you'll be hard put to find a warning that they should not be used during pregnancy. The point is that even over-the-counter medications may pose problems for the pregnant woman. For example, a nonprescription antinausea drug called **Marezine** (cyclizine) has been shown to cause birth defects in rats. It and a similar compound called **Antivert** (meclizine) were widely used for nausea and vomiting in pregnancy prior to the thalidomide tragedy of 1956. Sporadic cases of congenital defects were soon reported in offspring of women who had received the drugs.[27] A woman who did not realize she was pregnant might easily try such an OTC medication as **Marezine** to control her nausea. Unwittingly, she could be exposing her baby to a dangerous chemical, even though it's considered safe enough to be sold without a prescription.

Since **Bendectin** was the only drug approved by the FDA for treating nausea in pregnant women, doctors and their pregnant patients are limited in their options. They can try nondrug treatments such as eating soda crackers or popcorn, following a bland diet, drinking plenty of fluids, etc., or experiment with other antinausea drugs. Unfortunately, we know little about their potential to cause birth defects.

In considering this dilemma one expert concluded that "Drugs should be prescribed only when the risk of damage to the mother and fetus from the complications of nausea and vomiting is greater than the risk of teratogenic [birth defect] effects."[28]

## Drugs and the Nursing Mother

The newborn baby is not safe from dangerous side effects after delivery. Far from it. Many drugs can be transmitted from the mother to her baby through breast milk.

Picture the following situation. A woman bears her fourth child and decides she doesn't want more children. After two or three months, she begins taking birth-control pills again, never thinking to ask if her oral contraceptive might be dangerous to her nursing baby. Neither her obstetrician nor the child's pediatrician mentions complications. Yet an American Medical Association consultant had this to say: "It is neither wise nor advisable to prescribe oral contraceptives to nursing mothers."[29]

Part of the problem lies with nutrition. The Pill reduces the mother's milk supply and adversely affects its protein, fat, and vitamin content. There has also been concern raised that the hormones in birth-control pills may cause feminization of male babies.[30]

This is just one example. It applies to many other commonly prescribed medications. Table 2 at the end of this chapter provides a list of drugs that may be hazardous to nursing infants.

As in many other matters having to do with mother and child, this is not an area of cut-and-dried clinical conclusions. What we know for certain is that in many cases drugs given the mother will show up in her breast milk. But we don't often know exactly how that may affect her nursing baby.

**Valium** (diazepam) is a widely used antianxiety drug. It shows up in breast milk. Is the baby adversely affected by being administered **Valium**? If enough infants are exposed, will some suffer difficulties in getting off the drug, just as some adults seem to find themselves "hooked" on **Valium**? Nobody knows.

Perhaps the most important point is that many drugs and their by-products show up in a mother's milk in unpredictable quantities. Once again both doctor and patient are in the position of conducting an experiment in which the baby is the one at risk of adverse effects.

## Cautions for Kids

Once a newborn baby survives all the pitfalls and dangers of the first few months of life, you would think the worst is over. Not so.

Take something as seemingly benign as baby powder. Many new mothers and fathers get tremendous satisfaction out of liberally shaking out great clouds of talcum powder all over a baby's bottom, especially after bathing or changing a diaper.

How could something as American as apple pie, motherhood, or baby powder be dangerous? The answer is that poison control centers have documented side effects such as vomiting, coughing, difficulty breathing, and occasionally pneumonia and even death in children who have accidentally inhaled large amounts of baby powder.

Granted, this happens primarily when the infant gets hold of the bottle, shakes or drops it, and breathes large amounts of powder. Parents who use restraint while powdering, and who keep the container out of a toddler's inquisitive reach will generally be safe. But why tempt fate? In most instances baby powder is totally unnecessary.

Young children are vulnerable to all sorts of drugs and even to the way in which those drugs are given. Because it's virtually impossible to get a very young child to swallow a pill, doctors often resort to injections. One of the favorite shots is an IM, or intramuscular, injection. This involves placing—or trying to place—the drug between layers of muscle, where an ample supply of small capillaries guarantees the drug a quick route to the bloodstream.

Unfortunately, there's always the risk of hitting a nerve or blood vessel, and in children the risk is heightened because they have proportionally less muscle mass. Children, especially infants, should *never* receive an injection in the buttocks. There isn't enough muscle there yet to fully protect the delicate sciatic nerve. In the past, deformaties or limps were often attributed to polio when the real cause was a misplaced injection.

The proper location for an IM shot is the triceps muscle of the arm or the outer surface of the thigh muscle, which is both safer and less painful.

What really counts most, of course, is what the patient is getting. At the risk of beating a dead horse, I cannot resist mentioning tetracycline once more. Kids are subject to a whole lot of minor infections, and in past years it has been almost a reflex for the doctor to prescribe tetracycline, usually under one of its fancy (and thus more expensive) brand names. The problem with this reflex is that it runs the not-inconsiderable risk of causing a permanent and disfiguring discoloration of the teeth in children.

In a study of the prescribing patterns of 1,947 Tennessee physicians, it was discovered that 27 percent had given tetracycline to children younger than eight.[31] This despite the admonition by the Committee on Drugs of the American Academy of Pediatrics that "There are few if any reasons for using tetracycline drugs in children less than 8 years old."[32] The authors of the study stated:

> **The use of tetracycline in this age group is associated with a number of adverse effects, including dental staining, enamel hypoplasia, inhibition of bone growth, the "bulging fontanel syndrome" [abnormal skull growth], *Candida albicans* [yeast] superinfection, gastroenteritis, phototoxicity, and rashes, among others. These complications have been known for years; a warning listing these problems has been included in the official labeling (package insert) since 1970. . . . Yet tetracycline continues to be prescribed widely for young children.[33]**

Doctors aren't the only ones at fault. Well-meaning parents often badger physicians for an antibiotic when little Jonathan has a cold, even though viral infections won't benefit from such medication.

Parents are also guilty of administering incorrect or hazardous medicines to their children. A study conducted by Georgetown

University in 1975 revealed that as many as 20 percent of kids under two received potentially dangerous nonprescription drugs. Something as simple and seemingly harmless as aspirin can be quite hazardous to a youngster if given in anything but a properly reduced dose. So shape up, Mom and Dad, you should be as cautious (or more so) about the drugs you give the kids as you are about the ones you take. And we hope that by now you're quite cautious about those.

## Common Childhood Problems

Parents of young children may sometimes feel that their kids bounce from one health crisis to another. If it's not an ear infection, it's a sore throat, a tummyache, or a runny nose. Naturally, any parent wants to help a child feel better as soon as possible. But while it doesn't make sense to delay treatment, it's important not to overreact and possibly make matters worse.

- *Diarrhea*—As day-care centers have become more and more the norm through the 1970s and early 1980s, epidemiologists (those who study the pattern of disease in the population) have noted a rise in the reported incidence of childhood diarrhea. A bit of detective work soon made it clear that infections were being spread at child-care centers when hurried workers failed to wash their hands carefully after diapering infants. Their hands, sometimes contaminated with fecal bacteria, then became the vehicle for spreading the infection to other youngsters.

  Diarrhea may seem more an annoyance than a life-threatening disease, and that's generally true, but you should be aware that its risks are greater for children. It's pretty easy for a child to become dehydrated, or to lose large amounts of the electrolytes (sodium, potassium, chloride, etc.), which are responsible for keeping the proper cellular rhythms going. For that reason diarrhea in a child should always be taken seriously. And you should double that dose of caution when you're talking about an infant.

In most cases the cure will simply consist of withholding food temporarily while the child is given clear liquids. Normally, I encourage parents to banish soft drinks from their houses, but there are times when I break down and actually suggest a cola beverage or ginger ale if it will tempt an under-the-weather child to take a few sips. If you want to use what the pediatricians recommend, you will want to invest in **Pedialyte** or **Lytren**. These special liquid supplements are designed to replenish electrolytes in the proper balance.

You will definitely want to *avoid* **Lomotil** (diphenoxylate and atropine). This adult diarrhea medicine can be especially dangerous for children. It requires very careful supervision by a physician if it is to be administered at all. One OTC medication that has been reported to be safe and effective is **Mitrolan** (polycarbophil).[34] It should not be used if abdominal obstruction is suspected, but otherwise this drug is quite benign. The dose for children six to twelve years old is one tablet (500 mg) twice a day. The tablet is chewed before swallowing and is designed to restore a more proper water balance in the stool.

Diarrhea that doesn't go away by itself in twenty-four hours probably deserves medical attention. It could be a symptom of serious infection, appendicitis, food poisoning, or goodness knows what.

- *Ear infections*—If there is one, classic disease of childhood it would certainly be *otitis media*—middle-ear infections. Sometimes it seems children are born with ear infections, and they often have a hard time escaping them.

Chronic ear infections are uncomfortable for the child, distressing for the parents, and potentially dangerous. Yet there remains tremendous controversy over what to do about the garden-variety ear infection.

Some doctors favor aggressive drug therapy, others opt for insertion of a tiny tube to aid in drainage of infected material, and still others give minimal treatment and just wait for the child to outgrow the problem.

The last course is, in my opinion, totally unacceptable since it runs the very real risk of leading to hearing damage. It's a risk we don't think can be justified in view of good evidence that antibiotic treatment *will* help clear these stubborn infections.

But selecting the right antibiotic has become something of an art form. The problem is drug resistance. It used to be that simple penicillin would clear up most ear infections. But today there are all sorts of microscopic beasties roaming around, and many seem capable of withstanding drugs like penicillin, ampicillin, and amoxicillin. Pediatricians often have to resort to newer and more expensive broad-spectrum agents like **Ceclor** (cefaclor), or **Bactrim** or **Septra** (trimethoprim and sulfamethoxazole).

These drugs usually do the trick, but parents and pediatricians must treat them with respect. While safe for most children during short-term therapy, complications occasionally occur. A grandmother who read our newspaper column wrote to report the following tragedy:

**Last year our 6-year-old grandson was put on Septra for a month because of ear problems. He took the prescribed medicine for three weeks, when he developed a severe rash, terrible itching and hemorrhaging under the skin. His doctor sent him to an allergist. He was admitted to Children's Hospital with Stevens-Johnson Syndrome and died soon after. His liver, they said, was totally destroyed. Please warn other parents and spare some other child the agony he went through.**

What a heartbreaking story. We have no way of knowing for sure whether this drug really was responsible in this case. But there are instances in the medical literature of such severe symptoms occurring. Once again we are reminded that even "safe" drugs can occasionally cause severe, even life-threatening reactions. The FDA reports a number of deaths in children associated with these kinds of medications. Side effects have ranged from devastating damage to the skin, to blood and liver damage. Parents must be especially vigilant when giving medicine to children. ANY unusual behavior or side effects (especially skin rash) should be reported to the physician immediately!

- *Bed-wetting*—To the doctor it's "nocturnal enuresis." To the parent it's "bed-wetting." And to the child it's mortifying, distressing, and sometimes psychologically disabling.

  It's estimated that twenty million American youngsters over the age of five are bed-wetters.[35] In our society, where we often expect instant relief for everything that bothers us, it's no surprise that both doctors and patients (actually, parents of patients) are quick to look to drugs as the magic solution. But I'm here to tell you that there are no magic pills, and in most cases there probably shouldn't be any pills at all.

  Unfortunately, when Mom says, "She still wets the bed, Doctor," the physician's reaction is often to prescribe. As the *British Medical Journal* put it in an editorial, "Use of the word *enuresis* has raised bed-wetting to the status of a disease that requires a drug to cure it—when in fact in most cases the child is normal."[36]

  If the doctor does prescribe, there's a high likelihood the drug will be **Tofranil** (imipramine), which is primarily an antidepressant for adults. Once again we have a case where a drug is prescribed because of its side effects. A child gets **Tofranil** not because of its antidepressant activity, but because it leads to urinary retention.

  Several studies show that imipramine does work, in the sense that it reduces the frequency of bed-wetting. But the price may be high. "Between one in five and one in ten of the children treated with imipramine are said to have become nervous and irritable and to have had difficulty sleeping. Other adverse effects include restlessness, tearfulness, dizziness, nausea, and difficulty with concentration on schoolwork.''[37]

Even worse is the danger of poisoning inherent in offering such potent medication to young children. One report tells of two school-aged boys who took an overdose of imipramine. One eight-year-old had been dry for a while, then awoke wet one morning. He went to the medicine chest, got the imipramine, and took an estimated forty pills. He died twelve hours after being rushed to the hospital.[38]

The second victim was seven years old. He was promised a new belt if he'd stay dry four nights in a row. He'd taken imipramine unsuccessfully before, and his older sister was still being treated with it, so he took ten of her pills and wound up in the hospital semiconscious and with hallucinations.

Hardly seems worth it, does it?

Parents of bed-wetters often fail to realize that a good many children just don't have the physical maturity to have complete bladder control until they're a bit older. While many make it by age five, about a quarter won't. Becoming anxious, angry, demanding, or demeaning (or sometimes all of those) compounds the child's physical problem and adds a psychological one.

Experts in the field are convinced that much bed-wetting results from emotional stress in the first place. Arrival of a new baby, difficulty in school, or parental disharmony can all aggravate the situation. With luck, enuresis of this type will disappear all by itself when the psychological environment improves.

There are lots of stops along the way before drug treatment should even be considered. Just living patiently with the problem for a while will often be the cure. You may be able to speed the process along by offering encouragement and prizes for dry nights, but not in such a way as to create the situation mentioned above. The child should have the responsibility for keeping a chart of dry and wet nights and should receive lots of praise, accompanied with gold stars and a special treat, for each success.

The young person should also have the responsibility for changing wet sheets and seeing that they are placed in an appropriate place for washing. In this way the idea is transmitted—without punishment—that the child is responsible for his actions. It may also be of some benefit to cut down on fluid intake well before bedtime and have Mom or Dad wake up the child at various intervals throughout the night to go to the bathroom.

For those who must intervene, a variety of alarm systems that help the child help himself have proved relatively effective over the years. Products with hokey names like **Wee Alarm** and **Wee-Alert** are effective conditioners. Conditioning involves the use of a battery-operated apparatus that sounds an alarm when a small amount of urine touches two electrodes and closes a circuit. If placed under the child's sheet, it will wake him up at the first sign of wetting.

In order to work effectively, the child should be encouraged not to wear pajama bottoms. Lots of reassurance should be provided in the beginning, because kids can be frightened by the mystery or complexity of the thing. Each child should be taught how to set the alarm himself and what is expected—that whenever the buzzer goes off he or she is expected to get up and go to the bathroom and then reset the alarm.

Mom and Dad should be prepared to wake the child up at the sound of the ring during the first few weeks of treatment until he gets the hang of things. If the conditioning process is continued for about a month after a cure is first established, the chances of relapse should be significantly reduced.

- *Hyperactivity*—Yes, I know, it seems like *all* kids are hyperactive. But what we're talking about here are children who suffer from an almost constant fever pitch of motion that hurts their ability to concentrate in school, interactions with playmates, and almost everything else.

This is a "disease" which has itself had a long and difficult course. For a while, hyperactivity became one of those fad diseases we seem to have forced upon us every few years. Quicker than you could say Ritalin, tens of thousands of normal-but-excitable kids were being labeled "hyperactive" and crammed with amphetaminelike drugs which do have the paradoxical property of calming truly hyperactive children.

Reacting to the overdiagnosis, the medical community coined new terms for the problem. It became "minimal brain disfunction," and later "attention deficit disorder."

Make no mistake. Hyperactivity exists, and for the families faced with the problem, it can really be hell. The child suffers, siblings suffer, the parents suffer. While there's evidence that most children simply outgrow the problem by early teenagerhood, the havoc wreaked on the family and the victim is great.

That's why many parents and doctors resort to powerful drugs such as **Ritalin** (methylphenidate), **Cylert** (pemoline), **Dexedrine** (dextroamphetamine), and **Benzedrine** (amphetamine). Administered carefully, and supervised by a doctor who will take the time to see that the dosage is adjusted to need, the stimulant drugs can make a tremendous difference in the lives of the families. Children who formerly faced only frustration at school can suddenly attend and get their work done. They can sit still long enough to play with other children, eat dinner, and lead a normal life.

However these *are* very powerful drugs. They can cause insomnia, reduce appetite, cause weight loss, and retard growth. Stomachache, skin rashes, headache, irritability, and hallucinations may be associated with such therapy. And since long-term effects are still unknown, many feel hesitant about committing a child to a ten- or fifteen-year diet of stimulants.

That may account for the almost messianic mission of Dr. Bruce Feingold, who became convinced that the real problem in hyperactivity was diet, specifically the artificial flavors and colors found in a high percentage of the foods consumed by children.

Much research has been done on the "Feingold Diet," and when all the evidence is weighed the regimen is not as convincing as it once seemed. While a small percentage of hyperactive children improve on the diet, the numbers are not spectacular. It's a long way from being a general purpose cure but it probably leads to children eating better balanced meals, and nobody can complain about that.

Both the cause and cure of hyperactivity remain shrouded at the moment. The available drug treatments deal with the symptoms, but they do *not* cure the problem. Our best hope is that continuing research into hyperactivity will eventually yield clues that allow us to replace the current drug treatments with something both more specific and safer.

## Children and Drug Safety

Medicine can be a valuable tool in the fight against childhood illness. It can also turn, in an instant, from savior to killer.

It's difficult to say anything about childhood drug poisoning that parents don't know. Yet in spite of the obvious dangers and obvious solutions, more than three million children under the age of five will be poisoned this year, many of them on drugs left within easy reach.

Childproof caps have helped cut the toll, but in order to be even partially effective they have to be used. Sometimes people with children in the house request non-childproof caps on their prescription medications for convenience. They *are* easier to get open. For anyone.

And a surprising number of poisonings happen because somebody left the cap off the medicine, and/or left it within easy reach. Keep in mind that to a child the pills may look like candy, being brightly colored as they often are. In one recent incident eight children between the ages of two and four were poisoned when they found half a dozen discarded bottles of rheumatism and heart medications in a garbage can. "The children," said the news story, "thought the tablets contained candy."

Children are also great imitators. They learn to walk and talk by seeing adults do those things, so we shouldn't be surprised when they take a pill just like they've seen their parents do. It's hard for a young child to understand that the pill Mom or Dad just took with impunity could be a fatal overdose for her.

We'd hate to think that any of our readers will ever suffer the agony of having their child poisoned on medications intended to relieve discomfort. The best defense is a good offense. To help prevent drug poisoning in children, do the following:

- *Do a Drug Audit*—Go through the medicine chest right now. First, properly dispose of any drugs that aren't current and needed (we'll talk about proper disposal in a second). Think of every drug in your medicine chest as a poisoning opportunity for a child.

  Second, check and make certain that each and every drug is stored in a childproof container. While many parents think the tricky caps are more adultproof than childproof, the evidence is overwhelming: Childhood poisoning incidents have decreased considerably since the safety caps were mandated.

  Third, consider putting a lock on the medicine cabinet or moving medications someplace where they can be kept under lock and key. It may seem like an inconvenience, but remember, there is no limit to either the curiosity of a child or to his or her ability to get into things when your back is turned. By the way, that goes double for household chemicals like cleaning fluids, detergents, drain cleaners, paint thinners, fuels, or whatever. NEVER store them under the sink or in an accessible cupboard. That's just asking for trouble!

- *Dispose of drugs properly*—In the case we just mentioned

above, children wound up in danger because someone just threw unwanted drugs in the trash rather than disposing of them carefully.

By carefully I mean seeing the liquids are poured down the drain, capsules emptied of their contents, and pills crushed into powder and flushed. "Crush and flush" is a good rule to remember and an easy one to follow. It will take only seconds to render your potent medication truly childproof.

- *Do some drug education*—Keep in mind that children want more than anything to please. So let them know you'll be most pleased if they understand how carefully we must all use pills, and how they themselves should never take *anything* unless an adult is there to help them.

For the very young, you might agree on a danger symbol such as a red $X$ and then put that on pill bottles. Make it a rule that the child may not even touch anything with the red $X$.

In spite of everyone's best efforts, children will still manage to poison themselves—if not on drugs then perhaps on common household substances. Every household with a child in it should be stocked with the basics to treat poisoning.

First on the list is the telephone number of the local Poison Control Center. Next comes ipecac syrup. Properly and promptly administered, this will cause the child to vomit, which in most cases is the best first aid since it eliminates the majority of the poisonous substance from the stomach before it's absorbed. The exception is in cases where what's been swallowed (such as lye, acid, cleaning fluid, petroleum-based products, and other caustic substances) will do more damage coming back up than if it remains in the system. **Before taking any action, however, call your local Poison Control Center just to be safe.**

In order to do the job, ipecac must be given properly. That means administering a couple of glasses of water along with the syrup and, according to one of our consultants, getting the child in motion. Seems that shaking everything together gets the job done better. Best way to do this is by gently jiggling the child, walking him, or putting him on a swing.

Driving also works nicely (take along a bucket and some towels), which is what you should probably do anyway, since every case of suspected poisoning should be attended to at the emergency room or in a doctor's office.

Poisoning is a complex problem, and one where prompt, competent treatment can make all the difference in the world. This is definitely *not* a do-it-yourself job. Call the Poison Control Center nearest you no matter what! And no matter how great the young person looks after vomiting (which probably won't be all that great, to tell you the truth), get the child to competent medical help immediately.

Kids are people too. Unfortunately, they are at the mercy of parents, doctors, and drug companies who show varying degrees of interest in and responsiveness to their special medication needs. Although little is known about the way in which medications affect children, even less is being done to correct our ignorance. Until the gap is filled by research, parents will have to remain the vigilant guardians of their children's right to safe medication.

# References

1. "General Guidelines for the Valuation of Drugs to Be Approved for Use During Pregnancy and for Treatment of Infants and Children." A Report of the Committee on Drugs, American Academy of Pediatrics, 1974.

2. Sankey, R. J.; Nunn, A. J.; and Sills, J. A. "Visual Halluncinations in Children Receiving Decongestants." *Brit. Med. J.* 288(6427):1369, 1984.

3. Ibid.

4. Ibid.

5. Hecht, Annabel. "What's That Alcohol Doing in My Medicine?" *FDA Consumer* 18(9):12–16, 1984.

6. Ibid.

7. Committee on Drugs, American Academy of Pediatrics.

"Ethanol in Liquid Preparations Intended for Children." *Pediatrics* 73:-405–407, 1984.

8. Wingert, Willis, et al. "A Study of the Quality of Prescriptions Issued in a Busy Pediatric Emergency Room." *Public Health Reports* 90(5):402, 1975.

9. Ibid.

10. Ibid.

11. Cohlan, S. Q. "Fetal and Neonatal Hazards from Drugs Administered during Pregnancy." *N.Y. State J. Med.* 64:493–499, 1964.

12. Doering, P. L., and Stewart, R. B. "The Extent and Character of Drug Consumption during Pregnancy." *JAMA* 239:843–846, 1978.

13. Rodriguez, S. V., et. al. "Neonatal Thrombocytopenia Associated with Ante-Partum Administration of Thiazide Drugs." *N. Engl. J. Med.* 270:881–884, 1964.

14. Brody, Jane E. "Most Pregnant Women Found Taking Excess Drugs." *New York Times,* March 18, 1973.

15. Berlin, Cheston M., et al. "Assessing Effects of Maternal Drug Use." *Patient Care,* May 30, 1980, pp. 68–111.

16. Blake, Jean P., et al. "Drugs in Pregnancy: Weighing the Risks." *Patient Care,* May 30, 1980, pp. 22–37.

17. Gal, Peter, and Sharpless, Martha K. "Fetal Drug Exposure—Behavioral Teratogenesis." *Drug Int. and Clin. Pharm.* 18(3):186–201, 1984.

18. Jones, Pat. "Liquor Linked to Pregnancy Woes." *The Durham Sun,* Apr. 27, 1984, p. 1-C.

19. Basgall, Monte. "Moderate-Drinking Pregnant Women May Not Hurt Babies, Study Shows." *Raleigh News and Observer,* May 20, 1984.

20. Gal, op. cit.

21. Sexton, Mary, and Hebel, J. Richard. "A Clinical Trial of Change in Maternal Smoking and Its Effect on Birth Weight." *JAMA* 251(7):-911–915, 1984.

22. Ibid.

23. Hill, Reba M., and Stern, Leo. "Drugs in Pregnancy: Effects on the Fetus and Newborn." *Drugs* 17:182–197, 1979.

24. Weathersbee, P. S.; Olsen, L. K.; and Lodge, J. R. "Caffeine and Pregnancy—A Retrospective Survey." *Postgraduate Med.* 62(3):64–69, 1977.

25. Montouris, Georgia D., et al. "The Pregnant Epileptic." *Arch. Neurol.* 36:601–603, 1979.

26. "Merrell Dow Ceases Production of Bendectin—'Burden Too Heavy.'" *Med. World News,* Jul. 11, 1984, pp. 55–56.

27. Dipalma, Joseph R. "Drugs for Nausea and Vomiting of Pregnancy." *American Family Physician* 28(4):272–274, 1983.

28. Ibid.

29. Spellacy, W. N. "Oral Contraceptives Contraindicated for Nursing Mother." *JAMA* 221:1415, 1972.

30. White, Gregory, J., and White, Mary. "Breastfeeding and Drugs in Human Milk." *Veterinary and Human Toxicology* 26(Suppl 1):11, 1984.

31. Ray, Wayne A., et al. "Prescribing of Tetracycline to Children Less than 8 Years Old." *JAMA* 237:2069–2074, 1977.

32. Ibid.

33. Ibid.

34. Rutledge, Mary Louise, et al. "Clinical Comparison of Calcium Polycarbophil and Kaolin-Pectin Suspension in the Treatment of Acute Childhood Diarrhea." *Cur. Ther. Res.* 23:443–447, 1978.

35. Olness, Karen. "How to Help the Wet Child—and the Frustrated Parents." *Mod. Med.,* Sep. 30, 1977, pp. 42–46.

36. Editorial. "Poisoning and Enuresis." *Brit. Med. J.* 1:705–706, Mar. 17, 1979.

37. Stewart, Mark A. "Treatment of Bedwetting." *JAMA* 232:281–283, 1975.

38. Herson, Victor C., et al. "Magical Thinking and Imipramine Poisoning in Two School-aged Children." *JAMA* 241:1926–1927, 1979.

## TABLE 1
## Prescription Drugs That May Be Dangerous During Pregnancy

The following table lists some prescription medications for which one or more studies have raised concern about use during pregnancy. The degree of danger varies and in some cases may be virtually nil. But any woman who is pregnant and has any of these drugs prescribed for her should not be shy about discussing the issue with her doctor.

This list is far from complete. Since absolutely safe use in pregnancy is rarely established for any drug, most prescription (and nonprescription) drugs pose *some* risk to the fetus. Usually this risk is higher during the first trimester (first three months).

Women who are pregnant should make every effort to avoid all medications whenever possible. But when necessary for her health or the health of the growing baby, some drugs can be lifesavers. Please keep in mind that not all children exposed to these drugs will show any effects. In some cases, the statistical probability of complications is extremely low.

Just because a drug is not included in this list does not guarantee its safety for the unborn child. ALWAYS consult your doctor. Our goal in presenting this table is to help improve communication between physicians and parents.

## ANTIBIOTICS

Many of the antibiotic drugs cause problems related to the liver. Be particularly cautious about any drugs in the sulfa or tetracycline categories.

**Achromycin** (tetracycline)— Damages, discolors tooth enamel; possible disturbance of bone growth.
**Amphotericin B**— Physical deformities, abortion.
**Aralen** (chloroquine)— Deafness, eye damage, death.
**Azo-Gantanol** (sulfa drug)— Can produce a form of

**Antibiotics** *cont.*

> jaundice in the newborn which may lead to liver or brain damage. This seems to be a problem only during the last trimester of pregnancy and should not be of great concern during the first six months.

**Azo-Gantrisin** (sulfa drug)— Same problem as with **Azo-Gantanol.**

**Bactrim** (sulfa drug)— Same problem as with **Azo-Gantanol.** Animal studies have shown a higher incidence of cleft palate and other defects.

**Chloromycetin** (chloramphenicol)— Heart disturbances, bone-marrow suppression.

**Streptomycin**— Hearing loss due to nerve damage; skeletal abnormalities.

## ANTICONVULSANTS (EPILEPSY DRUGS)

In general, most anticonvulsants pose a risk. The incidence of cleft palate, cleft lip, heart defects, and spontaneous abortion is two to three times higher when mothers have taken some of the most common anticonvulsants. Among the drugs involved are **Dilantin** (phenytoin), **Tridione** (trimethadione), and **Depakene** (valproic acid).

## HEART AND BLOOD-PRESSURE MEDICATIONS

**Inderal** (propranolol)— Retardation of fetal growth; low heart rate and low heart output; respiratory depression.

**Reserpine (Demi-Regroton, Diupres, Diutensen-R, Hydromox-R, Hydropres, Metatensin, Naquival, Regroton, Renese-R, Salutensin, Ser-Ap-Es, Serpasil, Unipres,** etc.)— Disruption of temperature regulation in newborn; low heart rate.

## DIURETICS ("WATER PILLS")

**Diamox** (acetazolamide)— Animal data suggests this drug may be teratogenic, but human studies have not confirmed this. We could only find one report of a physical abnormality in the clinical literature.

**Diuril** (chlorothiazide)— The use of thiazide diuretics like **Diuril** or **HydroDIURIL** during pregnancy has been somewhat controversial over the years. They were once thought to be helpful against preeclampsia/toxemia and edema of the extremities but such therapy has fallen into disrepute. May cause potassium depletion, blood irregularities.

**Edecrine** (ethacrynic acid)— Can cause sodium depletion. May also have a negative effect on hearing.

**HydroDIURIL** (hydrochlorothiazide; also found in: **Aldactazide, Aldoril, Dyazide, Esidrix, Esimil, Hydralazide, Hydropres, Hydro-Serp, HyperSerp, Inderide, Lexor, Moduretic, Oretic, Oreticyl, Salupres, Ser-Ap-Es, Thiuretic, Timolide,** and **Unipres**)— See **Diuril** above.

**Lasix** (furosemide)— Can be given to pregnant women who are in grave danger from congestive heart failure or have serious kidney disease and have to use a diuretic. It must be prescribed with great care, however, since fluid volume, blood flow to the uterus, and sodium levels may all change and have an adverse effect on the fetus.

## TRANQUILIZERS AND SEDATIVES

**Equanil** (meprobamate)— A higher-than-normal rate of birth defects has been reported in several studies. The package insert states that "Because use of these drugs is rarely a matter of urgency, their use during this period should almost always be avoided."

**Haldol** (haloperidol)— limb deformations reported, but a causal relationship has not been established.

## Tranquilizers and Sedatives *cont.*

**Librax** (chlordiazepoxide and clidinium)— See **Equanil** above.

**Libritabs** (chlordiazepoxide)— See **Equanil** above.

**Librium** (chlordiazepoxide)— See **Equanil** above.

**Limbitrol** (chlordiazepoxide and amitriptyline)— See **Equanil** above.

**Lithium**—This is a difficult one. Women who suffer manic depression may need medication through pregnancy, but there are reports **Lithium** may increase the risk of heart irregularities, low heart rate, jaundice, and cyanosis in the newborn. If absolutely necessary the drug should be used in the lowest dose possible, and preferably not during the first trimester.

**Methadone**— Severe withdrawal symptoms in newborn.

**Narcotics**— Withdrawal symptoms; convulsions; death.

**Phenobarbital**— Bleeding disorders after birth are a possibility.

**Tofranil** (imipramine)— Deformities have been reported, but a causal relationship to the drug has not been established.

**Thorazine** (chlorpromazine)— There are reports of jaundice, mild sedation, and neurological disturbances immediately after delivery. These should disappear. But safety during pregnancy has not been established.

**Valium** (diazepam)— See **Equanil** above.

## HORMONES

These are powerful chemical substances with a substantial danger of affecting the fetus physically and possibly psychologically. Unless absolutely necessary for the health of mother or baby, they should probably be avoided.

**Estrogens**— DES (diethylstilbestrol), a synthetic estrogen hormone, has caused an increased incidence of cancer in the female offspring of women who received

**Hormones** *cont.*

> it during their pregnancies. Estrogen exposure in utero may increase the risk of limb defects.
>
> **Methyltestosterone, testosterone**— Can cause masculinization of a female fetus.

## DIABETIC DRUGS

> **Diabinese** (chlorpropamide)— Low blood sugar in newborn.
>
> **Orinase** (tolbutamide)— There is a lack of information on the safety and usefulness of this drug during pregnancy. In very high doses it has caused problems in animals.

## APPETITE SUPPRESSANTS

> **Amphetamines**— May cause malformations.

## BLOOD-THINNING DRUGS

With the possible exception of heparin, all anticoagulant drugs appear to present a significant risk due to fetal hemorrhage.

> **Coumadin** (warfarin)— Abortion, stillbirth, physical deformities, hemorrhage.
>
> **Dicumarol** (bishydroxycoumarin)— Intrauterine hemorrhage, fetal death.

## CANCER DRUGS

The very nature of cancer chemotherapy involves administering large doses of extremely potent drugs in an attempt to kill tumor cells without doing too much damage to normal

## Cancer Drugs *cont.*

tissue. It comes as no surprise, then, that most anticancer drugs have great potential for doing serious damage to anything so sensitive as a developing baby. Virtually all the major chemotherapeutic drugs have been associated with increased risk of birth defects. Among those known to cause difficulties are **Methotrexate, Leukeran** (chlorambucil), **Mitomycin C, Cosmegen** (dactinomycin), **Purinethol** (mercaptopurine), **Nolvadex** (tamoxifen citrate), **Velban** (vinblastine sulfate), and **Oncovin** (vincristine sulfate).

## THYROID PREPARATIONS

**Iodides**— Can cause goiter and thyroid enlargement.

**Tapazole** (methimazole)— Goiter; thyroid enlargement. If absolutely essential during pregnancy, the dose should be the lowest possible that is still sufficient to regulate the thyroid.

## NONSTEROIDAL ANTI-INFLAMMATORY DRUGS (NSAIDs)

**Indocin** (indomethacin)— Not recommended due to potential danger to fetus.

**Salicylates** (aspirin-containing drugs)— In large doses may lead to hemorrhage; prolonged gestation; complicated deliveries.

## VACCINES

In general, any necessary vaccination should be attended to before a woman becomes pregnant.

**Flu**— Can lead to spontaneous abortion.

**Diphtheria**— Can cause fever reaction in mother.

**Vaccines** *cont.*

**Measles**— Avoid during pregnancy.
**Pertussis (whooping cough)**— Can cause fever in
   mother.
**Rubella**— Pregnancy should be avoided for two months
   to three months after vaccination.
**Smallpox**— Risk of vaccinia.
**Tuberculosis**— May infect fetus. Avoid.


## VITAMINS

Many pregnant women will have modest vitamin preparations
prescribed for them during pregnancy, and in anything approaching a normal dose, vitamins are okay, even essential.
However, in megadoses, vitamins can cause problems.

Vitamin A— In large doses may cause cleft palate; eye
   injury.
Vitamin C— In megadoses may cause scurvy in newborn
   when Vitamin C level suddenly drops. If baby is breast-
   fed and mother continues Vitamin C this may be less
   of a problem.
Vitamin D— In large doses may lead to high calcium
   level; narrowing of heart vessels.
Vitamin K— Can cause form of jaundice in newborn.


## MISCELLANEOUS OTHER DRUGS

**Antabuse** (disulfiram)— Reports of limb deformities.
**Antivert** (meclizine)— Possible danger, but original reports not confirmed.
Cortisone, hydrocortisone— Mild adrenal suppression,
   insufficiency; possible low blood sugar.
**Flagyl** (metronidazole)— Reports conflict; possible chro-
   mosome abnormalities. Avoid if possible.

## Miscellaneous Other Drugs *cont.*

Prednisone, prednisolone— Mild adrenal suppression;
possible low blood sugar; reports of fetal distress.
**Symmetrel** (amantadine)— May cause heart lesions.

## TABLE 2
## Drugs and Breast Feeding

Many drugs will make their way from the mother's circulation
into her breast milk. The implications of that for the infant,
however, are often very difficult to discern. The type and amount
of drug taken by the mother, her body's breakdown of the drug,
fluid intake, and many other factors all affect the concentration
of drug which may eventually be found in her milk. And in many
cases we simply don't know the effects on infants receiving small
doses of drugs.

What follows is a partial list of drugs known to be excreted
in breast milk. Those with the symbol * may cause problems and
should be used with great care if at all; those marked *** have
known adverse effects on the baby and should not be taken by
a lactating woman unless a physician specifically prescribes them
with full knowledge of the consequences.

The other drugs on this list represent an unknown risk and
should be used only with extreme caution by nursing mothers
and only after careful consultation with their physicians.

Alcohol
*Amantadine **(Symmetrel)**
Aminophylline
Amitriptyline **(Elavil)**
Amoxapine **(Asendin)**
Amoxicillin
*Amphetamines (**Benzedrine** and other brand names)
*Ampicillin

**Drugs and Breast Feeding** *cont.*

   **Acetaminophen (Tylenol** and many other brand
     names)
   Aspirin
   Atropine
   Barbiturates **(Amytal, Brevital,** Phenobarbital, **Seconal,**
**Pentothal)**
  *Bismuth (found in some nipple creams)
   Brompheniramine **(Dimetane)**
***Cancer drugs
   Caffeine
***Cannabis (marijuana)
  *Chloramphenicol **(Chloromycetin)**
   Chloroform
  *Cimetidine **(Tagamet)**
***Contraceptives, oral
  *Danazol
   Dextroamphetamine **(Dexedrine** and other brand
     names)
  *Diazepam **(Valium)**
   Dicumarol
  *Diethystilbestrol
   Diphenhydramine **(Benadryl)**
   Ephedrine
  *Ergot **(Cafergot, Ergomar, Gynergen, Hydergine,**
    **Migral)**
   Erythromycin
   Ether
   Hydantoin
***Isoniazid (many brand names)
  *Indomethacin **(Indocin)**
***Iodine, radioactive
  *Iodophor (vaginal gel)
  *Kanamycin **(Kantrex)**
   Laxatives (many)
   Levopropoxyphene **(Novrad)**

**Drugs and Breast Feeding** *cont.*

**Mandelic acid**
**Mefenamic acid (Ponstel)**
Mephenoxalone **(Trepidone)**
Methadone
Methocarbamol **(Robaxin)**
*Metronidazole **(Flagyl)**
Morphine
Nalidixic acid **(NegGram)**
Naproxen **(Naprosyn)**
Neomycin **(Neobiotic, Mycifradin)**
Nicotine
Novobiocin **(Albamycin, Cathomycin)**
Nortriptyline
*Oxyphenbutazone **(Oxalid, Tandearil)**
Papaverine
Penicillin G
*Phenylbutazone **(Butazolidin, Azolid)**
Pseudoephedrine **(Sudafed** and many others**)**
Phenacetin
Phenytoin **(Dilantin)**
***Progesterone
*Propoxyphene **(Darvon, Dolene)**
Propylthiouracil
Pyrimethamine **(Daraprim)**
Quinidine
Quinine
Reserpine (many trade names including
**Butiserpazide, Diupres, Diutensen-R, Exna-R,**
**Hydromox-R, Hydropres, Metatensin, Naquival,**
**Rau-Sed, Regroton, Renese-R, Salutensin,**
**Ser-Ap-Es, Serpasil)**
Salicylates (aspirin)
Scopolamine
Sodium chloride (salt)
Streptomycin

**Drugs and Breast Feeding** *cont.*

**Sulfonamides (sulfa drugs, many brands including
    Gantanol, Azo-Gantanol, Azo-Gantrisin,
    Azulfidine, Bactrim, Gantrisin, Septra,
    SK-Soxazole, Terfonyl, Thiosulfil, Urobiotic-250)**
Tetracyclines (**Achromycin** and many other brand
    names)
Thiazides (many brands)
Thiouracil
Thyroid preparations
Tranquilizers (many, including **Thorazine, Atarax,
    Vistaril, Ultran,
    Stelazine)**
Vitamins
Warfarin

# Table References

Blake, Jean. "Drugs in Pregnancy: Charting Proved and Suspected Drug Toxicity." *Patient Care,* May 30, 1980.

Martin, Eric. *Hazards of Medications.* Philadelphia: J. B. Lippincott, 1971, p. 275.

Overbach, Avrin, and Rodman, Morton. *Drugs Used with Neonates and During Pregnancy.* Medical Economics Company, 1975.

Berkowitz, Richard L.; Coustan, Donald R.; and Mochizuki, Tara K. *Handbook for Prescribing Medications During Pregnancy.* New York: Little, Brown and Company, 1981.

Rayburn, William F.; Zuspan, Frederick P.; and Fitzgerald. Jeanne T. *Every Woman's Pharmacy.* St. Louis: C. V. Mosby Company, 1983.

White, Gregory J., and White, Mary. "Breastfeeding and Drugs in Human Milk." *Vet. and Human Toxicology.* 26 (supp. 1):1–25, 1984.

Knowles, John A. "Drugs Excreted into Breast Milk." *Pediatric Therapy.* 3d ed. St. Louis: C. V. Mosby, 1968.

# 11

# Preventing High Blood Pressure and Heart Attack with and without Drugs

*Groping for the causes • High blood pressure • Determining hypertension is trickier than you think • Home blood pressure devices can be helpful • Medical self-care • How high is too high? • Mild hypertension • Nondrug approaches • Medicine for hypertension • Drugs that contain thiazide diuretics • Adding beta blockers • Fixed-combination formulations containing reserpine-type drugs • Other drugs for blood pressure • What causes a heart attack? • The esoteric earlobe crease: Is it an early warning sign of heart disease? • The cholesterol controversy heats up again.*

Next to cancer, nothing strikes fear into people's minds quite so fast as a diagnosis of heart disease. And well it might. In the United States of America, Public Health Enemy Number One is still heart disease and other cardiovascular problems. Over one million people die from heart attacks, strokes, and related vascular complications each year.[1]

That is not to mention the thirty-seven million who suffer from high blood pressure. It has been guesstimated by reliable medical authorities that as many as 20 percent of all adults in North America suffer from blood pressure above the normal range. If you think about that for a moment, it means that one out of every five of your friends probably has hypertension (the medical term for high blood pressure), and quite possibly you do, too. But by now you do not need to be reminded of the problem. The barrage of scary publicity put out by the AMA and the American Heart Association most likely has you uptight enough already. The question is, what do we know about heart trouble and high blood pressure, how do you prevent such problems in the first place, and what should you do about them once you've got them?

The fact of the matter is that we are still a very long way from unlocking the secrets behind these common conditions. Although your doctor may pretend that he is on top of the situation, the truth is more like the blind leading the blind. That goes for high blood pressure, heart attack, arteriosclerosis, thrombophlebitis, heart-rate irregularities, and the rest of this bag of worms.

Hard to believe, isn't it? Just ask your physician what causes any of the above problems and see what he says. He will either tell you straight out that we don't really know very much, or he will cook up such a complicated story that it would confuse your average politician. You'll probably hear about high-density lipoprotein, low-density lipoprotein, and very-low-density lipoproteins. If your doctor really pulls out all the stops, he may mention apolipoprotein A-I.[2] But even though billions of dollars have been poured down the research tubes, we are still a long way from solving the riddles of heart disease.

Unfortunately, the medical profession is like a dinosaur. It takes a long time for the messages to get from the brain to the tail and even longer to slow the beast down once it has gotten started. I have already belabored the point that doctors are slow to discard outmoded medical techniques. (Bloodletting lasted for centuries, and many doctors still insist that ulcer patients should follow a bland diet, even though there is no sound scientific evidence to support this regimen.)

Despite the fact that your physician is still groping for the causes of heart attack, stroke, and high blood pressure, chances are good that he has you on some high-powered medications or a special diet. Take cholesterol, for example—a dastardly demon if ever there was one. Lots of doctors decry this evil substance and love to put their patients on medication or a low-cholesterol diet in order to reduce it. Yet eliminating cholesterol per se won't do much good if it isn't accompanied by a program to reduce *total* dietary fat. Just substituting gobs of margarine and polyunsaturated oil for butter is not going to solve the problem. And cutting back on eggs won't help a lot if you still go in for lunches laden with pizza, burgers, and fries.

Cholesterol is not the only villain in the heart-disease story. There are lots of other favorite culprits still floating around. Sugar has been implicated, as has lack of exercise, coffee consumption, pollution, cigarette smoking, soft water, sluggish thyroid gland, lack of vitamins, and psychological stress. Emotion, prejudice, and fad seem to play as great a role as hard scientific evidence in determining which of the contradictory theories your doctor will accept or reject. It is unlikely that any one of these "enemies" is solely responsible, but a good case can be made for a combination of factors.

This chapter contains straight talk. I am going to explain the stuff that doctors don't tell you about, especially when it comes to the drugs they prescribe for high blood pressure, high cholesterol, and heart disease. We are going to destroy some myths and explore some revolutionary new ideas.

## High Blood Pressure

Let's start with high blood pressure to get the ball rolling. So what is blood pressure, anyway? At the risk of getting too simplistic, try thinking of the cardiovascular system as a pump and a set of pipes. The pressure in the system at any given moment depends upon the power of the pump and the diameter of the pipes. The thrust of the blood pushing against the walls of the pipes, or arteries, creates your blood pressure.

Your heart acts much like an on-off pump since it contracts and relaxes, on the average, seventy-two times per minute. The pressure actually varies between a high point at the moment of contraction, called the *systolic pressure,* and a low point. When the heart relaxes between beats, the pressure drops to its lowest level, or *diastolic pressure.* On average, a young adult has a blood pressure of about 120/80. This means that when the heart contracts, the pressure reaches 120 millimeters of mercury; when it relaxes, the pressure drops to 80 millimeters of mercury. Don't let the metric units freak you out. Just think of it as a measure of pressure not unlike the pounds per square inch used to measure tire pressure.

If all this seems confusing, let me give you an analogy. Imagine you are taking a glorious shower. The water is streaming down with lots of force because the pressure in the pipes is at its peak (approximately fifty pounds). Then some fool strolls into the bathroom and decides to flush the toilet while you're still taking a shower. You know what happens. The pressure in the system temporarily drops to a lower level. Or imagine that you're washing pots and pans at the same time you have the dishwasher running. Every time the cycle changes (for water to be pumped into the dishwasher), the pressure at your spigot drops off. Although the analogy isn't perfect because the blood in the vascular system is not diverted, a similar falloff in pressure occurs in the arteries when the body's pump, the heart, is resting between beats.

Okay, that sort of explains the two different blood-pressure readings—systolic and diastolic—that alternate with each heartbeat. But why is it that your blood pressure varies from one hour of the day to another, or from one period of your life to another?

Since the pumper of a person at rest does not vary very much in the amount of force it exerts with each contraction, what really regulates the pressure is the diameter of the pipe. Just as you can regulate the pressure in your garden hose by adjusting the size of the nozzle, so too your body can regulate your blood pressure by varying the diameter of the blood vessels.

Not only does blood pressure vary between high and low points during contraction and relaxation, it varies depending upon lots of environmental conditions. The arteries change their diameter dramatically depending upon your activity. When you are sleeping, they increase their diameter and the blood pressure drops. During excitement, such as lovemaking, the diameter narrows and pressure shoots up. Thus, a normal person could start the day off in bed with a pressure of 110/75 and end up with a pressure of 150/90 during an argument with the boss.

Although some variation in blood pressure is normal and even necessary for proper physiological function, some folks maintain a level that is almost always greater than it should be. That is called hypertension. High blood pressure can strike anyone. Sure, older folks are more susceptible, but youth is no guarantee that you are safe. In fact, it is the young hypertensive patient who suffers the most.

People who are overweight are good candidates for raised pressure, and for some inexplicable reason black people are more vulnerable to this disease than whites. A study carried out in the metropolitan Washington, D.C., area in 1975 uncovered the startling fact that as many as "one half of the black adult outpatients attending clinics might be expected to have elevated blood pressures."[3]

The thing to remember is that no one is immune. Well, so what? What's a little high blood pressure among friends, anyway? While it is true that a little high blood pressure may not be too serious for older folks (some medical authorities have been tempted to speculate that small increases in blood pressure after the age of sixty or seventy may be a natural part of the aging process), hypertension cannot be shrugged off easily.

The problem is that high blood pressure can go undetected for long periods of time without producing any obvious symptoms. Many people who go for ten or fifteen years with elevated pressure don't notice specific difficulties. During that time, however, insidious and often irreversible damage can be done to the body.

Hypertension forces the heart to work harder in order to circulate the blood adequately around your system. The heart may become weakened over this period of time and lose some of its pumping power. Congestive heart failure is more common in patients with high blood pressure. The blood vessels also suffer from the constant battering that they receive from blood cruising along at higher than normal pressure. Deposits of fat somehow accumulate in the walls of arteries, leading to arteriosclerosis, often referred to as "hardening of the arteries." Researchers believe that arteriosclerosis increases the risk of heart attack.

The accumulation of fat and cholesterol in arteries is not restricted to the vessels in the heart. This "hardening" process may occur simultaneously in the brain and increase a person's likelihood of being hit by a stroke. (People with hypertension are three to five times as prone to strokes as people with normal pressure.) Other organs are not immune from the ravages of high blood pressure; the kidney and even the eye can be damaged.

By now it should be obvious that elevated blood pressure is not something to ignore. On the other hand, it is not something to get all panicky over. A lot depends upon the degree of hypertension, the age when it becomes apparent and, most important, what is done to correct the situation. In years gone by, all too many doctors ignored or downplayed the significance of high blood pressure. Treatment was often initiated only reluctantly. Nowadays doctors are better informed, but they may overreact by resorting to powerful medications before carefully evaluating their patient or considering the drug's potential for serious side effects.

The very first thing that you have to learn is how to take your own blood pressure. The detection of hypertension is too important to be left entirely to your doctor during periodic checkups, and that goes for its presence as well as its absence. For all kinds of reasons, a blood-pressure determination in a doctor's office may not reflect the true state of your cardiovascular system. The very act of entering a doctor's office can raise your pressure over the "normal" limits. And when the doctor walks into the room, wowee zowee!

Doctors in Milan, Italy, decided to actually measure the effect the doctor can have on patients' blood pressure.[4] What they found was incredible! Within two minutes of walking into a room the doctor caused an elevation of approximately 27 points in systolic pressure and 15 points in diastolic pressure. Heart rate also jumped up.

What's so fascinating about this research is that it included both hypertensive and normal patients. I know that I get pretty anxious when I visit my doctor, and that in itself can send the pressure up.

Lots of studies have demonstrated that home determinations are usually lower than "official" office measurements and can be more reliable in determining the effectiveness of treatment.[5-7] All too many physicians are ready and willing to begin treatment on the basis of just one or two elevated readings. How unfortunate it would be if unnecessary therapy were started due to anxiety artificially induced by the trip to the doctor. It is also true, however, that sometimes a patient, by doing it at home, may pick up a case of high blood pressure that a doctor has missed.

There is an easy way for you to determine whether or not you have high blood pressure—learn how to take it yourself. For one thing, you can do it in the peace and quiet of your own house, an atmosphere more reflective of your regular blood pressure anyway. Second, and even more important, you will be able to record your pressure frequently over a long period of time in order to chart fluctuation. You may spend a good part of the day at work, so you should also take periodic readings there. Since it is not the occasional increase in pressure but rather the sustained elevation that is of concern, who but you yourself is best equipped to monitor blood pressure frequently?

Unfortunately, few doctors are willing to take the time or effort to teach the patient self-monitoring techniques. Other medics object to patient involvement on "philosophical grounds," as witness the following exchange between three doctors during a medical symposium on high blood pressure:

DR. PAGE:   Do you think that home blood pressures are worth doing?

DR. DUSTAN:   Yes, but the usefulness of the entire population is limited because home readings require from the patient a continued commitment to help maintain his health and not all patients can do this. It requires of the physician continuing interest even though the patient's problem seems to be solved by treatment, and not all physicians are capable of this.

DR. PAGE:   Roughly how many people among your practice do you think are capable of taking their own pressures?

DR. DUSTAN:   All of them, and all of them do.

DR. WILKINS:   I do not agree. Only a minority of my patients take their own blood pressures. Why? Maybe this is philosophical, but I believe the emotional burden of disease should not be borne by the patient but by the physician, the family, or other supporting elements. In some patients, the emotional stimulus of taking one's own blood pressure may have adverse influences. He becomes anxious about the reading, about the procedure—

DR. DUSTAN:   One's attitude toward home reading, I think, depends to a considerable degree on how much experience one has had with them. As far as an emotional burden is concerned, somewhere along the way the patient has to realize it is his illness, and he is only being asked to assist in obtaining the information the doctor needs to treat him better.[8]

I must say that I am on Dr. Dustan's team as far as this argument is concerned. It is time doctors started to realize that patients are intelligent human beings, capable of participating in their own treatment programs. Home determinations not only enable the patient and the doctor to establish the presence or absence of high blood pressure, but allow for excellent analysis of the success or failure of medical therapy.

A blood-pressure monitoring device should be as much a part of everyone's home as a thermometer. The pressure of your blood is just as important as the pressure in the tires of your car. You don't want to neglect either one.

It used to be that the only way you could measure your blood pressure properly was with a stethoscope and a sphygmomanometer—the inflatable arm cuff and pressure gauge used at the doctor's office. But using a stethoscope can be tricky. It requires perfect placement over the brachial artery which is right around the elbow where the fold is formed when the arm is bent. Then you have to listen carefully for subtle sounds of blood whooshing through that artery as air is slowly let out of the cuff. This isn't always easy, and even doctors and nurses can make mistakes.

Fortunately, times have changed. Over the last decade we have seen a revolution in electronic wizardry. Calculators that used to cost a bundle can now be purchased for ten bucks or less. Fancy digital blood pressure–monitoring devices that were sold to physicians for hundreds of dollars have also dropped dramatically and become affordable. What's more, they can be purchased in almost any pharmacy in the country. Digital monitors are also available in department stores, and through many mail-order catalogues. Familiar companies such as Timex and Norelco have hopped on the blood pressure–monitor bandwagon.

What makes such devices so helpful is that they are easy to use, are highly portable, and can be stored conveniently. Many come equipped with something called a "d ring," which enables people to wrap the cuff around an arm without any assistance. About the only tricky part of the whole operation is placing the built-in microphone found inside the cuff over the top of the brachial artery.

The microphone is usually marked with a circle or an arrow. You will need to take your index and middle finger and place them over the inside of your elbow. About one inch from the funny bone, and on the crease where your arm folds, you should

be able to feel a pulse. That is where the microphone needs to
be placed. You then pump up the cuff and wait for the results.
Most machines automatically deflate and give you a digital read-
out of systolic and diastolic pressure as well as heart rate.

Some of the fancier models actually inflate and deflate themselves and come equipped with a little printer that will provide
you with a permanent record of the time of day, the date, blood
pressure, and pulse. I used to think that the more bells and
whistles they put on these machines, the more things there were
to break down. That's true, of course, but I have used such a
device and have to confess that it is handy. Having a permanent
record that you can plot on a graph or just show your doctor is
very useful. In my experience the easier and more convenient
something is, the more likely it is to be used.

Unfortunately, these extras don't come cheap. You can buy a
stripped-down digital blood-pressure monitor for about $50 or
$60. The self-inflating models that come with a printer may cost
from $150 to $200, or more.

So how to choose the right machine? Well, you could zoom
off to your pharmacy or department store and try out some
different models to see which is easiest for you to use. You could
check out *The New People's Pharmacy—3*, where I discussed a
number of new models. Or you could write away for the Medical
Self Care Catalog. These folks have evaluated lots of different
blood-pressure equipment and offer a variety of devices, from a
basic digital model for about $75 to a fancy, paper readout,
self-inflating model for around $180. Their prices are about as
good as you will find anywhere, and in addition to the blood-
pressure monitors they have lots of other handy-dandy self-care
equipment. Their address is:

Medical Self Care Catalog
P.O. Box 999, Dept. P
Point Reyes, CA 94956

There is another option. You can always do what the doctor
does, and that is to buy a stethoscope and a mercury sphyg-

momanometer. It's awkward, the technique is tricky, and the machine's not easy to store. But it is accurate once you master the technique.

Here's how it works. When the cuff is blown up with a little rubber air bulb, it cuts off the circulation in your arm. In so doing, it prevents blood from being pumped to your lower arm and fingers. As air from the valve in the bulb is slowly released, the pressure in the cuff begins to drop. As the pressures of the cuff and your vessels equalize, blood will once again be able to flow. By placing a stethoscope over the artery in the crook of your arm, you will be able to hear the first sound of blood being pumped.

The first sound you hear represents the systolic, or peak blood pressure. If you continue to slowly let air out and lower the pressure in the temporary tourniquet, you will be able to hear the pulse beat regularly as it is recorded through the stethoscope. When the muffled sound of blood cruising through the artery begins to disappear or is no longer heard, the diastolic pressure has been reached and should be recorded. As mentioned earlier, the "normal" young adult reading should be around 120/80 (the 120 represents that point on the gauge where the first systolic sound is heard; and the 80 represents the place at which the sound disappears, in other words, the diastolic pressure). Your doctor should be more than willing to spend the few minutes necessary to teach you the proper technique for recording your own home blood pressure.

But as you can see, the stethoscope method is a whole heck of a lot more complicated than using an electronic device. For one thing, it usually requires the assistance of someone else. And there is always room for observer error. Hearing those whooshing sounds can be tricky. Then there's the problem of breakage. If you drop the glass column filled with mercury you will have a toxic substance rolling around on the floor. All in all, I think the digital devices make the most sense.

Okay, you have a blood pressure–monitoring device and you know how to use it. Now what? Well, the first thing to do is record your pressure regularly, on a daily basis (it should become a habit just like brushing your teeth, once in the morning and once in the afternoon or evening), and keep a chart so that you can show your doctor how you are doing. She will be able to use this information in order to determine whether or not your therapeutic program is successful.

When do you have hypertension? How high is too high? In the old days doctors usually did not start to worry unless the pressure reached 160/95. More recently, some have suggested that therapy should be initiated a little sooner. In point of fact, there is a great controversy within the medical community as to when a patient should be considered hypertensive and treatment started. It used to be that diastolic pressure was the only thing that concerned doctors, but lately they are paying careful attention to both systolic and diastolic readings.

A systolic pressure below 130 and a diastolic pressure below 90 is normal, whatever that means. If you are over forty and have a blood pressure of 130/90 or less, you should consider yourself lucky because you must be doing something very right. A systolic pressure between 130 and 140 accompanied by a diastolic pressure between 90 and 100 is no reason for panic. It is reason to keep an eye out and monitor the pressure frequently, particularly if you are under forty-five. Check with your physician to see if he wants to consider the possibility of treatment, especially nondrug treatment.

Once diastolic pressure gets between 100 and 110, you can be considered a moderate hypertensive, and treatment should definitely be proposed. If diastolic pressure gets much over 115, the problem is very serious indeed and requires careful medical attention.

It would appear from what I have just said that the question of high blood pressure is a simple matter. If the pressure goes over the "normal" limit, it should be treated. Unfortunately, it is not nearly so straightforward. Hypertension is probably not one simple disease. There are many factors that should be considered before drug therapy is begun. First and foremost is whether or not the blood pressure is consistently high. One reading, or even a couple of readings, over the "safe" level is no call to start with drugs unless it is so high as to be considered serious. It is sustained high blood pressure that requires attention. Secondly, the age of the patient and the degree of hypertension must be taken into account. Finally, a lot depends on where your doctor's head is at.

Some physicians believe you must vigorously treat mild high blood pressure come hell or high water. To them anything over a diastolic reading of 85 is considered a problem and they often start prescribing drugs to keep it down as close to 80 as possible. Other doctors worry about side effects from blood-pressure medication and are much more cautious and conservative about starting therapy. They may wait till the pressure climbs above 90 or 95 diastolic before calling in the cavalry.

As far as I am concerned, the conservatives have the edge in this debate. Naturally, I would like to see the blood-pressure numbers stay as low as possible, but the quality of life is also important. Older people often react badly to blood-pressure drugs that may cause diarrhea, fatigue, depression, or memory loss. If mild hypertension isn't detected until age sixty or later, I am not convinced one has to get it down to 120/80 or even 130/90.

Of course, only your doctor will be able to make the final decision about this complicated issue. You would do best to discuss it with him and hope he is keeping up with the controversy.

Once blood pressure creeps over the mild to moderate limits and stays there, almost everyone would agree that it is time to do something. More often than not, doctors immediately stick their hypertensive patients on some form of drug therapy. Getting blood pressure down with drugs may not always be the best way to start off. Although doctors rarely pursue them, there are other initial alternatives to pharmacological treatment.

Numero uno in a program of blood-pressure control should be weight reduction. Being overweight has been well established to be a contributing factor in the elevation of blood pressure.[9-11] In other words, getting rid of those love handles tends to lower blood pressure.[12]

Of course, losing weight is always easier said than done. I have been trying to get rid of my spare tire for about ten years and only in the last six months have I seen the beginning of success.

My secret? I realized that I couldn't shed excess pounds without help. I found a registered nutritionist who had experience in modifying eating behavior. She taught me how to change nasty old habits—like always eating everything on my plate. Now I keep a diary of my daily intake and am happy to report a loss of fourteen pounds. And I seem to be keeping them off. Hooray! Because my blood pressure is down too. As I write these words it stands at 118/61 as measured by a self-inflating Norelco HC-3500 electronic monitor. That ain't half bad for an almost-forty-year-old pharmacologist. So Blood Pressure Law Number 1 is: Lose excess weight!

It used to be that restriction of salt intake was the second most important part of any program of blood-pressure control. I was one of the loudest shouters when it came to telling people to throw away the saltshaker. I still believe we eat far too much salt, and I have eliminated sodium from my diet as much as possible. But in recent years the salt connection has become far more controversial than it used to be.

Dr. David McCarron, associate professor of medicine and director of the Oregon Hypertension Program, has shaken up the medical establishment with some amazing observations:

1. There are predictable nutritional differences between individuals with high blood pressure and those with normal blood pressure.

2. Deficiencies rather than excesses are the principal nutritional patterns that characterize the hypertensive person in America.

3. Reduced consumption of calcium and potassium is the primary nutritional marker of hypertension, with reductions in vitamins A and C also being noted.

4. Dairy products are the food group for which reduced consumption is most closely related to high blood pressure in the United States.

**5.** These observations are largely independent of age, race, sex, body mass index [ratio of lean to fat], and alcohol consumption.

**6.** Diets low in sodium are associated with higher blood pressure, while high-sodium diets are associated with the lowest blood pressure.[13]

Now that is beyond incredible! What Dr. McCarron did was analyze the diets of more than ten thousand people. He found that those with low salt intake had higher blood pressure, and individuals who consumed the most salt had the lowest blood pressure. That runs counter to everything we have been told for the last twenty years.

Before you make a beeline for the pickles, pretzels, and sauerkraut, however, you had better know that lots of hypertension experts disagree with Dr. McCarron's findings. And he himself would not advocate increasing salt intake. He merely reported a fascinating association.

But what is really interesting in his report is the observation that certain dietary deficiencies may be more important in hypertension than most physicians or patients realize. Remember that he found low calcium and potassium intake among the people with high blood pressure. There is a growing belief that extra calcium and potassium could help lower blood pressure.[14-16]

So how much do you need? That is still unclear. If you are conscientious and really do eat a well-balanced diet, the chances are that you don't need dietary supplements. But most adults I know do not eat enough dairy products. I myself do not drink anywhere near a quart of skim milk a day, which is what I would need to approach the 800 mg RDA (Recommended Dietary Allowance). So I take a calcium-magnesium supplement that gives me about 800 to 1,000 mg of calcium.

I do not take a potassium supplement, because too much potassium may be dangerous for the heart. It can cause palpitations and abnormal heart rhythms, weakness, confusion, numbness, and difficulty breathing. I do, however, eat foods high in potassium. (Turn to page 436 for a list of high-potassium foods.) In addition I use a salt substitute at the table. These products contain potassium chloride instead of sodium chloride and are a good way to get extra potassium as long as you don't overdo.[17]

So Blood Pressure Laws numbers 2 and 3 are: Consume adequate amounts of calcium and potassium. I also make sure to eat at least one or two carrots every day for that missing Vitamin A, and I take in extra Vitamin C, just to be on the safe side. And since I still believe most people should do without extra salt, Blood Pressure Law Number 4 still is: Fight the urge to reach for the saltshaker. If you can keep total salt intake less than one teaspoon a day, you can't go wrong. That's not easy, though, since sodium is found in so many foods. Just do your best.

Another important nondrug approach for hypertension is physical activity. While an increase in blood pressure seems to be an inevitable concomitant of aging in highly developed societies such as ours, many "primitive" cultures do not demonstrate this kind of maladaptation.[18]

Primitive peoples are almost always more active than we are, and high blood pressure seems to be a disease they can avoid. A comprehensive investigation carried out a while back in the United States also seems to confirm the observation that habitual physical activity may militate against high blood pressure.[19]

After assessing the physical activity and general health of about seventeen hundred men in Tecumseh, Michigan, researchers concluded that the more active the men, the lower their blood pressure, both systolic and diastolic. Interestingly, the difference in pressure between active and inactive men occurred regardless of age.

Two recent studies confirm these results. Investigators at the University of South Carolina put 6,039 healthy men and women with normal blood pressure on treadmill testing equipment to determine their level of physical fitness. As you would expect, some were in great shape, while others were physically unfit. Four years later the researchers tested everyone's blood pressure again. They found that the physically unfit had a higher elevation of blood pressure and "were at four times greater risk of hypertension than highly fit subjects with low baseline pressures."[20]

Exercise and physical conditioning should definitely be a crucial part of any program designed to lower blood pressure. Numerous scientific investigations have determined that after a period of medically supervised physical training, blood pressure can drop dramatically.[21-24]

Now don't rush out to start jogging a mile every day. The quickest way to a heart attack is unsupervised and overdone physical activity. Medical supervision is a must, and your doctor should be more than willing to recommend a safe program of exercise after he has done a complete medical checkup in order to determine your capabilities.

The best exercise program is one that schedules regular activity. At least three sessions should be planned each week. Thirty minutes to one hour should be sufficient to provide adequate conditioning. After a brief period of warm-up calisthenics, get into a total body exercise such as bicycling, vigorous walking, jogging (moderate), or swimming. Don't be a dummy and start exercising in hot weather or after a meal. That is a quick way to end up flat on your back. It is also wise to avoid a superhot shower right after your workout, since that can put a strain on the cardiovascular system. Just cool down slowly for ten or fifteen minutes and then take a moderately warm shower.

Some doctors recommend that modest activity should be interspersed with brief periods of strenuous exercise. If chest pains develop at any point, it is reason to reduce the degree of exertion and have your doctor reevaluate the exercise program, but it is not necessarily a reason to discontinue the program unless your doctor advises you to.

If you are not in good shape to begin with, do not start out your physical training as if you were trying to make up for lost time. A gradually intensified program is the most beneficial and safest method to good health. One more caveat. Skip the weight training and the isometric (or static) exercises. Your heart rate and blood pressure can skyrocket when you pull, push, or lift too much, too fast.

Before high-powered drugs are employed to reduce high blood pressure, a program of exercise and weight control should be tried. Any half-intelligent human being should value her or his life enough to make this kind of effort for a healthy heart and cardiovascular system. Therefore, Blood Pressure Law Number 5 is: Exercise.

Perhaps the most provocative new approach to the control of blood pressure involves biofeedback and techniques of mental relaxation. The science of biofeedback offers an exciting new method for the management of many disease processes. By providing continuous visual or auditory information about the state of the internal physiology, a person is able to learn how to control things like heart rate, brain waves, or blood pressure, processes that were once considered involuntary bodily functions beyond conscious human control.

Some studies indicate that an individual may be capable of reversing many maladaptive disease syndromes such as Raynaud's disease (cold, tingling extremities) or migraine headaches through biofeedback. Coupled with a program of mental relaxation, reductions in elevated blood pressure may be possible.

One medical investigation carried out in England, combining a yoga relaxation technique and a "relaxometer" biofeedback apparatus, produced amazing results. Of the twenty hypertensive patients studied, sixteen demonstrated improvement. "Their average systolic pressure fell from 160 to 134 mm Hg [mercury] and their average diastolic pressure fell from 102 to 86 mm Hg."[25] Not only did these people drop into normal blood-pressure ranges, but many were able to reduce or eliminate completely their use of blood-pressure medications. A follow-up study indicated that improvement was sustained over the course of more than a year.[26]

More recent research has confirmed that biofeedback and muscle-relaxation programs can indeed help lower blood pressure.[27-29] I am convinced that our minds can have a profound influence on our bodies, and that if we can learn how to relax and control bodily functions, we might be able to eliminate a surprisingly large number of drugs.

Unfortunately, most doctors scorn such "unscientific" techniques as yoga, muscle relaxation, meditation, or biofeedback. No course in these areas is taught in medical school, and doctors understand little about them. However, Dr. Herbert Benson, an associate professor of medicine at Harvard University and director of the Hypertension Section at Best Hospital in Boston, has produced solid scientific evidence that blood pressure can be controlled through mental processes.

Originally, Dr. Benson concentrated his efforts on animals, training monkeys by systematic rewards and punishments to regulate their own blood pressure either upward or downward. This work was extended to people through biofeedback technology, and similar results were obtained.

During the course of his work, Dr. Benson considered applying techniques of mental relaxation to see if comparable reductions were achievable. Students who practiced transcendental meditation had approached Benson and offered to participate in his study. Dr. Benson confided, "At first I didn't want to get involved with them. The whole thing seemed a bit far out, and somewhat peripheral to the traditional study of medicine. But they were persistent, and so finally I did agree to study them."[30]

Fortunately, because Dr. Benson was open-minded, he discovered something exciting. Although blood pressure did not drop during the meditation period, other important physiological processes did vary. "What we found," said Benson, "was that during the meditation itself there were distinct changes. The essence of these changes could be, I think, summarized by saying that the whole body's metabolism slows down. And it slows down to a degree that would be seen otherwise only after several hours of sleep. In this case, however, the changes occur within a few minutes of starting what I now like to call the 'relaxation response.'"[31]

It was not long after this startling discovery that Dr. Benson wrote his now well-regarded book, *The Relaxation Response.* He found that it was not necessarily transcendental meditation that helped, but generalized mental relaxation that seems to enable people to calm down and lower blood pressure.

Although transcendental meditation, or TM as it came to be called, appears to be an effective method of mental relaxation, it probably has no advantages over any other meditative techniques, whether they be Zen or yoga or what-have-you. Dr. Benson has in fact developed his own "nonreligious" program of mental relaxation. His procedure goes as follows:

1. In a quiet environment, sit in a comfortable position.
2. Deeply relax all your muscles, beginning at your feet and progressing up to your face—feet, calves, thighs, lower torso, chest, shoulders, neck, head. Allow them to remain deeply relaxed.
3. Breathe through your nose. Become aware of your breathing. As you breathe out, say the word *"one"* silently to yourself. Thus: breathe in . . . breathe out, with *"one."* In . . . out, with *"one"* . . .
4. Continue this practice for ten to twenty minutes. You may open your eyes to check the time, but do not use an alarm. When you finish, sit quietly for several minutes, at first with your eyes closed and later with eyes open.[32]

If that sounds complicated, I've got another suggestion. Dr. Emmett Miller has one of the world's most soothing voices. He has put together a number of relaxing audio tapes that are absolutely extraordinary. If Dr. Miller can't calm you down, you're in big trouble.

You can order Dr. Miller's tapes by writing to P.O. Box W, Dept. P, Stanford, CA 94305. You will receive a brochure describing various cassettes. My personal favorites include "Healing Journey," "Letting Go of Stress," "Rainbow Butterfly," "Easing into Sleep," and "10-Minute Stress Manager." Each tape costs around $11.00 plus postage and handling.

Unfortunately, as noted earlier, the medical profession has been slow to accept revolutionary approaches; they have been conditioned to believe in the tried-and-true value of drug therapy. As a pharmacologist, I should be on their side, but as a person concerned about our overmedicated society, I always prefer to seek alternatives to drugs whenever possible. Mental-relaxation techniques will probably be helpful whether they be transcendental meditation, yoga, Zen, Dr. Benson's simple breathing exercise, or Dr. Miller's audio cassettes. By measuring your own blood pressure, you will be able to determine how you are doing. So Blood Pressure Law Number 6 is: Learn How to Relax.

Okay, you have cut down your salt intake, increased calcium and potassium in your diet, gotten rid of your spare tire, established a regular pattern of exercise, and incorporated mental relaxation into your daily regimen. Great! But your blood pressure is still too high. Then it is time to get that blood pressure down with drugs.

## Medicine for Hypertension

Drugs *can* make a difference. They can save your life! Just because I advocate starting out with other forms of therapy, do not get the idea that I am simply against using drugs. If you cannot control your blood pressure with any of the previously mentioned methods, or if it is diagnosed as being very high, it is absolutely imperative that you get the pressure down with medication. A decrease in moderate to severe high blood pressure will reduce serious illness and prolong life. The sooner therapy is initiated, the better are the chances of preventing a heart attack or a stroke.

The goal of antihypertensive therapy should be to achieve the best results possible. That should not, however, be done at the expense of the well-being of the patient. All too often doctors feel compelled to seek textbook solutions to the problems of hypertension. They raise drug dosages or move up to more potent medication in their never-ceasing quest for normalization. This may lead to adverse reactions that are not well tolerated by the patient.

Since most people will have to take their medicine for the rest of their lives, serious side effects may prove so discouraging that the patients decide to eliminate drugs altogether. This can be a terrible mistake. Research has shown that even if blood pressure cannot be brought down to completely normal levels, modest improvement will afford some protection against serious cardiovascular complications. If you are not comfortable with your drug regimen, discuss the problems with your physician. He or she may be able to change your program.

There is no ideal drug for the treatment of high blood pressure. Each agent is capable of producing side effects. Since people vary in their responses to hypertensive medication, the only truly effective treatment is one that is individualized for each and every patient.

It is not enough for your doctor to stick you on some drug, tell you to take it twice a day, and then make another appointment three months in the future. There has to be constant monitoring of blood-pressure levels (this is where home determinations come in handy) and excellent communication between doctor and patient. The first few days in a new drug treatment program are critical in order to find out how well the patient is doing and whether there are any adverse reactions. There are no shortcuts to successful therapy.

The most frequently prescribed drug in this country is *not* **Valium**, and it's not **Tagamet**. The most commonly prescribed medication by far is a hard-to-pronounce, little known compound called hydrochlorothiazide, sometimes abbreviated HCTZ. According to the FDA's fourth annual review of drug use in the United States, almost eighty million prescriptions are filled each year for drugs that contain hydrochlorothiazide.[33] It can be found alone or in combination with other antihypertensive agents in such brand-name compounds as **Aldoril, Aldactazide, Apresazide, Apresodex, Aquazide, Chlorzide, Diaqua, Diu-Scrip, Dyazide, Esidrix, Esimil, Hydralazide, Hydrap-Es, HydroDIURIL, Hydromal, Hydropres, Hydro-Serp, Hydroserpine, Hydro-T, Hydrotensin, Hydro-Z, Hyper-Serp, Inderide, Lexor, Maxzide, Moduretic, Oretic, Salupres, Serpasil-Esidrix,**

**Ser-Ap-Es, SK-Hydrochlorothiazide, Thiuretic, Timolide, Unipres,** and **Zide.**

Hydrochlorothiazide belongs to a class of compounds known as thiazide diuretics, or "water pills" as my mother calls them. Other drugs that contain thiazide diuretics include:

| | |
|---|---|
| **Aldoclor** | (chlorothiazide) |
| **Anhydron** | (cyclothiazide) |
| **Aquastat** | (benzthiazide) |
| **Aquatag** | (benzthiazide) |
| **Aquex** | (benzthiazide) |
| **Diupres** | (chlorothiazide) |
| **Diuril** | (chlorothiazide) |
| **Enduron** | (methyclothiazide) |
| **Exna** | (benzthiazide) |
| **Fluidil** | (cyclothiazide) |
| **Metahydrin** | (trichlormethiazide) |
| **Metatensin** | (trichlormethiazide) |
| **Naqua** | (trichlormethiazide) |
| **Naquival** | (trichlormethiazide) |
| **Naturetin** | (bendroflumethiazide) |
| **Rauzide** | (bendroflumethiazide) |
| **Renese** | (polythiazide) |

As far as I am concerned, there are few differences among these various diuretics. Therefore, it would be to your advantage to have your physician prescribe generically, given the fact that you may be taking this kind of medication for a very long time. For example, **HydroDIURIL, Esidrix,** and **Oretic** are brand-name versions of hydrochlorothiazide. In most cases a generic is available at one fourth the cost of the brand-name product, and in some instances the savings can be even greater.

Most physicians start their patients on diuretic therapy as the first step in any treatment program because the drugs are considered quite effective for mild to moderate high blood pressure, and because side effects are thought to be minimal. After a week or so, blood pressure usually drops between ten and fifteen points, which is about all that can be expected for this introductory stage of treatment.

In recent years, however, a controversy has arisen over the long-term safety of such drugs, and a few doctors are beginning to reevaluate routine use in primary therapy. Although it is certainly true that you lower the risk of heart attack and stroke by reducing blood pressure, there is fear that certain biochemical changes brought on by such medicines may actually increase the risk of cardiovascular disease.[34] In other words, you may be working at cross-purposes.

Let's get specific. Thiazide diuretics have been reported to have a negative effect on the balance of blood fats.[35] That is, they may raise certain kinds of blood cholesterol levels that could, *if sustained,* increase the risk of arteriosclorosis in the long run. I emphasize "if sustained" because other researchers report that serum cholesterol levels return to normal after a year or less on the drug.[36, 37] While this issue is still somewhat up in the air, I would have to say that at this writing the risk seems minimal and probably nonexistent.

Such drugs may also increase blood-glucose levels. It is unclear whether this is truly a problem, but I am sure there have been individuals falsely labeled as diabetics because of the results of lab tests showing high sugar. Other biochemical changes include increased uric-acid levels (which may lead to gout), lowered magnesium levels, and the risk of zinc deficiency. One set of researchers warns that patients who experience a reduced sense of taste and smell, difficulty with wound healing, skin problems, impotence, and difficulty adapting to the dark may have developed a zinc deficiency from their diuretics.[38] Although few physicians ever call for a zinc test, it should be performed periodically, and if serum zinc levels fall below 80 $\mu g$/dl (micrograms per deciliter) a daily supplement of at least 50 mg might have to be considered.

By far the most common, and potentially the most serious, side effect of thiazide diuretics is potassium depletion. These drugs kick potassium out of the system, and that can lead to big trouble. Muscle cramps and fatigue may crop up as the only symptoms a patient notices. But often there are no signs of a potassium problem unless you go in for a blood test.

So what's the big deal about potassium anyway? There is growing fear that potassium depletion may lead to cardiac arrhythmias (irregular or abnormal heart rhythms).[39] This is probably not a hazard for people with healthy hearts. But anyone taking digitalis-type medication such as **Lanoxin** (digoxin) or who has a record of an abnormal electrocardiogram, lowered potassium levels could be life-threatening.

Unless patients make a special effort to make sure their diet is high in foods containing this mineral, they could end up in deep trouble. Unfortunately, most doctors do not know which foods to recommend (due to a serious lack of training in nutrition), and so they often resort to prescribing potassium chloride supplements in the form of pills, syrup, or salt substitutes. These preparations are less satisfactory than proper diet unless the patient also happens to be on digitalis-type medication, which requires an extra amount of potassium.

The problem with potassium supplements is that they are poorly tolerated. Stomach irritation, abdominal cramps, nausea, diarrhea, ulcers, and a terrible taste are some of the more frequent complications. An evaluation of the use of these special preparations cautions against routine use and suggests that overzealous prescribing of potassium by physicians should be questioned.[40] Whenever feasible, a diet high in potassium-containing foods should be the first line of defense against diuretics. The list on page 436 should prove invaluable for the patient on water pills because it offers not only relative concentrations of potassium but nutritional value as well.

Even if you do make a conscious effort to eat lots of different potassium-containing foods on a regular basis, that doesn't necessarily guarantee protection. Large doses of diuretics can undermine the best nutritional game plan. And some people are more susceptible than others to this problem.

Since there is only one way to find out what your potassium levels are, make sure you have a blood test done *before* therapy is started. Each month thereafter an evaluation of the blood

## High-Potassium Foods (per three-ounce portion)

|  | Calories | Potassium (mg/100gm) |
|---|---|---|
| Almonds | 598 | 773 |
| Apricots (dried) | 332 | 1,260 |
| Apples (dried) | 353 | 730 |
| Avocados | 167 | 604 |
| Bananas | 58 | 370 |
| Beef (hamburger, lean) | 219 | 558 |
| Cocoa powder (plain) | 300 | 1,500 |
| Cress (garden) | 32 | 606 |
| Dates | 274 | 648 |
| Figs | 274 | 640 |
| Flounder | 202 | 587 |
| Halibut (broiled) | 171 | 525 |
| Horseradish (raw) | 87 | 564 |
| Lichees (dried) | 277 | 1,100 |
| Molasses (light) | 252 | 917 |
| Molasses (blackstrap) | 213 | 2,927 |
| Oranges | 36 | 200 |
| Peaches (dried) | 262 | 950 |
| Peanuts (roasted) | 582 | 701 |
| Peanut butter | 581 | 670 |
| Pecans | 687 | 603 |
| Potato (baked, with skin) | 93 | 503 |
| Prunes | 255 | 694 |
| Raisins | 289 | 763 |
| Rye wafers, whole grain | 344 | 600 |
| Sesame seeds | 563 | 725 |
| Soybean flours | 350 | 1,750 |
| Squash (butternut) | 68 | 609 |
| Sunflower seeds | 560 | 920 |
| Wheat germ | 363 | 827 |
| Yeast (brewer's) | 283 | 1,894 |
| Yeast (torula) | 277 | 2,046 |

(Source: Composition of Foods, Agriculture Handbook 8, Agricultural Research Service, U.S. Department of Agriculture, Washington, D.C.)

chemistry should be made until the doctor is satisfied that there are no complications. At regular intervals during the year, additional lab tests should be carried out.

Several diuretics do not deplete potassium levels as much as those previously mentioned. These so-called potassium-sparing medications include **Dyazide** and **Maxzide** (hydrochlorothiazide and triamterene combined), **Moduretic** (amiloride and hydrochlorothiazide), and **Aldactazide** (spironolactone and hydrochlorothiazide).

All of these drugs have something in common—they contain hydrochlorothiazide as one component. You remember good old HCTZ, the most frequently prescribed drug in the country. It's a diuretic that depletes or wastes potassium. In order to counterbalance that effect an additional ingredient that "spares" or preserves potassium is added. The combination of two such diuretics in one pill would appear ideal, since effective blood-pressure-lowering ability was added to potassium preservation. And judging from sales figures over the last several years, these formulations have been big winners in the marketplace.

**Dyazide** has captured the lion's share of the business. At this writing, approximately eight million people swallow at least one red-and-white **Dyazide** capsule every day. That makes it one of the hottest drugs on the doctor's hit parade, with sales in excess of $200 million annually.

Unfortunately, **Dyazide** has had a little problem over the years. Unbeknownst to most doctors, the product was not well formulated. What that means is that the ingredients in **Dyazide** (as originally compounded) did not get into the body as well as they might have. Compared to other drugs with the same amount of hydrochlorothiazide, **Dyazide** delivers about 50 percent less. This means that a patient taking **Dyazide** might have received only half as much medicine as his doctor thought he prescribed. It would be a little like buying a twelve-ounce bottle of Coke, only to discover when you drank it that you only got six ounces instead.

SmithKline claims that lower doses of HCTZ are perfectly adequate to control most hypertensive patients, but as of early

1985 they were scrambling to bring out a new and improved **Dyazide** formulation that provides optimum absorption. That's because another drug company, Mylan Pharmaceuticals, beat them to the punch with a better mousetrap—a **Dyazide**-like preparation called **Maxzide** that appears to deliver exactly what is promised.

Of course, it won't be long before SmithKline has a "new" **Dyazide** on the market which is also 100-percent bioavailable—providing patients with exactly as much medicine as it claims. Then it will be up to the doctors to decide whether they think **Maxzide, Dyazide, Moduretic,** or **Aldactazide** is the best potassium preserver. By the way, my least favorite of the group is **Aldactazide**, since it has been found to cause tumors in rats.

Well, what about the patient? Which diuretic is best? Are these drugs worth the extra expense? They certainly are a lot more costly than generic HCTZ. Unfortunately, it's not a simple yes or no answer. For someone who can get by with generic HCTZ and keep the potassium levels up, the answer is probably no. If, on the other hand, potassium starts to drop, then one of these drugs may be worth the investment. If you are put on a diuretic, you will definitely want to talk about these important issues with your physician.

While you are at it, you should also be aware of the other side effects associated with water pills. Although uncommon, occasionally there may be some problems associated with the use of the milder thiazide diuretics. Some patients develop skin rashes, especially after exposure to the sun. Weakness and anemia have been reported occasionally. There may be some digestive upset, nausea, or diarrhea. Dryness of the mouth and sometimes an unpleasant aftertaste may be part of the price the hypertensive must pay to get his blood pressure down. None of these side effects is particularly dangerous, though any unusual reaction should always be reported to your physician.

Once a doctor has evaluated a hypertensive patient's progress, he or she may decide that a diuretic is not sufficient to do the job. At this point it is not uncommon for a physician to add an additional drug. These days it is more than likely to be something called a beta blocker. In fact, many physicians are turning to these agents as first-line treatments. They work in part by blocking the actions of adrenalin (epinephrine) on the heart. In this way they can prevent the heart from over-working. That's why they may also be useful for treating angina and certain irregular heart rhythms. They also lower blood pressure quite nicely.

Examples of beta blockers include **Inderal** (propranolol), **Blocadren** (timolol), **Corgard** (nadolol), **Lopressor** (metoprolol), **Tenormin** (atenolol), **Trandate** and **Normodyne** (labetalol), and **Visken** (pindolol). While there are subtle differences between these beta blockers, they all work in pretty much the same way and for the most part have similar side effects. Fatigue, slowed heart rate, reduced ability to exercise, depression, digestive-tract disturbance (nausea and diarrhea), Raynaud's phenomenon (numb, tingling, painful extremities), nightmares or vivid dreams, forgetfulness, disorientation, and hair loss have been reported with **Inderal** and many of the other beta blockers as well.

Anyone with asthma must avoid such medications because they can make breathing problems worse. And no one should ever stop taking a beta blocker suddenly. It may bring on an attack of angina or even a heart attack.

All that sounds gruesome. I have to admit that beta blockers are *not* my favorite drugs. Nevertheless, they do get blood pressure down quite impressively for many patients, and I am surprised at how well tolerated they seem to be with that kind of adverse-reaction profile. Well over thirty million prescriptions are filled for **Inderal** alone in this country every year.

Which beta blocker would I choose? I guess my favorite would have to be **Tenormin**. Reports from physicians I trust lead me to believe that it is well tolerated and may produce far fewer psychological problems than **Inderal**. Other drugs may be less likely to slow heart rate, such as **Visken**. All in all, you will probably get the drug your physician has the most experience with and therefore feels most comfortable with. What you need to do is let your doctor know how comfortable *you* feel. If you start to go into a slump and experience depression, not to mention fatigue or forgetfulness, ask about trying another compound. Not all beta blockers are created equal, and some people do better on one than another.

Another blood-pressure-lowering drug that has become quite popular of late is **Minipress** (prazosin). It dilates arteries and veins and therefore is far less likely to cause cold hands and feet than beta blockers. The trickiest part of taking **Minipress** occurs during the first day or so of use. There is often a sudden drop in blood pressure that can make people terribly dizzy and faint about thirty minutes after taking their first dose. The best thing to do is take the drug and lie down for about three hours until the body adjusts. Then very slowly get up and see if the dizziness and vertigo have disappeared. If not, get right back into bed.

After the first day or so, this problem should wear off and the drug should be much easier to tolerate. It may cause headache and fatigue, aggravate symptoms of angina, and cause palpitations and fluid retention (edema), but in general, **Minipress** is often easier to handle than many other blood-pressure medications. It also does *not* increase cholesterol levels, something that may be a problem with some of the beta blockers.

Another second-line blood-pressure drug is often reserpine. This drug is sold either generically, as reserpine, or as a brand-name product called **Serpasil** or **Rau-Sed**. It is also available as a primary ingredient in many blood-pressure preparations.

Reserpine has one thing going for it. The drug is definitely cheap. And it often works well to bring down mild to moderately high blood pressure, especially in combination with a diuretic. But reserpine produces some unpleasant side effects. Drowsiness, diarrhea, nausea, sedation, fatigue, stomach ulceration, slow heartbeat, nasal congestion, muscular rigidity, nightmares, and psychological depression (sometimes severe enough to lead to thoughts of suicide) are some of the more common adverse reactions people may experience.

A gain in weight is not unusual, due to accumulation of fluids

## Fixed-Combination Formulations Containing Reserpine-type Drugs

| | |
|---|---|
| **Butiserpazide** | **Raudixin** |
| **Diupres** | **Rauwiloid** |
| **Diutensen-R** | **Rauzide** |
| **Enduronyl** | **Regroton** |
| **Exna-R** | **Salutensin** |
| **Hydromox R** | **Sandril** |
| **Hydropres** | **Ser-Ap-Es** |
| **Hydroserpine** | **Serpalan** |
| **Hydrotensin** | **Serpasil** |
| **Metatensin** | **Serpasil-Esidrix** |
| **Naquival** | **Serpate** |
| **Oreticyl** | **SK-Reserpine** |

and an increased appetite. Although medics rarely mention it, impotence or decreased libido has occasionally been known to occur. A review article published in the *New England Journal of Medicine* over a decade ago noted the following: "The high frequency of depressive reactions that may be insidious and easily rationalized or passed unnoticed both by the patient and his physician make rauwolfia alkaloids [reserpine] less desirable than oral diuretics for long-term treatment of hypertension."[41] I find little today that would change my opinion. Given the fact that reserpine offers few advantages over other second-line agents, it would appear that its use is not justified except in special situations.

One drug that used to be considered a mainstay in the medical management of most degrees of hypertension was **Aldomet** (methyldopa). When combined with a diuretic, as in the case of **Aldoclor** (methyldopa and chlorthiazide) and **Aldoril** (methyldopa and hydrochlorothiazide), its effectiveness is increased, and it can be beneficial for folks with moderate to severe hypertension. In patients with some kidney damage, **Aldomet** can be particularly useful, since it does not damage this vital organ, something some other drugs may do.

But methyldopa has lost some of its luster in recent years. Although it is still one of the most commonly prescribed blood-pressure medications, physicians are more aware of side effects with drugs like **Aldomet** and **Aldoril** than they were a decade ago. It can cause sedation and lethargy, not to mention depression and forgetfulness. I have heard a fair number of reports that people can develop difficulty concentrating while on methyldopa. When people stand up suddenly, they may feel dizzy and faint. Skin eruptions, nasal congestion, reduction of sexual desire, and drug fever have also been noted. Digestive-tract upset —including constipation, cramps, and colitis—may become a problem for some patients, and doctors must be especially vigilant to make sure there are no blood disorders or liver damage. While quite a few folks do just fine on methyldopa, many will not feel all that terrific. It will be up to you and your doctor to decide if the benefits outweigh the risks.

A newer drug that has gained in popularity in recent years is **Catapres** (clonidine). It is similar in antihypertensive effect to **Aldomet** but may be slightly better tolerated. It can cause drowsiness, dry mouth, constipation, slow heart rate, and dizziness when you get up suddenly. And the drug may NOT be discontinued abruptly. People can have a severe increase in blood pressure if the drug is stopped too suddenly. They may also experience irregular heartbeats.

One of the newer discoveries with **Catapres** is that the drug seems to have some unexpected effects. There have been reports that it could offer a golden parachute for drug addiction of different sorts. By that I mean it may dramatically reduce the withdrawal symptoms associated with breaking a narcotic addiction.[42] And a more recent study suggests that **Catapres** may make it much easier for heavy smokers to quit cigarettes.[43] In that study, the drug suppressed the anxiety, tension, irritability, and restlessness that are so common in people when they stop smoking. So if you have high blood pressure and also smoke, you might want to discuss **Catapres** with your doctor. It just might be a good high-blood-pressure medicine for you if you would like some help in quitting those nasty ciggies.

A newer drug called **Wytensin** (guanabenz) is comparable in some respects to **Aldomet** and **Catapres**. Appropriate for mild to moderate hypertensives, **Wytensin** may have the added benefit of slightly lowering cholesterol levels. Common side effects include dry mouth, drowsiness and dizziness. As with **Catapres** you should never stop **Wytensin** abruptly as it could lead to rapid elevation in blood pressure, anxiety and palpitations.

If a combination of a diuretic and one of the other drugs listed above does not control blood pressure adequately, many doctors will add **Apresoline** (hydralazine) or **Ismelin** (guanethidine). Both drugs are effective but they have a high incidence of side effects.

**Apresoline** can cause with nausea, diarrhea, dizziness, headache, loss of appetite, and heart palpitations. Less frequently, the drug may produce fluid retention, nasal congestion, dry mouth, anxiety, angina, and psychological disturbances. If drug fever or a generalized, arthritislike achey feeling develops, the drug should be discontinued with a doctor's supervision.

**Ismelin** is usually reserved for the management of severe high blood pressure. It can produce quite a few unwanted adverse reactions. Besides making the patient dizzy every time he or she stands up quickly (especially in the morning), **Ismelin** commonly causes weakness, severe diarrhea, slow heartbeat, nasal congestion, aggravation of asthma, loss of sexual potency, and inhibition of ejaculation in males. As unpleasant as these reactions may be, it could be necessary to put up with them in order to reduce dangerously high levels of blood pressure. Remember, your life is at stake. Sometimes the dose can be reduced when this drug is combined with other medications, such as a diuretic or second-line drug.

Newer drugs for severe hypertension include **Loniten** and **Capoten**. They are usually reserved for moderate to severe high blood pressure because of some serious side effects. **Loniten** (minoxidil) can cause rapid heart rate and can aggravate angina. It may also produce severe fluid retention (edema) and has the unique effect of causing hair to thicken and grow. This can be quite disturbing for women, since the hair growth often appears on the temples, between the eyebrows, in the sideburn area, on the back, arms, and legs.

**Capoten** (captopril), a relatively new compound with a different mode of action from other blood pressure medications was originally approved only for moderate to severe hypertension, but new research has shown that it can be effective even for milder cases.[44] While less likely to produce sexual side effects, fatigue and mental confusion **Capoten** can cause dizziness when you stand suddenly, especially when therapy is first started. Other side effects include loss of taste, rash, vertigo, headache and rapid pulse. Serious blood disorders and kidney problems have also been reported but they are relatively rare at lower doses if patients are in good general health. Sore throat or fever must be reported promptly to a doctor. All in all **Capoten** is an exciting new approach to blood pressure control.

An even newer drug has come along on **Capoten's** heels. **Vasotec** (enalapril) is quite similar to **Capoten** in most respects though it may be a little less likely to cause rash or taste disturbances. Once a day dosing makes it slightly more convenient. Both **Vasotec** and **Capoten** represent important advances in the treatment of hypertension.

To summarize, then, remember that whatever drug your doctor selects for the treatment of your high blood pressure, continuous monitoring of blood pressure is mandatory. The current wisdom seems to be that a beta blocker should be added to a diuretic, and if that doesn't do the trick **Apresoline** gets the nod.[45] Treatment should be individually tailored to each patient, and the dose should be adjusted frequently in order to correspond to changing medical conditions. Weight reduction, salt restriction, mental relaxation techniques, and exercise may in themselves be capable of reducing blood pressure and are always worth trying before drugs are prescribed.

## Heart Attack

So much has been written about heart attacks that there may seem to be very little new to discuss, yet there are so many misconceptions, controversies, and downright contradictions floating around that it would be criminal if some attempt were not made to set the record straight.

The first question to be answered is: What the devil is a heart attack, anyway? Usually, a heart attack occurs when a blood clot lodges in one of the major arteries that feed the heart itself with blood. As the circulation to the heart is reduced, damage occurs and part of the heart "dies." Life-threatening complications set in, and the greatest hazard is that the heart will start beating irregularly or perhaps even stop altogether.

What causes a heart attack? That is the million-dollar question. Although there are lots of theories, no one can say for sure what causes a blood clot to break loose and gum up the works. The best guess is that atherosclerosis gunks up the arteries, and that promotes clotting. What starts the whole process remains a mystery, but we do know that there are certain risk factors that can predispose an individual to a heart attack.

Heredity, high blood pressure, overweight, cigarette smoking, psychological stress, physical inactivity, improper diets, high cholesterol, a sluggish thyroid gland, soft water, excessive coffee consumption, and pollution have all been implicated in one way or another as contributing factors to heart attack. As already mentioned, probably no one thing causes a heart attack; rather, a combination of many of the foregoing elements can increase your chances significantly.

How can you tell if you are eligible for a coronary? There is no simple test that reveals susceptibility. Obviously, untreated high blood pressure is important. If you carry around a spare tire, if you sit on your butt all day, if you smoke like a fiend, if you are under a lot of tension, and if you feel hostile and mad at the world a lot of the time, your life insurance salesman is not going to be very happy.

Physicians like to run expensive electrocardiogram (ECG) tests to measure the state of the heart. Unfortunately, a single office ECG is a poor predictor of heart capability; it is impossible to tell from this whether an individual is at risk for a heart attack. But an exercise electrocardiogram, or stress test, is a valuable tool in the diagnosis of heart disease. By recording heart activity

during exercise, often on a treadmill, it is possible for a trained
clinician to detect many coronary abnormalities well before they
cause a heart attack.

According to an article sponsored by the American Heart
Association and published in *JAMA,* "Exercise testing should
be performed routinely in all men who reach thirty-five years of
age, especially in those with coronary risk factors, in order to
maximize the benefits of early preventive and therapeutic inter-
ventions. The exercise test should be repeated at least every five
years in those over thirty-five, and yearly in those who demonstrate an ischemic response [reduced blood flow]."[46]

It is unfortunate that few internists or cardiologists are
equipped to run an exercise electrocardiogram in their offices.
They should, however, insist that their patients have such a
treadmill test done at the nearest clinic or hospital. If your
doctor does not suggest it, then you should request it. Such a
stress test should always be done before a patient embarks on an
ambitious physical fitness program, in order to determine true
capabilities.

Another test that is much simpler is only as far away as your
nearest mirror. Over a decade ago, doctors from the Division of
Cardiology at the Mount Sinai School of Medicine in New York
discovered that patients with coronary artery disease frequently
showed up with a "diagonal earlobe crease."[47] What was that
again? You read right. Earlobe crease. For reasons that are not
entirely clear (genetic? physiological? hormonal?), people with
clogged arteries seem to have a greater chance of having a diagonal fold, crease, or wrinkle in one or both of their earlobes.

What is so amazing is that the association has held up for over
ten years in study after study. A report in the *New England
Journal of Medicine* (November 15, 1984) confirms once again
that earlobe creases and perhaps even ear-canal hair may be
markers for heart disease:

**The earlobe crease has been demonstrated to be signifi-
cantly associated with coronary-artery disease in specific
populations. Patterns of hair growth have previously been**

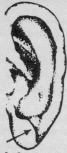

suspected as possible risk factors for coronary-artery disease. We investigated both the earlobe crease and ear-canal hair . . .

The earlobe crease was found to be significantly associated with coronary-artery disease and a significant difference was seen between men with and without coronary-artery disease in the presence of ear-canal hair. . . . The combined presence of ear-canal hair and the earlobe crease was found to be significantly associated with coronary-artery disease. Moreover, combining the earlobe crease and ear-canal hair yielded the greatest sensitivity (90 percent) and the lowest false-negative rate (10 percent).[48]

Now this is *not* to say that everyone with a crease is a candidate for a coronary, just that it could serve as an early warning sign of coronary artery disease and might merit further study. Why not schedule a talk with a cardiologist, just to be on the safe side. But don't let him whip you in for triple-bypass surgery just on the basis of an earlobe crease. That's not the point of this esoteric information.

Even if your electrocardiogram is perfectly normal and you do not have this weird earlobe thing, you are still not immune from arteriosclerosis, heart disease, or a heart attack. What can you do to prevent a mucked-up heart? Scientific studies over the past few years suggest strongly that regular physical activity may provide some protection against coronary heart disease. Not only does vigorous activity seem to reduce high blood pressure, help shed excess pounds, and increase the efficiency of the heart, it would appear that the chances of coming down with a heart attack may be diminished. Yes, I know that James Fixx, author of the best-selling *The Complete Book of Running,* died while running, but don't forget that he apparently had a genetic predisposition for heart disease, since his father died at a young age from a heart attack.

One of the most comprehensive investigations into the relationship between physical activity and coronary heart mortality was carried out among longshoremen in the San Francisco Bay area from 1951 to 1972.[49] A total of 6,351 workers were studied in order to determine whether the type of work a man did could influence the health of his heart. It was discovered that those longshoremen whose jobs required vigorous physical exercise had a lower rate of heart attacks than other longshoremen who were less active. The authors concluded that heavy, energy-expending work can serve as a protective mechanism against the development of coronary artery disease.

Not everyone has the "luxury" of a physically demanding job. Since most of us have occupations that do not require the kind of protective exertion that longshoremen get, does that mean we are condemned to die from a heart attack? Absolutely not! Recreational physical exercise may not be as regular or sustained as on-the-job activity, but it can serve a protective function and make us feel better about ourselves to boot.

But short bursts of exercise at lunchtime or occasional sports activity are not enough to do the job. A round of golf on weekends or a leisurely set of mixed doubles hardly gets the heart beating. What you need is a regular program of physical exercise that is planned and supervised by a physician.

Before starting out, remember to have a stress test done in order to evaluate the condition of the heart. Then start out nice and easy, and slowly work up to a rigorous workout. You can find some excellent suggestions about designing an exercise program in Covert Bailey's book *Fit or Fat.* Each session should begin with a brief period of warm-up calisthenics (five to ten minutes) followed by thirty to sixty minutes of regular exercise. Take another ten to fifteen minutes to cool down and relax.

This kind of activity should be scheduled at least three times a week. Jogging, bicycle riding, swimming, tennis, or even a brisk walk can all be effective forms of exercise. Group exercise sessions may be more practical, and if you can get into such a program, so much the better. Avoid isometric exercise, such as weight lifting, since it may cause dangerous increases in blood pressure. Once you have started an exercise program, you should plan on maintaining it for the rest of your life, since stopping may be worse than not starting at all.

Lack of exercise is not the only important factor that can predispose an individual to a coronary. Until recently, psychological stress and personality type had been pretty much ignored in the search for evil demons. However, over the last decade or so some heart experts have begun to look more closely at the state of mind of an individual than at physical factors. We have heard a lot about the so-called Type A personality. It has been challenged in recent years, but there still seems to be a kernel of truth in there somewhere. Experts I have spoken to believe that hostility may be one of the most important psychological triggers for heart disease. The person who is convinced that the world is out to get him and distrusts everyone or is ready to pick a fight at the drop of a hat may be at an increased risk of a heart attack. Personality traits are hard to change, but with help the task *can* be accomplished.

Well, what about diet? Doctors hate cholesterol. They are convinced that it is a primary cause of coronary heart disease, and they have managed to scare millions of Americans into eliminating eggs from their morning breakfasts. When they fail to bring down blood cholesterol in this manner, physicians frequently resort to drug therapy. But cholesterol is an essential biochemical necessary for the development of new cells and tissue. Just because it has received a bad press does not make it any less important. It is manufactured by your own body (bet you didn't know that), and without it you would be in bad shape.

Cholesterol has many indispensible physiological functions, one of which is to increase the solubility of absorbed fats (from foods) and assist in the transport of these fats from your stomach to storage depots in other parts of your body. The cholesterol that you eat in your food is not nearly as responsible for raising your blood cholesterol as is that made by your own body in response to the fat consumed in meat and other foods. Therefore, if you merely eliminated cholesterol from your diet without cutting down significantly on saturated fats, you would do little to lower your serum cholesterol.

Even more important is the question whether diet will actually prevent heart attacks. Solid scientific evidence supporting this view is downright puny. An article in *Science* (January 4, 1985) summarizes the controversy:

> To many observers, the recent National Institutes of Health consensus panel report seemed merely to restate the conventional wisdom. The panel announced on 13 December [1984] . . . that high concentrations of blood cholesterol cause heart disease. In addition, . . . "lowering cholesterol can reduce the incidence of coronary artery disease and save lives." The panel recommended that all Americans, from age two onward, reduce their consumption of saturated fats and cholesterol and suggested a diet like the American Heart Association's prudent diet, which emphasizes fruit and vegetables, restricts egg yolks to no more than two a week, and specifies lean meat, skim milk, and low-fat cheeses.[50]

So what's the big deal? You've heard all that before, right? Well be patient. Here comes the juicy part:

> But despite what the panel said, there is no irrefutable evidence from clinical trials that cholesterol-lowering saves lives. And it is not as though no one has tried to get evidence.

Over the past 20 years, there have been nearly two dozen clinical trials of cholesterol-lowering. These trials involved at least 50,000 people at high risk for heart disease, selected so that they would be most likely to benefit from lowered blood cholesterol if it helps at all. But these trials failed to show that cholesterol-lowering prevents deaths from heart disease. Moreover, if you lump all the trials together and look for an effect, you still do not see one.[51]

Holy Moly! That, my friend, is earthshaking. We're talking very big numbers here. You would think the case would be closed, but clearly it is as controversial as ever. Does that mean you should pig out on pizza, milk shakes, steak, and salami? Of course not. A prudent diet is certainly appropriate. Saturated fats should be reduced as much as possible. While it must be admitted that there is no guarantee that diet can help prevent death from coronary artery disease, it cannot hurt, and may be well worth the effort. If it aids in reducing excess pounds, then for sure it has succeeded.

There is one other heart attack–prevention program that must be mentioned. Why not consider plain old aspirin?

That may not be as silly as it sounds. In 1974 a comprehensive British research project discovered that a single aspirin tablet taken daily could improve life expectancy by 25 percent in men who had already suffered one heart attack.[52] That is truly incredible. The Boston Collaborative Drug Surveillance Group undertook an even larger investigation comparing 776 patients hospitalized for heart attack with almost 14,000 patients who had been hospitalized with other disorders. It was found that people who took aspirin regularly had a significantly lower incidence of fatal heart attacks.[53]

There is sound theoretical evidence to support the theory that aspirin could help prevent heart attacks. It is well known that acetylsalicylic acid (aspirin) can reduce clotting factors in blood, specifically platelet aggregation. Because the thing that causes a heart attack is a blood clot, it is only logical to concentrate on this stage of the problem. While doctors have concentrated on earlier steps, such as serum cholesterol and arteriosclerosis, it would appear to me that the problem worth studying is blood clotting, and aspirin may be the solution.

It is interesting to note that as far back as 1953 evidence appeared to indicate that aspirin could be beneficial.[54] Dr. Sidney Cobb "found that only 4 percent of 191 patients with prolonged rheumatoid arthritis had died from myocardial infarction [heart attack], compared with the 31 percent of deaths in the general population of the U.S.A. from this cause. This may not be a statistically appropriate comparison, but it does suggest that the continuous taking of aspirin as an analgesic may have unexpectedly reduced deaths from atherosclerotic heart disease."[55] A more recent look at rheumatoid arthritis seems to confirm the observation that patients with this disease have considerably less sickness and death due to heart attacks even though they have just as much coronary arteriosclerosis as everyone else.[56] This just adds more support to the theory that aspirin may prevent the last and most important step in the development of a heart attack: blood clots. Maybe arthritis victims have something to cheer about after all.

On the basis of preliminary evidence, even before the British and Boston studies were published, one heart specialist saw fit to write the following commentary in *Lancet:*

> I suggest that men over the age of twenty and women over the age of forty should take one aspirin tablet (0.325 g.) a day on a chronic, long term basis in the hope that this will lessen the severity of arterial thrombosis and atherosclerosis. Exceptions to this would be people with bleeding disorders, aspirin allergy, uncontrolled hypertension, and those with a history of bleeding lesions of the gastrointestinal tract [ulcers] or other organ system. . . . The treatment I advise may turn out to be completely ineffective but the financial cost will have been slight. However, to me the rationale for this regimen seems sound, the risks small, and the possible benefits enormous.[57]

Dr. Lee Wood made that statement in 1972, before the British and Boston studies had even been completed. Nothing in the intervening years has contradicted him. On the contrary, evidence has accumulated to support his point of view.

A recent study confirmed that one aspirin a day reduced the incidence of heart attacks in high-risk patients (those with something called unstable angina) by over 50 percent.[58] There are even suggestions that less is best, and that one quarter or one eighth of an aspirin tablet may be effective. If you are at increased risk, why not discuss the aspirin story with your physician. You may be surprised at what you hear.

Well dear reader, that is about all I have to say about high blood pressure and heart attacks. Keep in mind the following points and you will improve your chances quite significantly:

**Exercise may be good—overweight may be bad bad bad.**

**Controlled blood pressure may be good—high blood pressure may be bad.**

**Diet may be good—atherosclerosis may be bad.**

**Biofeedback may be good—psychological stress may be bad.**

**Aspirin may be good—smoking may be bad.**

**Tea may be good—coffee may be bad.**

**Hard water may be good—soft water may be bad.**

**Active thyroid gland may be good—sluggish thyroid may be bad.**

**Mental relaxation may be good—Type A behavior pattern and hostility may be bad.**

# References

1. *Heart Facts,* American Heart Association, Dallas, Texas, 1983, pp. 1–3.

2. Maciejko, James J., et al. "Apolipoprotein A-I as a Marker of Angiographically Assessed Coronary-Artery Disease." *N. Engl. J. Med.* 309:385–389, 1983.

3. Mroczek, William J., et al. "Detection of Hypertension Blood Pressure Determination in Outpatient Clinics of Medical School-Affiliated Training Programs." *JAMA* 231:1264–1266, 1975.

4. Mancia, Giuseppe, et al. "Effects of Blood-Pressure Measurement by the Doctor on Patient's Blood Pressure and Heart Rate." *Lancet* 2:695–698, 1983.

5. Perloff, Dorothee, et al. "The Prognostic Value of Ambulatory Blood Pressure." *JAMA* 249:2792–2798, 1983.

6. Rowlands, D. B., et al. "Assessment of Left Ventricular Mass and Its Response to Antihypertensive Treatment." *Lancet* 1:467–470, 1982.

7. News. "At-Home BP Readings Prove Best in Drug Trials." *Medical World News* 24(19):52, 1983.

8. "Symposium on Hypertension: The Treatment of Essential and Malignant Hypertension." *Mod. Med.* 40(6):75–113, 1972.

9. Messerli, F. H. "Cardiovascular Effects of Obesity and Hypertension." *Lancet* 1:1165–1168, 1982.

10. Stamler, R., et al. "Weight and Blood Pressure. Findings in Hypertension Screening in One Million Americans." *JAMA* 240:1607–1611, 1982.

11. Messerli, Franz F. "Obesity in Hypertension: How Innocent a Bystander?" *Am. J. Med.* 77:1077–1082, 1984.

12. Reisin, E., et al. "Cardiovascular Changes after Weight Reduction in Obesity Hypertension." *Ann. Intern. Med.* 98:315–319, 1983.

13. McCarron, David A., et al. "Blood Pressure and Nutrient Intake in the United States." *Science* 224:1392–1398, 1984.

14. Skrabel, F., et al. "Low Sodium/High Potassium Diet for Prevention of Hypertension: Probable Mechanisms of Action." *Lancet* 2:895–900, 1981.

15. Henningsen, Nels-Christian, et al. "Potassium/Sodium Ratio and Thermogenes." *Lancet* 1:591–592, 1983.

16. Belizam, Jose M. "Reduction of Blood Pressure with Calcium Supplementation in Young Adults." *JAMA* 249:1161–1165, 1983.

17. Sopko, Joseph A., and Freeman, Richard M. "Salt Substitutes as a Source of Potassium." *JAMA* 236:608–610, 1977.

18. Epstein, F. H., and Eckhoff, R. D. "The Epidemiology of High Blood Pressure—Geographic Distributions and Etiologic Factors." In *The Epidemiology of Hypertension.* J. Stamler and R. Stamler, eds. New York: Grune & Stratton, 1967, pp. 155–166.

19. Choquette, Gaston, and Ferguson, Ronald J. "Blood Pressure Reduction in Borderline Hypertensives Following Physical Training." *Can. Med. Assoc. J.* 108:699–703, 1973.

20. News Front. "More Support for Regular Exercise." *Mod. Med.* 52(10):53, 1984.

21. Montoyle, Henry J., et al. "Habitual Physical Activity and Blood Pressure." *Medicine and Science in Sports* 4(4):175–181, 1972.

22. Boyer, J. L., and Kasch, F. W. "Exercise Therapy in Hypertensive Men." *JAMA* 211:1688, 1970.

23. Bjorntorp, P. "Hypertension and Exercise." *Hypertension* 4 (suppl III):III56–59, 1982.

24. Hagberg, J. M., et al. "Effect of Exercise Training on the Blood Pressure and Hemodynamic Features of Hypertensive Adolescents." *Am. J. Cardiol.* 52:763–768, 1983.

25. Patel, C. H. "Yoga and Bio-Feedback in the Management of Hypertension." *Lancet* 2:1053–1055, 1973.

26. Patel, C. H. "12-Month Follow-up of Yoga and Bio-feedback in Management of Hypertension." *Lancet* 1:62–63, 1975.

27. Patel, C. H., et al. "Controlled Trial of Biofeedback-Aided Behavioural Methods in Reducing Mild Hypertension." *Br. Med. J.* 282:2005–2008, 1981.

28. Engel, B. T., et al. "Behavioral Treatment of High Blood Pressure. III. Follow-up Results and Treatment." *Psychosom. Med.* 45:23–29, 1983.

29. Andrews, G., et al. "Hypertension: Comparison of Drug and Non-drug Treatments." *Br. Med. J.* 284:1523–1526, 1982.

30. Scarf, Maggie. "Tuning Down with TM." *New York Times Mag.* Feb. 9, 1975, p. 27.

31. Ibid.

32. Ibid.

33. Updates. "Diuretics Most Prescribed." *FDA Consumer* 18(5):6–7, 1984.

34. Kaplan, Norman M. "New Choices for the Initial Drug Therapy of Hypertension." *Am. J. Cardiol.* 51:1786–1788, 1983.

35. Editorial. "Antihypertensive Drugs, Plasma Lipids, and Coronary Disease." *Lancet* 2:19–20, 1980.

36. Veterans Administration Cooperative Study Group on Antihypertensive Agents: "Comparison of Propranolol and Hydrochlorothiazide for the Initial Treatment of Hypertension." *JAMA* 248:1996–2011, 1982.

37. Williams, W. R., et al. "The Relationship between Diuretics and Serum Cholesterol in HDFP Participants." Presented at the American College of Cardiology, Mar. 20–24, 1983, New Orleans.

38. Reyes, A. J. "Diuretics and Zinc." *S. Afr. Med. J.* 62:373–375, 1982.

39. "New Trial Tightens Link between Thiazides and Cardiac Arrhythmia." *Medical World News,* Jan. 24, 1983, p. 32.

40. Wilkinson, P. R. "Total Body and Serum Potassium During Prolonged Thiazide Therapy for Essential Hypertension." *Lancet* 1:759–762, 1975.

41. Page, Lot B., and Sidd, James J. "Medical Management of Primary Hypertension II." *N. Engl. J. Med.* 287:1018–1022, 1972.

42. Washton, Arnold M., et al. "Lofexidine, a Clonidine Analogue Effective in Opiate Withdrawal." *Lancet* 1:992–993, 1981.

43. Glassman, Alexander H., et al. "Cigarette Craving, Smoking Withdrawal, and Clonidine." *Science* 226:864–866, 1984.

44. "Drugs for Hypertension." *Medical Letter* 26:107–112, 1984.

45. Ibid.

46. DeBusk, Robert. "The Value of Exercise Stress Testing." *JAMA* 232:956–958, 1975.

47. Lichstein, Edgar, et al. "Diagonal Ear-Lobe Crease: Prevalence and Implications as a Coronary Risk Factor." *N. Engl. J. Med.* 290:-615–616, 1974.

48. Wagner, A. U., et al. "Ear-Canal Hair and the Ear-Lobe Crease as Predictors for Coronary-Artery Disease." *N. Engl. J. Med.* 311:-1317–1318, 1984

49. Paffenbarger, Ralph S., Jr., and Hale, Wayne E. "Work Activity and Coronary Heart Mortality." *N. Engl. J. Med.* 292:545–550, 1975.

50. Kolata, Gina. "Heart Panel's Conclusions Questioned." *Science* 227:40–41, 1985.

51. Ibid.

52. Elwood, P. C. "A Randomized Controlled Trial of Acetylsalicylic Acid in the Secondary Prevention of Mortality from Myocardial Infarction." *Br. Med. J.* 1:436–440, 1974.

53. Boston Collaborative Drug Surveillance Group. "Regular Aspirin Intake and Acute Myocardial Infarction." *Br. Med. J.* 1:440–443, 1974.

54. Cobb, Sidney, et al. "Length of Life and Cause of Death in Rheumatoid Arthritis." *N. Engl. J. Med.* 249:533–536, 1953.

55. Editorial. "Aspirin and Atherosclerosis." *Br. Med. J.* 1:408, 1974.

56. Davis, R. D., and Engelman, E. G. "Incidence of Myocardial Infarction in Patients with Rheumatoid Arthritis." *Arthritis Rheum.* 17:527–533, 1974.

57. Wood, Lee. "Treatment of Atherosclerosis and Thrombosis with Aspirin." *Lancet* 2:532–533, 1972.

58. Lewis, H. Daniel. "Protective Effects of Aspirin against Acute Myocardial Infarction and Death in Men with Unstable Angina." *N. Engl. J. Med.* 309:396–403, 1983.

# 12

## How to Save Money on Prescription Drugs

---

*New drugs can be expensive • The doctor's prescription: How to make sense out of gobbledygook • What is the difference between generic and brand names? • Saving money is harder than you think • Are generics equivalent? • Who makes aspirin?: One of the best-kept secrets in the pharmaceutical industry! • All the rules have changed: Truce in a nasty little drug war • The economics of prescription drugs • Your best-priced prescription • Table 1: Off-Patent Brand-Name Drugs and Their Generic Equivalents • Table 2: Brand-Name Drugs That Will Be Coming Off Patent.*

---

Have you been to the drugstore lately? If you've had to pay for a prescription in the last several months, you know that the price of many medicines is skyrocketing and could soon be astronomical.

Take the teenager with cystic acne. Her dermatologist prescribed **Accutane** (isotretinoin), which he assured her would be a miracle cure for her severe skin problem. What he didn't tell her was how much it would cost. When the pharmacist handed her a three-month supply of **Accutane** and a bill for $300, she almost fainted.

While this may be an extreme case, more and more of the new medications being prescribed are extremely expensive. People with arthritis may find their monthly bill runs between $20 and $30 for drugs like **Feldene** (piroxicam), **Clinoril** (sulindac), **Naprosyn** (naproxen), or **Tolectin** (tolmetin). If you also have to take high-blood-pressure pills such as **Corgard** (nadolol) and **Dyazide** (triamterene and hydrochlorothiazide) you can add another $25 or so, bringing your monthly medicine bill to $50 or more.

The tragedy is that older people are most likely to need more medications, and they are exactly the ones who often find it most difficult to pay the tab. But anyone who needs to watch the budget carefully may have to make hard decisions. A letter we received from a pharmacist drives home this point.

> **I'm a pharmacist with a lot of older customers.** It broke my heart yesterday when one of them burst into tears as I handed her the refill for her blood-pressure medicine.
> I had to tell her the price had gone up and her bill was over $30. She sobbed that they were going to cut off her lights if she didn't pay her electric bill, and it would have to be either that bill or this medicine. The electric bill won.
> Why don't doctors realize some patients can't afford the fanciest, newest medications?

An unemployed factory worker wrote to us about his wife's antidepressant:

> **My wife suffers from severe depression.** Twice in the past five years she's tried to commit suicide. Luckily, she was saved both times, but you can imagine that when she gets depressed it scares me.

Her doctor has her on a medicine called Elavil. It's been working well, but this drug really strains our limited budget. A month's supply costs over $15.

The last time we got it refilled, the pharmacist told us this drug is available much cheaper—under $6 for the same amount. The trouble is, she can't dispense this generic medicine without the doctor's permission. But when I asked him, he said the generic does not work as well. Is this true? Saving money would be a big help, but I don't want to take a risk with my wife's life.

And there, my friend, are the two biggest obstacles to saving money in the drugstore. Some doctors like to prescribe the newest, fanciest brand-name products on the market. They may think that this makes them appear up with the latest technological developments, but such drugs are almost inevitably more expensive than older tried-and-true therapies.

In addition, many physicians have been sold a bill of goods by the huge pharmaceutical firms. They are often told that generic drugs are inferior to brand-name versions. Doctors then pass the same message on to the patient and as a result people may end up paying two hundred or three hundred percent more for a brand-name drug.

Well, I'm here to tell you it doesn't have to be that way. You *can* save money on prescription medications. Lots of money! But it will require some effort on your part.

In this chapter I'll tell you a bit about how and why the cost of medicine is sometimes so high, and then I'll write you a prescription for getting yourself the best possible deal on the drugs you purchase.

One of the first things you'll have to do is change the way you think about drugs. You see, most of us tend to treat medicine as if it were sacred. If the doctor prescribes Brand X, then that's what we think we must take, even though a generic version may be only half the price. And if we see an ad on television for **Actifed** or **Pepto-Bismol**, then those are the brands we look for, rather than some unfamiliar-sounding chemical name.

But attitudes must change if we're going to save any money. Many familiar medications come in several different brands, sold by lots of different companies. It's up to you, the patient, to shop around a bit and make the best deal on the product you need.

I'm going to give you lots of ammunition for the war on excessive drug costs, but you are going to have to be willing to use it and use it aggressively if you expect to translate that information into more money in your pocket. Judging from past behavior, your doctor and perhaps even your pharmacist will resist feeble attempts to reduce drug costs.

Nevertheless, there is a way to beat the game and come away with significant savings on many medications. But you'll have to start out well prepared, and be determined. If you are willing to take on these bastions of the medical establishment, read on. By the time you finish this chapter you are going to know more than your physician about prices and how to save some big bucks in the murky world of prescription drugs.

## The Doctor's Prescription

The first thing that the consumer (a patient is really nothing other than a health consumer) must learn is how to read a prescription. If your doctor will not tell you exactly what medication he has prescribed, then it is up to you to figure it out for yourself.

Although the pharmacist and the physician have long had a secret code (usually composed of Latin abbreviations), it is an easy nut to crack, especially with regard to the information required for saving money. Basically, all you need to know is the name of the drug, the form (tablets, capsules, elixir, etc.), the potency (100 milligrams, or whatever), and the amount you are to receive (40 tablets, 100 capsules, etc.). Check out the handy-dandy example and see if you can get the hang of it.

The term *modern medicine* is something of a cliché. It presumably implies state-of-the-art medical knowledge, with all the vast, high-technology resources we wonder at. That's one of the things that makes prescriptions almost quaint, because they retain elements of medicine's hocus-pocus past.

Far too many physicians still specialize in writing illegibly. They may also resort to such abbreviations as *disp., cap.* (easily figured out to mean *dispense, capsule*), or less comprehensible jargon such as *Sig.: 5 gtt., t.i.d., p.c.* Such abbreviations come from a "dead" language (Latin). That's modern medicine? The pharmacist translates this secret message to mean "label the prescription: 5 drops, three times a day, after meals."

But I ask a simple question: Why? Why is it necessary to use such a code? If it seems to you like the doctor and pharmacist are trying to hide something, I wouldn't argue. It certainly is no way to establish good communication between a physician and a patient.

---

**John Doe, M.D.**
777 Medical Rip-Off Center
Anywhere, U.S.A.
Telephone: HElp 7-1234

Name John Q. Public                      Date Mayday 1986
Address Brokeville                            Age 40
        Rx


Ampicillin Capsules, 250 mg
Dispense 100 capsules
Label: Take one capsule three times a day

*John Doe, M.D.*

---

Basically a prescription is a very simple thing—the doctor's order to provide you with a certain quantity of a particular drug, and to label the package with certain instructions. Just why this straightforward act needs to be accompanied by ancient Latin chants and incantations is a mystery, which may be exactly what the medical people hope to keep it. Writing a prescription is the outcome of most visits to the doctor, and having it appear to be a very important, complex, and significant task adds to the mystique of doctoring.

It would certainly simplify life for everyone if physicians printed out prescriptions in plain English. It would give you a chance to question the doctor about his instructions and would cut down on mistakes. But even if your doctor is unreformable, that doesn't mean you're out of luck. Fortunately, it is not necessary for you to be able to understand the nonsense syllables scribbled on a prescription form, since the pharmacist will hopefully write them out in English on the label.

Okay, so you know what medication you are supposed to take, but in the quagmire of prescription drugs there can be an awful lot in a name. By now most people have heard the word *generic* batted around and are aware that it has something to do with reduced prices. Unfortunately, it has not helped many patients save money. That is because generic prescribing is misunderstood and rarely exploited to full advantage.

Whenever a pharmaceutical manufacturing company develops a new drug in the lab, the product receives a number. For months, and often years, it's known only by this number.

Once it reaches the clinical testing phase the drug gets an official name. This is the *generic,* "scientific," or nonproprietary name. It's created by a quasi-official organization under the direction of the American Medical Association and the American Pharmaceutical Association, among others.

The drug acquires, along the way, two important things in addition to its generic name. First, a patent, which assures the drug company approximately seventeen years of protection against competition, and second, a *trade name* (also called *proprietary name*). This easily promoted brand name is quite different from the official generic title, which is often hard to spell, difficult to remember, and practically impossible to pronounce.

Let's take a look at a few examples. **Dyazide** is one of the most commonly prescribed medications in the country. It is a diuretic that lowers blood pressure without depleting the body of potassium. Its ingredients, *hydrochlorothiazide* and *triamterene,* hardly come tripping lightly to the tongue. Or how about **Bactrim**? This antibacterial agent is used for everything from urinary-tract infections to earaches and traveler's diarrhea. Just try to remember or pronounce its generic components: *sulfamethoxazole* and *trimethoprim.*

Or how about such familiar favorites as **Librium** *(chlordiazepoxide),* **Darvocet-N** *(propoxyphene napsylate),* and **Dilantin** *(phenytoin)*? Is it any wonder doctors tend to stick with snappy brand names they can spell and pronounce with ease? And don't forget, the drug companies are putting plenty of bucks into promoting these catchy names.

For the life of the patent (and even long afterward) glossy full-color ads in medical journals will tout the drug's abilities and emphasize its trade name. The doctor will be visited by assertive drug detail reps who will bombard him with free samples, notepads, pens, rulers, calendars, and all other manner of geegaws. Each of these samples and goodies bears a drug's trade name.

This goes on for about seventeen years. At the end of that time the drug "comes off patent." This means other companies, after establishing their ability to produce a chemically identical product, can manufacture the same stuff and sell it under either the generic name or under a new trade name they create.

Or, we should say, they can *attempt* to sell it. Here's the doctor, stuffed with years of being told **Valium** is what to write when a patient needs a minor tranquilizer. Although **Valium** has recently come off patent and generic houses are ready to put out their own versions of *diazepam,* when the doctor goes to write a prescription for a minor tranquilizer, what do you think he or she is most likely to put down on that prescription blank?

Now all this wouldn't make much difference if diazepam and **Valium** cost the same. But a generic drug is almost always cheaper than its trade-name rival. After all, somebody has to pay for not only the original research leading to the drug's discovery, but also for all that advertising, the drug reps on the road, the imprinted pencils and pads, etc. Pharmaceutical manufacturers spend over a billion dollars a year just promoting their drugs to doctors. All this adds up, and as we'll see in a bit, the differences in drug costs to the consumer are often unbelievable.

It would seem that saving money on drugs should be easy. Just get the generic version of the medicine and you're home free. Unfortunately, it's not that simple.

First, even if your doctor has written you a generic prescription, that does not mean the medicine is available generically. Many medications are available only under their trade names because the seventeen-year patent period hasn't expired, or because the market wasn't large enough to entice a generic manufacturer to take up production.

But let's imagine that your medicine is indeed available from both the original manufacturer and from generic suppliers at significant savings. You haven't won the battle by a long shot.

Your physician can do one of three things. He can write a brand-name prescription such as **Valium** or its generic counterpart diazepam. In most states that wouldn't matter, since the pharmacist has the option to substitute a generic product even when the doctor writes a brand name, *unless* the doctor specifies that substitution isn't permissible.

It is this third option that can cost you money. When the physician writes "dispense as written" or "do not substitute," the pharmacist has no leeway. The drug *must* be dispensed exactly as called for, which usually means by a specific brand name.

Why would the doctor do that? Two reasons. First, because he or she has absolute, scientific knowledge that one company's preparation of a drug acts differently in the body than another company's. Or, second, because the doctor has been convinced that's true *without* any real scientific information to support that conclusion.

We'd all like to think that our physicians are careful, rational, logical, analytical, and well informed. And they mostly are. But when it comes to drugs, marketing is a very strong force. Think about this for a second. Why do you use the brand of catsup or beer that you use? Possibly because it tastes best to you. Or, more possibly, because you were persuaded of its virtues by a heavy barrage of television, magazine, and newspaper advertising. Well, the doctor faces a similarly intense marketing effort on behalf of trade-name drugs.

Now you may be getting indignant right about here. Perhaps you've tried Dole pineapples and you say they are better than the house brand. Or maybe it's Kleenex brand facial tissues that you favor over the generics. Well, I can understand that, because the makers of house-brand generic products do not have to meet the identical standards of the brand-name versions. No one says that el cheapo toilet paper has to be as soft and firm as the advertised brands.

But when it comes to drugs, the generics must *by law* be identical! The FDA does not allow one company to market medicine that is only 80 percent as effective as the original product.

Once a drug goes off patent, part of the marketing effort of the big pharmaceutical manufacturers goes to convincing doctors there is a significant difference between the brand-name drug and its generic equivalent. Ads will exhort the doctor to order the brand-name version rather than any generic equal, and imply something is wrong with the generics. For example, in a recent issue of the *Journal of the American Medical Association* we find an ad for Pfizer's **Vibra-Tabs Vibramycin**, a brand-name version of the drug doxycycline. "Protect your choice by writing Dispense as Written" urges the ad. What the doctor is really protecting, perhaps without meaning to do so, is the drug company's profits.

## Generic vs. Brand-Name

The argument your doctor will almost always resort to when defending his practice of prescribing expensive brands is that they are superior in quality to the generic varieties. Since nobody wants a prescription for bad medicine, this approach usually shuts a patient up pretty fast. By the time the doctor is done, you'll probably apologize for mentioning the subject.

If your doctor hands you this tired line, he or she is fooling you in the worst way. The inequality-of-drugs routine is usually just plain untrue. There have been some very rare exceptions, but it is almost 100 percent true that generic drugs are every bit the equal of their brand-name twins. On occasion they're even a bit better.

This isn't really surprising when you consider how closely regulated the manufacturing and distribution of prescription drugs is. The FDA holds every manufacturer—brand-name and generic alike—to high standards designed to assure consumers that the final product is what it's supposed to be in terms of dose, potency, cleanliness, and other critical factors.

But don't take my word for it. Listen to what the experts have to say. Let's start with antibiotics, because they're prescribed with great regularity. Guess what? Many of the most commonly prescribed classes of antibiotics are made by a few major firms, which resell the drugs to other pharmaceutical suppliers for distribution!

Brand A and Brand B may not only be equal in therapeutic effect, they may be absolutely identical because they're the same pill, made by the same manufacturer, in the same factory, at virtually the same time!

The Council on Economic Priorities (CEP) did a fascinating little study of drugs and their pricing. One of the things they found was that more than seventy companies *supply* the antibiotic tetracycline, but "Only four firms manufacture the bulk ingredient within the United States according to the U.S. Tariff Commission. No more than ten firms manufacture the final dosage form."[1]

There you have it. Four firms made the tetracycline, ten pressed it into tablets, and seventy sold it. Some of those seventy claim theirs is better, and charge more because of it. Are you going to swallow that?

The story is the same for lots of other drugs. The Council on Economic Priorities study reported some years ago that:

It is a widespread practice for one firm to manufacture a product and sell that product to different firms, which in turn sell at different prices under different brand names. For example, taking into account only the major firms, we find that Mylan Laboratories manufactures final dose form *Erythromycin* for SmithKline, Pfizer, Parke-Davis, Squibb, and Wyeth, each of which sells the *Erythromycin* under its own name. Bristol Laboratories manufactures *Ampicillin* for itself as well as for Smith Kline, Robins, Parke-Davis, and Wyeth. Beecham sells *Ampicillin* to Pfizer, Lederle and Ayerst. Not only do each of these firms sell each of these products at different prices, but small generic houses purchase final dose form antibiotics from the same manufacturers.[2]

Exasperating as it is to learn that numerous pharmaceutical suppliers charge different prices for the same product, it is even more disturbing to hear that the *same* company often charges wildly variable prices for its own, identical product! At the time of the CEP study, a company called ICN Pharmaceuticals sold 100 ampicillin (250 mg) tablets for $7.50. It sold the same ampicillin under the brand name **Acillin**. The price? $14.50!

If all that sounds confusing, let's take a look at a popular nonprescription product for just a minute. One of the best-kept secrets in the pharmaceutical industry is who makes aspirin. Though most people assume that the company that sells an over-the-counter product has manufactured it, that's often not the case at all. Just as with prescription medicine, many firms purchase ready-made tablets from another source and just stick their labels on the bottles. Hard as it is to believe, the acetylsalicylic acid in most of the four hundred brands of aspirin on the market comes from only two manufacturers: Dow and Monsanto. By the way, Norwich-Eaton does make its own aspirin, as does Sterling, the manufacturer of **Bayer Aspirin.**

Pain relievers are a billion-dollar business, and in this highly competitive market each advertiser does its best to make its brand stand out from all the others. One commercial insists its analgesic has more pain reliever than any of the other leading brands, while another product is hyped as faster-acting. Companies will claim they have ingredients that are gentler to the stomach or repeat unmercifully that popular refrain—"the most potent pain reliever you can buy without a prescription."

Since the primary ingredient in such products is aspirin, knowledgeable people have long been skeptical that these differences are important except in commercials. And in fact, researchers at Consumers Union have reconfirmed that there are no significant variations among nine widely purchased brands of plain aspirin.[3]

It didn't matter whether they tested the big boys like Bayer or Squibb, or cheaper house brands put out by K-Mart or Kroger. The researchers found that strict government standards were being met in all cases and that each tablet was practically identical in the amount of aspirin it contained. The tablets also dissolved at virtually the same rate, ensuring that they would be absorbed into the bloodstream equally. The conclusion—"All aspirin is pretty much the same."[4]

Still don't believe that brand-name drugs and their generic counterparts are created equal? Here's what a former director of the FDA's Bureau of Drugs, Dr. Henry Simmons, has to say on the matter: "Based on many years of experience with this program we are confident that there is no significant difference between so-called generic and brand-name antibiotic products on the American market."[5]

But what about other classes of medicines? To settle the question once and for all, Congress got into the act through an investigation by the Office of Technology Assessment. The study group was headed by the dean of the Yale University School of Medicine, Dr. Robert Berliner. *Consumer Reports* summarized the panel's findings by saying, "The OTA panel concluded that the great proportion of chemically equivalent products—85 to 90 percent, according to Dr. Berliner's estimate—presents no problems of therapeutic equivalency and could be used interchangeably. 'Most drugs ought to be prescribed generically,' Dr. Berliner told Consumers Union."[6]

They certainly should be. And they finally may be, thanks to a new law that came along in 1984.

## All the Rules Have Changed

In 1984 a nasty little drug war broke out in Washington, D.C. It wasn't the war against illicit drugs, but a war between brand-name and generic medications. What the politicians and drug companies were fighting for was your pocketbook.

At issue were two questions. First, when in a drug's development stage would the seventeen-year patent period be measured from, and second, how much testing and certification would a generic drug have to go through?

These two issues came to be linked because of proposed changes in legislation that has long governed the drug industry. Patent protection extends from the time the patent application is granted. For almost any other product, that means the item gets marketed and makes money from that time on. With drugs, however, the period of premarketing testing and review by the FDA is often years long, and the big companies have long complained they don't get seventeen years of profitable sales out of their seventeen-year patents.

The generic manufacturers, in turn, had their own gripes. The law, strongly influenced by the big, brand-name manufacturers, made these companies go through almost the entire process of proving the drug was safe and effective. This, even though the drug was coming off patent after seventeen years of use. The generic manufacturers felt, and rightly so, that this was absurd. They were willing to prove they could produce a chemically equivalent product. They wanted the right to submit the drug's existing history of use to show it worked.

The two groups, each represented by some pretty hefty lobbying muscle, went at it tooth and nail. Each hoped to extract the most and give up the least. The biggies wanted their seventeen-year run extended by the length of time the drug was in the testing and approval process, but they didn't want to give the generic manufacturers any easier access to the market.

It was as bloody a political battle as we've seen fought in a long time. Not only was there a lot of money at stake, but the big companies even fell to fighting among themselves about how much to compromise. The political tide, though, was running heavily against the brand-name manufacturers. Health-care costs are a hot topic now, and nobody wanted to vote for anything that would raise the tab.

In the end, there emerged a compromise that will save you the consumer an estimated billion dollars in the next ten years. The brand-name manufacturers get a flat five-year extension of their patent protection, to make up for the time lost to premarketing delays. And the generic manufacturers get a vastly simplified process for gaining approval to market their products once the original manufacturer's patent protection ends. In fact, they even get to start the paperwork process before a drug comes off patent, so they can be up and running on the day they are given the green light.

A lot of very important and widely used drugs have already or soon will come off patent in the next few years, including such hall-of-famers as **Valium, Aldomet, Aldoril, Ativan, Dalmane, Diabinese, Motrin, Inderal, Intal, Ludiomil, Triavil,** and **Desyrel**. Many, if not all of them, will now acquire generic competitors promptly, much to the economic benefit of long-suffering patients.

## The Economics of Prescription Drugs

Make no mistake about it. Drug companies are in business and their pricing policies reflect that. Often there is an extraordinary spread between the cost of making the drugs and their price.

Even the drug companies admit this. One Squibb Corporation vice president said, "Drugs are priced to assure a cash flow, to provide the kind of return needed to support new research and to attract capital and talent."[7] The company's **Corgard** high-blood-pressure medication went up in price by 22 percent between September of 1983 and May of 1984, said the executive, because, "There is a market out there, and **Corgard** is priced at what the market can bear."[8] Ouch. That's our pocketbook the man is talking about. There's very little consideration for the consumer who can't afford to keep up with the "market price."

There are plenty of ways to economize when the budget is tight. Instead of steak, you buy chicken—or beans. You patch old clothes instead of buying new ones, and you learn to do without. But when it comes to medicine, everyone wants you to take it.

The public service announcements remind you constantly that high blood pressure is the "silent killer." You are exhorted to take your medicine. If you have heart disease or asthma, the pills are your lifeline. Doing without could be like committing suicide.

That's why generic drugs could save some people's lives. A brand-name medication may often cost two to three times as much as a generic copy. In one survey, one hundred tablets of the high-blood-pressure medication hydralazine cost $6.95, unless the doctor insisted on the brand-name version (**Apresoline**), in which case the tab would have been $15.12.[9] One price sampling in late 1984 found the diarrhea medicine **Lomotil** cost $8.79 for twenty tablets under its brand name, or $3.29 if prescribed generically as diphenoxylate.[10]

If those savings sound impressive, hold on to your hat. A reader of our syndicated newspaper column reported the following. "I used to pay $26.50 for 100 **Librium** capsules at the pharmacy. Now I buy the generic version through the American Association of Retired Persons for $3.45. My wife paid $12 for **Donnatal** for her digestive tract. She now gets 100 tablets of the generic version (hyoscyamine, atropine, and phenobarbital) for $1.95."

By now there should be no doubt that sometimes generic drugs can vary dramatically from their brand-name counterparts. But not everyone will benefit. Your pharmacist may not pass on the savings to you. The mark-up on an expensive brand-name medicine can be lots more than a cheaper generic, so the pharmacist may not be motivated to substitute. Or the pharmacist may provide a generic but pocket a substantial part of the savings for himself. After all, the pharmacists are also in business to make money. The only incentive to pass the savings along might be the threat that you'll take your busines elsewhere if they don't.

The point of all this is that it's going to take some careful planning on your part to get prescription drugs at the lowest possible price. The doctor won't necessarily write it right, and the pharmacist won't necessarily fill it the cheapest possible way. If you want the best deal, you'll have to work for it.

## Your Best-Priced Prescription

Okay, the doctor has done the exam, decided what you have, and is about to write a prescription. Leap into action right here or you'll lose all chance of saving money.

*Step #1—Ask what drug the doctor is prescribing, and whether the drug is available generically.* It is not enough to simply say, "What are you giving me, doctor?" The answer could well be a brand name. Ask if it is. If the drug is still patent-protected, ask if there is any acceptable alternative medicine that might be available generically. Sometimes a protected brand is all there is, and the doctor can't help out any further in the quest for the best savings.

However, if the doctor is preparing to write a brand-name prescription for something available generically, *ask for the doctor to write it generically.* If he balks, calmly explain that you are attempting to keep your medical costs as low as possible.

Be firm. The doctor might, as we described earlier, pull out the old "The brand name stuff is really better, trust me, I know all about these things" argument. Now you know this isn't true, so stand your ground. Suggest that he order a book from the Superintendent of Documents (Washington, D.C. 20402) called *Approved Prescription Drug Products*. This reference will tell the doctor which generic distributors have supplied the Food and Drug Administration with adequate proof their products are effective.

It may be difficult to be so assertive the first time (this gets easier with practice), but remember the doctor is almost never acting on firm information when he insists that a brand-name drug is somehow superior. Ask him for the evidence. I'll bet dollars to doughnuts the reason isn't a very scientific one. Then ask yourself—and the doctor—if it's enough reason for you to be spending two to three times as much on your prescription.

Doctors are often very surprised at what drugs cost. Many are only vaguely aware of the actual cost to a patient of a particular course of drug therapy, and even less aware that the price spread is as substantial as it is between brand-name and generic drugs. Help educate them. Many become considerably more cooperative when the actual numbers are brought to their attention. More and more doctors are finally taking cost into account when getting ready to write a prescription, and the cost factor has even become a selling point in some drug company ads of late.

Again, let the doctor know you both appreciate and expect his efforts to hold down the cost of your health care.

In the tables at the end of the chapter, you'll find a partial list of brand-name drugs that are available generically. It certainly wouldn't hurt to make a copy of the list and have it along when you go to the doctor's office. There are literally thousands of drugs, and it's entirely possible that even the most conscientious of doctors might be unaware of a drug's availability in generic form, especially if the switch has happened relatively recently. Remember, one of the reasons generics cost so much less is because they don't advertise and don't send around expensive road salesmen to hawk their wares. Don't be too surprised if the doctor asks you to leave a copy of the list for his use.

*Step #2—Ask the doctor for a free sample plus a prescription for enough medication to last a moderately long time.* As with most things, drugs are cheaper when purchased in larger quantities. But you don't want to get a prescription for a three-month supply only to find out after taking several pills that you are allergic to the medicine. The pharmacist won't take the bottle back and you'll be stuck with expensive pills you can't use.

If your doctor gives you a small free sample—enough to get you by for several days—you can find out if the medication agrees with you. If it does you can take the prescription in and get it filled at substantial savings. Prices often show discounts at quantities of 50 and 100, so if the prescription can reasonably be written for those amounts, ask the doctor to do it. Oh, and make sure the expiration date is written on the label. You don't want to get so much medicine that it will go bad before you have had a chance to use it.

The other consideration here, of course, is cash. If the medication is expensive, you might not want to fork over a large sum of money all at once in order to save a relatively small amount per pill. If the doctor has prescribed a large quantity and you find the total tab will be more than you want to spend at the moment, ask the pharmacist to dispense half the amount. He can and should do it without any problem.

*Step #3—Comparison shop. Do it by phone if at all possible.* Yes, there are going to be times when you feel utterly miserable and just want to get the prescription as quickly as possible. It may be worth it to pay a higher price in exchange for your comfort, especially when the total amount involved is relatively small or when the prescription is a one-shot deal.

If you know that's the situation, you might ask the doctor to write one small prescription and a second, larger one for the balance of the drug you'll need. Get the first day or two of pills wherever it's convenient. Then, when someone else is available to shop around for you, or when you feel a bit better, fill the rest of the prescription at the best possible price.

Where comparison shopping becomes very important is when you have a long-term prescription for a drug to be taken daily. This would include drugs for heart problems, high blood pressure, arthritis, and other chronic problems. The cost of some of these drugs can run to several dollars a day, and whether you pay top or bottom price can make a heck of a difference over the course of a year.

If nothing else, shopping around by phone will yield some very interesting information about drug prices. You'll find, first of all, that some drugstores don't want to quote over the phone. Why not? Because they know once you're in the door, the chances of your marching out without buying the drug you need are pretty small. This marketing reality is sometimes explained as dedication to some ethical standard. What bull! If the druggist won't give you a price by phone, it's either because he knows he's higher or because he wants you to go to so much trouble getting into his pharmacy that you're unlikely to leave in search of other prices. Don't fall for it.

You'll also find that drug prices vary a whole lot more for an identical item than almost any other consumer product. Normally, competition, advertising, and other market forces in an area act to keep most retail prices pretty close from store to store —the Ritz Emporium getting a few bucks more, the Dollarama Discount Palace a few bucks less. But I'm willing to bet the variation from store to store on a *particular* prescription will surprise you.

And there will be neither rhyme nor reason to it. The fanciest drugstore won't always have the highest price for everything, and the "discount" pharmacy won't always have the lowest. The store that's low on one may be high on another.

*Step #4—Talk to the pharmacist before the prescription is filled.* Don't be bashful. Say you want the prescription filled with a low-cost generic.

Ah, you thought the savings were all set just because you got to the pharmacy with a prescription written for a generic version of the drug. The opera isn't over until the fat lady sings, and your savings aren't in the piggybank until you walk out the pharmacy door.

No, generics are not all created equal when it comes to price. Often a pharmacy will stock both a brand-name and a generic equivalent, and sometimes that pharmacy will stock the brand name and two or more generics. Which you get, as noted earlier, might depend on the time of day, which bottle was closer to where the pharmacist was standing, or how much the pharmacist thinks you can afford to pay. Let him know early that you're shopping for the minimum price.

Once in a great while, minimum price might even mean favoring the brand name over a generic! This is a real switcheroo, and it won't happen more than once in a blue moon. This situation can occur because the generic is indeed normally priced higher, or it can happen because the pharmacist has gotten a particularly good deal on a batch of the brand-name drug. Maybe he purchased in a large quantity, or from a distributor who needed to turn over the inventory for one reason or another.

*Step #5—Consider shopping by mail.* This won't work if you need a one-shot prescription for some immediate illness. However, if you have a chronic problem that requires ongoing medication, shopping by mail can save you big bucks.

The reason is that there are a number of superdiscount pharmacies that operate mail-order services. Probably the largest and best known is the one run by the American Association of Retired Persons. You can get price information by writing to AARP Pharmacy Service, Dept. A, PO Box 1423, Alexandria, VA 22313.

Raised as we all are on the notion of going to the corner pharmacy to get a prescription filled, the notion of sending off for one's medication may seem a bit strange at first. But in reality it's a very simple, very easy process. In fact, it can be even easier than going to the local pharmacy. You just stick your prescription in an envelope (along with your name and address, written legibly, which the doctor won't have done on the prescription blank) and a check for the number of pills. Back comes the prescription, delivered to your door by the postal carrier. No muss, no fuss, and at rock-bottom prices.

Just because this is the cheapest option does not mean it's the best. There are a lot of good reasons for paying the difference and going to the handy-dandy pharmacy. In addition to immediate service, you get (or should get) the chance to consult personally with a licensed, qualified pharmacist who can provide information on the drug, how to take it, any possible adverse effects, interactions with other drugs, and so on.

You should, in fact, shop for a pharmacist the same way you shop for a lawyer, plumber, physician, electrician, or any other service professional. After all, the pharmacist is a highly trained health professional who can provide you with crucial information about your medicine and help you avoid serious mistakes.

If you've got a prescription for a new drug, having someone knowledgeable to talk with can be especially important, and the services of a competent, patient, and interested pharmacist can be invaluable. On the other hand, if it's your fortieth refill of a high-blood-pressure or heart medication, you probably don't need that much counseling any more.

The long-term medication user should definitely shop around, and do so carefully. Compare prices locally, and then compare the best of these against the mail-order places. It takes a little bit of planning to get the order in far enough ahead to keep yourself supplied, but the savings can be more than worth the effort.

If you've taken these five steps, chances are very good you'll walk out of the pharmacy with the best possible deal on your prescription. Whether you saved dimes or dollars, you did something else that's important—you helped impress upon the medical establishment the fact that we, as consumers, have an interest in the cost of our health care, and an absolute right to that interest.

# References

1. Brooke, Paul A. *Resistant Prices. A Study of Competitive Strains in the Antibiotic Markets.* New York: Council on Economic Priorities, 1975.

2. Ibid.

3. "Is Bayer Better?" *Consumer Reports,* 47:347, 1982.

4. Ibid.

5. "How to Pay Less for Prescription Drugs." *Consumer Reports,* 40:48–53, 1975.

6. Ibid.

7. Waldholz, Michael. "Prices of Prescription Drugs Soar after Years of Moderate Increases." *Wall Street Journal,* May 25, 1984, p. 31.

8. Ibid.

9. Alexander, Charles P. "Prescription for Cheap Drugs." *Time,* Sep. 17, 1984, p. 64.

10. Ibid.

## TABLE 1
## Off-Patent Brand-Name Drugs and Their Generic Equivalents

| | |
|---|---|
| Achromycin V | tetracycline |
| Actidil | triprolidine |
| Aldactazide | spironolactone with hydrochlorothiazide |
| Aldactone | spironolactone |
| Aldomet | methyldopa |
| Aldoril | methyldopa with hydrochlorothiazide |
| Alpen | ampicillin |
| Amcill | ampicillin |
| Amphicol | chloramphenicol |
| Antepar | piperazine |
| Antivert | meclizine |
| Anturane | sulfinpyrazone |
| Apresazide | hydralazine with hydrochlorothiazide |
| Apresoline | hydralazine |
| Aralen | chloroquine |
| Aristocort | triamcinolone |
| Arlidin | nylidrin |
| Artane | trihexyphenidyl |
| Atarax | hydroxyzine |
| Ativan | lorazepam |

**Off-Patent Brand-Name Drugs and Their Generic Equivalents** *cont.*

| | |
|---|---|
| **AVC** | sulfanilamide; aminacrine; allantoin |
| **Azulfidine** | sulfasalazine |
| **Bactocill** | oxacillin |
| **Bactrim** | sulfamethoxazole with trimethoprim |
| **Benadryl** | diphenhydramine |
| **Benemid** | probenecid |
| **Bentyl** | dicyclomine |
| **Betalin S** | thiamine |
| **Butazolidin** | phenylbutazone |
| **Butisol** | butabarbital |
| **Cafergot** | ergotamine with caffeine |
| **Chlor-Trimeton** | chlorpheniramine |
| **Chloromycetin** | chloramphenicol |
| **Choledyl** | oxtriphylline |
| **Cloxapen** | cloxacillin |
| **Compazine** | prochlorperazine |
| **Cyclospasmol** | cyclandelate |
| **Dalmane** | flurazepam |
| **Darvon** | propoxyphene |
| **Depakene** | valproic acid |
| **Dexedrine** | dextroamphetamine |
| **Diabinese** | chlorpropamide |
| **Diamox** | acetazolamide |
| **Dimetane** | brompheniramine |
| **Diuril** | chlorothiazide |
| **Doriden** | glutethimide |
| **Dymelor** | acetohexamide |
| **Dynapen** | dicloxacillin |
| **E.E.S.** | erythromycin ethylsuccinate |
| **Elavil** | amitriptyline |
| **Endep** | amitriptyline |
| **Enduron** | methyclothiazide |

**Off-Patent Brand-Name Drugs and Their Generic Equivalents** *cont.*

| | |
|---|---|
| Equanil | meprobamate |
| Esidrix | hydrochlorothiazide |
| Erythrocin | erythromycin stearate |
| Fastin | phentermine |
| Flagyl | metronidazole |
| Fiorinal | aspirin and caffeine with butalbital |
| Folvite | folic acid |
| Furadantin | nitrofurantoin |
| Gantanol | sulfamethoxazole |
| Gantrisin | sulfisoxazole |
| Garamycin | gentamicin |
| Hep-Lock | heparin |
| Hydergine | ergoloid mesylates |
| Hydrazid | isoniazid |
| HydroDIURIL | hydrochlorothiazide |
| Hygroton | chlorthalidone |
| Ilosone | erythromycin estolate |
| Inderal | propranolol |
| Isordil | isosorbide |
| Kenalog | triamcinolone |
| Kwell | lindane |
| Lanoxin | digoxin |
| Larotid | amoxicillin |
| Lasix | furosemide |
| Librax | chlordiazepoxide with clidinium |
| Librium | chlordiazepoxide |
| Lomotil | diphenoxylate with atropine sulfate |
| Marax | theophylline; ephedrine; hydroxyzine |
| Meclomen | meclofenamate |
| Megace | megestrol |

**Off-Patent Brand-Name Drugs and Their Generic Equivalents** *cont.*

| | |
|---|---|
| Mellaril | thioridazine |
| Miltown | meprobamate |
| Mycifradin | neomycin |
| Mycostatin | nystatin |
| Mysoline | primidone |
| Navane | thiothixene |
| Nembutal | pentobarbital |
| Nicolar | niacin |
| Norflex | orphenadrine |
| Omnipen | ampicillin |
| Oretic | hydrochlorothiazide |
| Orinase | tolbutamide |
| Paraflex | chlorzoxazone |
| Parafon Forte | chlorzoxazone with acetaminophen |
| PBZ | tripelennamine |
| Pentids | penicillin G |
| Pen-Vee K | penicillin V |
| Percocet-5 | acetaminophen with oxycodone |
| Percodan | aspirin with oxycodone |
| Periactin | cyproheptadine |
| Peritrate | pentaerythritol tetranitrate |
| Persantine | dipyridamole |
| Phenergan | promethazine |
| Plegine | phendimetrazine |
| Polycillin | ampicillin |
| Procan | procainamide |
| Pronestyl | procainamide |
| Prostaphlin | oxacillin |
| Principen | ampicillin |
| Pro-Banthine | propantheline |
| Quinaglute | quinidine |
| Quinora | quinidine |

**Off-Patent Brand-Name Drugs and Their Generic Equivalents** *cont.*

| | |
|---|---|
| Redisol | cyanocobalamin |
| Restoril | temazepam |
| Rimifon | isoniazid |
| Ritalin | methylphenidate |
| Robaxin | methocarbamol |
| Robaxisal | methocarbamol with aspirin |
| Robinul | glycopyrrolate |
| Saluron | hydroflumethiazide |
| Seconal | secobarbital |
| Septra | sulfamethoxazole with trimethoprim |
| Serax | oxazepam |
| Soma | carisoprodol |
| Stelazine | trifluoperazine |
| Synalar | fluocinolone |
| Tegopen | cloxacillin |
| Tenuate | diethylpropion |
| Tetracyn | tetracycline |
| Terramycin | oxytetracycline |
| Thorazine | chlorpromazine |
| Tofranil | imipramine |
| Trancopal | chlormezanone |
| Trimpex | trimethoprim |
| Tylenol with Codeine | acetaminophen with codeine |
| Urecholine | bethanecol |
| V-Cillin K | penicillin V |
| Valisone | betamethasone |
| Vasodilan | isoxsuprine |
| Vibramycin | doxycycline |
| Vistaril | hydroxyzine |
| Wygesic | acetaminophen with propoxyphene |
| Zaroxolyn | metolazone |

**TABLE 2**
**Brand-Name Drugs That Will Be Coming Off Patent**

| Year | Product |
|------|---------|
| 1985 | Valium |
| | Motrin |
| | Triavil |
| | Ludiomil |
| | Desyrel |
| | Intal |
| | Nubain |
| | Yutopar |
| 1986 | Haldol |
| | Catapres |
| | Zyloprim |
| | Sinequan |
| | Velosef |
| | Alupent |
| | Carafate |
| | Cephulac |
| | Bretylol |
| 1987 | Cleocin |
| | Tranxene |
| | Ancef |
| | Bactrim |
| | Septra |
| | Duricef |
| | Unipen |
| | Loxitane |
| 1988 | Feldene |
| | Adriamycin |
| | Nalfon |

**Brand-Name Drugs That Will Be Coming Off Patent** *cont.*

|  |  |
|---|---|
|  | Pavulon |
|  | NegGram |
| 1989 | Keflex |
|  | Clinoril |
|  | Nebcin |
|  | Amoxil |
|  | Proventil |
|  | Lotrimin |
|  | Blenoxane |
|  | Mutamycin |
|  | Asendin |
| 1990 | Zomax |
|  | Tolectin |
|  | Amikin |
|  | Parlodel |
|  | Dolobid |
|  | Imodium |
|  | Retin-A |
| 1991 | Procardia |
|  | Ovral |
|  | Sinemet |
|  | Monistat |
|  | Stadol |
| 1992 | Naprosyn |
|  | Ceclor |
|  | Flexeril |
|  | Spectrobid |
|  | Lorelco |
| 1993 | Lopressor |
|  | Corgard |

**Brand-Name Drugs That Will Be Coming Off Patent** *cont.*

|  |  |
|---|---|
|  | **Tenormin** |
|  | **Xanax** |
|  | **Dobutrex** |
| 1994 | **Tagamet** |
|  | **Mezlin** |
|  | **Bricanyl** |
| 1995 | **Minipress** |
|  | **Pipracil** |
|  | **Talwin** |
|  | **Capoten** |
|  | **Oraflex** |

# 13

---

# Self-Treatment: Hiking in the Himalayas, or What to Do When the Doctor Won't Come

---

*Drugs that don't cure anything • Preparing your own black bag for travel • Traveler's diarrhea • Urinary-tract infections • Nausea, vomiting, and motion sickness • Laxatives • Sunburn • Drugs that can lead to bad sunburn • Bites, stings, itches, and rashes • Fungus infections: Athlete's foot and jock itch • Cuts and scratches • Headache • Colds and allergies • Multipurpose medicines: Bactrim and Septra for traveler's diarrhea and urinary-tract infections • Codeine: Take it to a desert island • Recommended reference material • The Medicine Chest: A Practical Guide to Medications.*

---

This chapter is for anthropologists, adventurers, travelers, reporters, back-to-the-landers, Arctic explorers, and hermits.

In fact, this chapter is for anyone who may not have immediate access, or any access, to medical treatment. The information should *not* serve as a substitute for competent medical supervision, when that's available. It can, however, serve as a guide for anyone who, for some reason or another, is isolated from professional medical assistance. Then it's either do-it-yourself or it doesn't get done.

For the traveler, this chapter could help alleviate some of the suffering that goes with being sick while on the road. Whether it's a strain, a pain, or a case of Montezuma's Revenge (a.k.a. Delhi Belly, the Aztec Two-Step, Tokyo Trots, Casablanca Crud, and lots of less pleasant terms), any sickness is automatically worse when it happens away from home. For those who can't find conventional medical services, we present recommendations for stocking your very own little black travel bag.

If the notion of doctoring yourself sounds radical, take solace in the fact that Grandma did it more often than not, and got along quite well, thank you. Once upon a time, Americans were quite self-reliant. They knew how to care for themselves, find their own dinner in the wild, and take care of most of the rest of life's necessities. Today, we need (or think we need) a specialist to fix our car, do our hair, raise our food, install our plumbing, repair our appliances, and take care of us when we're sick.

Today we run to the doctor every time something looks like it might be a smidge out of sorts. It's been said that a majority of the illnesses in our modern, industrialized society are psychosomatic in nature, and there seems more than a little truth to that accusation. At the very least, we worry and overtreat a great many minor ailments. It's often a major case of much ado about nothing.

For most of the common, everyday things that go wrong it is hardly necessary to make a trip to the doctor. Too many of us are ready to zoom off to the physician with a headache, an ordinary blister, or a temperature that's two degrees higher than 98.6. The headache will usually go away with two aspirin, the blister can be treated with common sense, and there's good evidence that the fever serves a purpose in fighting infection.[1]

It's instructive to see how doctors treat us. If we look at the physician's hit parade of prescription products, we find a lot of medicines that don't cure anything. Don't believe me? Well, among the leading drug best-sellers are painkillers (**Tylenol with Codeine, Darvocet-N 100**), tranquilizers and sleeping pills (**Valium, Ativan, Dalmane, Tranxene,** and friends), and antihistamines (**Dimetapp, Ornade, Benadryl,** and lots of others).

Not a one of these drugs *cures* anything! Tranquilizers may put people far enough away from Planet Earth that they don't care about their problems for a while, but that's hardly solving the problem. Many painkillers are used in situations where a couple of aspirin would do about as well (and some of them do most of their work because they contain aspirin). And the antihistamines may slow the nasal dribble, but they certainly don't eliminate the allergy or other problem causing your nose to try and run away in the first place.

Now, please don't misunderstand me. This is not the Old West, and I'm not an advocate of the notion that pain and suffering is somehow morally uplifting. *The People's Pharmacy* does not encourage biting bullets as a means of coping. Many of these drugs do a fine job, and can be wonderful first aid. *But,* and this is a big but, the vast majority of drugs in these categories, and several others, are either overprescribed or misprescribed.

The reasons for this aren't too hard to understand, and it is *not* all the doctor's fault. Lots of studies show that we the people pretty much insist that the doctor do *something* every time we go into the office. There's a strong tendency on the part of most people to feel they really didn't get their thirty-five dollars' worth out of a doctor visit unless they go home with a prescription for something. Think about this for a second: Have you ever said, "Doctor, can't you give me something for this _____?" (fill in the blank with cold, backache, sore throat, flu, hangnail, or whatever was ailing you). You've done it, haven't you? We all have, and until we unlearn those habits, we'll continue being part of the problem.

Most doctors honestly want very badly to be helpful and to
cure you of whatever nastiness is making life less than pleasant.
It's hard for them to say no when you stand there insisting on
a pill or potion, even when they know there's nothing that will
cure the problem. It's often a case of "Do nothing and your cold
will be gone in a week, or you can take these and your cold will
last seven days."

Believe it or not, you, with zero years of medical school and
no stethoscope, are the best first line of defense when it comes
to taking care of your body. Why? Because by *not* running to the
doctor with every sniffle, and by *not* insisting on a prescription
just because you've made a trip to the doctor's office, you'll
contribute a lot to your overall health. Keep in mind, as we've
discussed throughout this book, that every drug, every treatment, has associated with it some risk of mistreatment, of adverse effects, of unexpected consequences. If something will go
away by itself, let it.

Part of being your own doctor means knowing when to quit.
That's good doctoring, too, just as it's good doctoring when the
family doctor realizes the outside edges of his playing field have
been reached and sends for a specialist. You're the doctor of first
resort. If something seems minor, try living with it for twenty-
four hours. If it's getting better, great. If it's standing still, or
getting slightly worse, think about treating it. If the course is
obviously downhill, it's time to call the doctor.

Use your noodle, now. Don't lie there with a heart attack for
twenty-four hours, waiting to see if it's getting better. Nobody
knows your body better than you. Think about what's wrong. If
it seems serious, and if in doubt, get help. If it seems trivial,
watch it closely.

Here are *The People's Pharmacy* candidates for do-it-yourself
diseases and drugs. We'll first discuss what might go along when
you're leaving home, and then some additional medications that
might usefully be added to the home medicine chest. With a bit
of preparation, and some cooperation from a sympathetic physician, you'll be in pretty good shape to cope with most of life's
minor ills.

## Traveler's Diarrhea

Let's get the number-one problem out in front and solved first. Traveler's diarrhea. Turista. King Tut Gut. The Ho Chi Minhs. You knew it as soon as you ate the food from that roadside stand, but it smelled so good, and somebody said there was no danger if the stuff had been heated, and . . .

Okay, the first thing to do is stop blaming yourself. One study found that people who ate only in four-star hotels suffered problems just as frequently as those who foraged at will.[2] Roadside food stands have been taking a beating for years, yet they may often be innocent. It appears that a fair number of people succumb to *turista* just because their systems don't adapt readily to the changes in food and water. It's not that the food and water necessarily harbor some dreadful bugs, just that it's a different set of bugs than your intestines are used to seeing. All the same, it hardly makes sense to court disaster by drinking the local water (and that includes the *ice* in your soda or mixed drink) or happily munching on unpeeled fruit or raw veggies in the midst of a picturesque outdoor market where sanitary standards may not be up to snuff.

A fair percentage of the time, there is evidence of a bacterial invader. One bacterium, *Escherichia coli,* is estimated to account for from 40 percent to 70 percent of the cases of traveler's diarrhea,[3] with a variety of other bacteria, viruses, and protozoans accounting for the rest. There are lots and lots of varieties of *E. coli,* and one or more strains are normal inhabitants of even the best-bred gut. When an unfamiliar type sets up housekeeping in your territory, though, it can run riot, producing a large quantity of toxins that cause fluid to be secreted in the intestines. It's downhill from there.

Before leaping to counterattack, be aware that most cases of *turista* will solve themselves in forty-eight to seventy-two hours. It won't be fun for two or three days, but you will live. About a third of the people with traveler's diarrhea will wind up in bed, and about 40 percent will have to change their plans somewhat to deal with their inconvenient problem.[4]

What's that? You're not going to just lie there and take it? Well then, let's try and deal with the belly of the beast.

A lot has changed in the treatment of the trots in the last few years. We now know of at least three things that work pretty well, though there's still controversy over whether these drugs should be used *before* a person gets sick (prophylactically) or only after the bug has struck.

Heading the list is an old friend, bismuth subsalicylate. Don't recognize it? I'll bet you do, because it's the active ingredient in **Pepto-Bismol**. Lots of studies show that this is a pretty effective stopper-upper, especially when the problem is *E. coli*. **Pepto-Bismol** is effective, cheap, and without known side effects for most people.

The major problem with **Pepto-Bismol** is the dose. It takes a fairly substantial swallow to get the job done—about two ounces four times a day. If **Pepto-Bismol** is available wherever trouble strikes, run right out (better yet, send someone) and get it. But it's pretty impractical to think anyone will actually pack the twenty-one 8-ounce bottles needed to supply a single person a daily protective dose during a three-week vacation.

Also note that **Pepto-Bismol** contains salicylate. That's awfully similar to aspirin, so anyone who is sensitive to aspirin or who is taking medicine that interacts with aspirin (**Coumadin, Methotrexate, Anturane, Benemid**), needs to steer clear. And never take aspirin at the same time you are taking **Pepto-Bismol** —that would be like doubling your aspirin dose.

A bit more convenient to tote is either **Vibramycin** (doxycycline) or **Bactrim** (a combination of the drugs trimethoprim and sulfamethoxazole, also sold under the brand name **Septra**). Both are pills and both have proved remarkably effective in field trials, reducing the incidence of traveler's diarrhea anywhere from 50 percent to 95 percent.[5]

Both drugs are relatively safe for short-term use. However, if you choose **Vibramycin**, do NOT combine it with **Pepto-Bismol** on the assumption you'll kill twice as many *E. coli*. The bismuth subsalicylate decreases the availability of the doxycycline by about half. Also watch your sun exposure if you're using **Vibra-**

**mycin**. Like most tetracycline drugs, it can make you a lot more sensitive to sun, so you could get a nasty burn in a remarkably short time.

As for **Bactrim** or **Septra**, about 20 percent of those taking this drug for a week or more will have a skin rash, and in about half those getting a rash, the outbreak will be severe enough to mandate getting off the drug. Again, sunlight may increase the risk, so stay inside and get well quickly.

For our money, the best bet is to go, enjoy yourself, and not swallow any medication until—and if—you get sick. Since all the drugs can cause problems of their own, and since there's a better-than-even chance you won't get even a slight case of traveler's diarrhea, why suffer the indignity of being made sick by something you were taking to stay well?

Once again we encounter the first principle of do-it-yourself medicine—whenever feasible, do nothing in order to do no harm. However, the second principle of do-it-yourself medicine is "be prepared." Both **Vibramycin** and **Septra** are prescription drugs, so see your doctor about getting some and keep one or the other on hand if you're headed into strange territory.

## Urinary-Tract Infections

While we're talking about **Bactrim** and **Septra**, let's talk about urinary-tract infections (UTIs), since these drugs can also work wonders in that department.

There seem to be two groups of women in the world—those who've had urinary-tract infections, and those who are going to get them. Many women suffer repeated infections. While men are occasionally afflicted, it's a pretty rare event for a male. Seems to have to do with the way the plumbing lines were designed, and there's evidence that birth-control pills further predispose some women to UTIs.

Anyone who's ever experienced the pain and discomfort of a UTI will remember the experience. For those fortunate enough to remain uninitiated, a UTI can have you running to the bathroom every few minutes, with each trip a separate experience in pain.

If a UTI strikes on a trip, especially in a foreign country, it can be particularly trying. First, it can really cramp your style. Second, it may be difficult to explain the trouble to a doctor who doesn't speak your language.

Before setting off to cure the problem, let's understand what can go wrong. Just like the name says, a urinary-tract infection is a bacterial infection of some portion of the urinary system. The kidneys produce urine and funnel it to the bladder, where it accumulates and passes by way of the urethra to the outside world. If the infection is way up in the kidney, you have pyelonephritis. If the infection has taken up residence in the bladder, the problem is referred to as cystitis. And if it's in the tubing leading from bladder to exit, it's urethritis. Regardless of where it is, it means pain and suffering.

The first problem is diagnosis. Not everything that causes painful or frequent urination is a urinary-tract infection. You may get some help here from a handy little chemically treated strip called **Microstix-Nitrite**. It's available at most pharmacies, and you don't even need a prescription. Dip the strip in a urine sample. If one part of the strip turns pink in thirty seconds, there's a pretty good likelihood a UTI lurks somewhere in the system. The same company makes a more sophisticated set of test strips called **N-Multistix**, which cover a wide variety of other things detectable in the urine. A similar product, made by another company, is **Chemstrip 8**.

By the way, the best urine sample is one taken midstream. The first part of the urine voided will contain a fair number of bacteria that normally live in the lower and external parts of the system. With those swept out of the way, the midstream sample gives a pretty good indication of what's really going on up there.

Some doctors will not be delighted with your self-diagnosis. They'll tell you that UTIs are a very complicated subject, and that can certainly be true. But if the problem arises while a woman is in the boonies somewhere, some information and a start on treatment is sure better than having neither information nor treatment. And the **Microstix** has been designed so that most anybody who reads the directions and follows them can get good results.

If the problem turns out to be a UTI, the chances are the offending organism is our old friend *E. coli.* Yes, the same *E. coli* of traveler's diarrhea fame. That's why it should come as no surprise that **Bactrim** and **Septra** again turn up as useful bacterial bashers to treat urinary-tract infections.

The strategy of attack has altered. For years, doctors have tinkered with varying doses and varying periods of administration, sometimes keeping women on the drugs for weeks. Now there's a definite trend towards a single-dose treatment. You swallow a couple tablets of **Bactrim** or **Septra**, or three grams of oral amoxicillin, or two grams of **Gantrisin** (sulfisoxazole) and very often that will have done the trick. All these are prescription drugs, and will require that the doctor cooperate in seeing that you're properly supplied with instructions for correct dosing.

While **Gantrisin** might be preferred because it costs less and is less likely to cause side effects, there's something neat and tidy about being able to carry **Bactrim** or **Septra** around and know that the drug does at least double duty, helping cure either traveler's diarrhea or UTIs. Whenever we can get two-for-one, we take it.

If the decision is to use **Gantrisin**, do not take large doses of Vitamin C at the same time, or drink humongous amounts of acidic fruit juices. Like all sulfa drugs, **Gantrisin** can damage the kidneys if the urine becomes acidic. You'll also want to stay out of the sun, since **Gantrisin** can sensitize the skin and produce instant sunburn.

You'll want to keep a running tab with the **Microstix** test to see if the bacterial beasties have been defeated. Keep in mind that the symptoms of UTI (including flank pain, pubic pain, frequent urination, or a sense of the need to urinate coming on very suddenly) can also be warning signs of other, more serious troubles, including kidney stones and venereal disease. Also, UTIs that are stubborn and persist for long periods can cause substantial damage to the kidney tissue, so this isn't something to mess around with. If it's a simple UTI and you can zap it quickly, great. If not, rev up the sled dogs and get help.

## Nausea, Vomiting, and Motion Sickness

Most of us aren't real keen on being sick to our stomachs. But that may be Mother Nature's way of saying what you sent down for lunch wasn't acceptable in either quality or quantity. The system has a remarkable capacity for knowing its own limits, and there's usually a good reason for rejects.

Very often, though, the cause of a traveler's vomiting is motion sickness. Whether it's a rough plane ride, the gentle rise-and-fall of a ship, or a car tour over twisting mountain roads, motion sickness can strike with amazing swiftness. And when it does, there are few things in the world as thoroughly miserable.

People who don't usually get motion sickness think, for reasons that I've never understood, that those of us who do are sissies or softies, and they seem to delight in telling the poor sufferer hanging over the rail that it's all in his or her head.

Hah. Explain that to our astronauts. About half of those sky explorers are getting sick on each space shuttle mission! NASA and the astronauts were so embarrassed, they renamed the problem "Space Adaptation Syndrome," and now refuse to divulge who on each mission is suffering the problem. (Apparently on a billion-dollar mission, nobody can get just plain old motion-sick.) But the evidence is in the bag. Call it whatever you want —looks like motion sickness to me.

If you know you're motion sickness–prone, but have every intention of getting on a boat to sail, ask the doctor for a prescription for **Transderm-Scop**. It's an adhesive patch containing the drug scopolamine, which has proved to be a pretty effective antinausea medication. You put the patch on behind your ear, and it can be left in place up to three days. The drug slowly seeps out of the patch and into your system, keeping lunches and dinners in their place.

**Transderm-Scop** has to be applied several hours before the ship (or whatever) starts swaying. Be very careful not to get anywhere near your eyes with the patch or with your fingers after you've handled the patch. Scopolamine can dilate pupils and cause blurred vision. Even though this effect is temporary, it could be scary while it lasts.

Like most motion-sickness medications, **Transderm-Scop** has some side effects. About two thirds of those using the patch will experience a dry mouth, and about one sixth report drowsiness.

Before subjecting yourself to that, you might give ginger a try. As we discussed in Chapter 4, this common household spice may be a good alternative for nausea and vomiting associated with motion sickness. In one study, ginger was even more effective than the old standby **Dramamine**.

## Laxatives

Americans are hung up on bowel function. Regularity has become a fetish. We sit on the altar and worship.

Incredible as it may seem, there are hundreds of laxatives sold in this country, to the tune of over half a billion dollars yearly. As part of its comprehensive review of over-the-counter medications, the FDA released a report in 1975 that said one out of every four ingredients used in OTC laxatives is either worthless or unsafe.

According to the FDA, "There is widespread misuse of self-prescribed laxatives. Prolonged laxative use can in some instances seriously impair normal bowel function." So watch out for advertisements claiming laxatives contain "natural ingredients." Taking a laxative isn't natural.

Whatever the state of your bowels, traveling can produce temporary shifts in regularity. The simultaneous change of food, drink, time zone, and place can cause the system to slow down.

The best cure? One more time—do nothing. Ignore it. No bowel movement today? Great. Maybe tomorrow. Go see the sights. Stop worrying about it. What went in will eventually come out. If you want to help the process, eat bulky, high-residue foods such as bran, vegetables, and fruits, and drink plenty of liquids.

We urge you to stay away from laxatives, especially local varieties. Many of these are not just laxatives, but extremely strong purgatives. Folk beliefs in some areas say that a person needs a regular "cleaning out," and believe me, some of these concoctions will really clean your closet. That can set in motion a very dangerous cycle of purge/constipation/purge. That's a merry-go-round you don't want to buy a ticket for.

Eat moderately and sensibly and let your bowels work on their own schedule.

## Sunburn

Travel and sunburn seem to go together, having formed some sort of unholy alliance dedicated to our pain and suffering. The problem, of course, is that most of us don't enjoy the luxury of lying about in the sun year-round. When opportunity knocks for a suntan, we don't just cautiously crack the door ajar—we fling it wide open. The result is usually one body baked to a brilliant, painful red.

Avoiding such problems has become considerably easier in recent years. Once upon a time, suntan lotions were concoctions of all sorts of crud. Some, but not much, actually screened out the sun's rays. What you mostly got was some sort of oil—cocoa butter, coconut oil, or mineral oil. About all they could do was help you fry instead of bake.

With the discovery of para-aminobenzoic acid (PABA), the suntan lotions were revolutionized. It was now possible to construct effective sun screens which would selectively admit as much (or as little) of the tanning ultraviolet rays as wanted.

This led the FDA to decree that manufacturers place on every bottle of suntan goo a rating called the Sun Protection Factor.

The numbers, which range from 2 to 15, allow you to compare the screening power of various suntan lotions.

A wise traveler would carry a bottle of SPF 15, to use whenever he or she has already had enough exposure, and then a bottle of suntan lotion appropriate to his or her particular skin sensitivity. Those who turn dark on merely seeing the sun can get by with something with an SPF of less than 8. Those who burn anytime after dawn better stay with the higher numbers.

If you've managed to get burned, I do not recommend that you use any of the creams, sprays, and dressings like **Americaine, Kip First Aid Spray, Medicone Dressing Cream, Morusan, Noxzema Sunburn Spray, Solarcaine, Unburn,** and **Unguentine Spray.** Yes, I know, the commercial promised you it would spray away the pain, and you're lying there suffering. But these concoctions all work because they contain a local anesthetic like benzocaine, which may for some people actually irritate the skin and thereby add to their woes.

Probably the best thing to do is take a bath in cool water. Then apply cool compresses of Burow's Solution (aluminum acetate) for about twenty minutes, three or four times a day. Topical steroids such as **Cortaid, CaldeCort, Clinicort,** or **Lanacort** may be helpful. Moisturizers like **Lubriderm, Nivea, Eucerin,** or **Vaseline** petroleum jelly may also be soothing. For the pain, you may want to take two aspirin every three to four hours, and promise yourself you won't leave home again without your SPF 15 suntan lotion.

A really bad burn probably requires oral steroids like cortisone or prednisone. Taken for only a few days such drugs can dramatically relieve the suffering with relatively few side effects. But it will be up to a dermatologist to decide if the problem is so severe that it requires the heavy artillery.

Many prescription medications can either sensitize the skin, making you more vulnerable to sunburn, or can make you more subject to heat stroke. If you are taking *any* prescription medication, it would be a good idea to check on its possible effects in the sun before venturing out. Among the drugs with a definite tendency to cause such problems are:

Amitriptyline (**Elavil**)
Cyclothiazide (**Anhydron**)
Chlorpromazine (**Thorazine**)
Chlorpropamide (**Diabinese**)
Chlortetracycline (**Aureomycin**)
Demeclocycline (**Declomycin**)
Desipramine (**Pertofrane, Norpramin**)
Diphenhydramine (**Benadryl**)
Doxepin (**Adapin, Sinequan**)
Doxycycline (**Vibramycin**)
Furosemide (**Lasix**)
Imipramine (**Tofranil**)
Nalidixic acid (**NegGram**)
Nortriptyline (**Aventyl, Pamelor**)
Oral contraceptives
Promethazine (**Phenergan**)
Protriptyline (**Vivactil**)
Sulfa drugs (including **Gantrisin, Gantanol, Azulfidine**)
Tetracycline drugs (**Achromycin, Cyclopar, Panmycin, Robitet, Sumycin,** and others)
Tolbutamide (**Orinase**)
Trimipramine (**Surmontil**)

## Bites, Stings, Itches, and Rashes

Nothing ruins a trip to the outside world faster than the discovery of things that go bite in the night. While not exactly life-threatening (usually), insect bites can be anything from mildly annoying to maddening. And some of those biters *do* carry diseases, most notably the malaria offered by our friend the mosquito.

As we mentioned in Chapter 4, finding an insect repellent used to be a real crapshoot. Each lotion and nostrum claimed it had the magic, super secret to repelling airborne invaders. There were enough strange ingredients in most bug repellents to keep a witch doctor happy for months.

The puzzle has become a lot easier to solve since diethyltoluamide or **DEET** has been given a vote of confidence by the United States Army. This makes shopping for an insect repellent relatively easy. Go into the backpacking store or pharmacy. Look at the labels on the bug juice. Use whatever has the highest percentage of DEET, unless you have a personal preference for one brand or another because of its scent or method of application.

Products with a big dose of DEET include **Muskol, Ben's 100, Jungle Plus, Maximum Strength Deep Woods Off!, Jungle Juice 100, Repel 100, Skram Insect Repellent, Space-Shield II Insect Repellent**, and **Sportsmate II Premium Insect Repellent Cream**.

Of course, no insect repellent yet invented is guaranteed to keep every last critter from grabbing a piece of the action . . . in this case, you. So there you are with an itching bite, or perhaps prickly heat, or maybe the aftermath of a losing battle with poison ivy. Now what?

On the theory that less is more, try hot water, as we discussed in Chapter 4. Running some hot water on the offending area for a few seconds can give up to several hours of relief. Remember, the water has to be warm enough to be mildly uncomfortable, but not so hot that it will burn.

When itching gets out of control and becomes generalized over the entire body, it's time for something special. Add one cup of **Aveeno Oatmeal** to a tub of lukewarm water and soak for ten to twenty minutes. Be careful—the bathtub could become very slippery. Put a towel on the bottom to keep you from breaking your neck. No sense getting hurt by the cure.

If there's no oatmeal at hand, you may want to try cornstarch. Just add one to two cups of cornstarch powder (such as **Linit**) to four cups of water and mix it into a paste. Then put the glop in a tub of lukewarm water, stir thoroughly, and crawl in. A twenty-to-thirty-minute soak is good for almost any inflammatory skin condition. It will help relieve rashes, itching, crotch irritation, or an allergic reaction. Once again be extra careful about slipping and sliding when getting in or out of the tub.

After drying, resist the urge to slather on one of the highly promoted topical ointments. Instead, make up a Burow's Solution of aluminum acetate. Dissolve one **Domeboro** tablet (available without a prescription at the pharmacy) in a pint of water and mix it well. Loosely bandage what itches, and then dribble the mixture over the bandage little by little, keeping the dressing wet. If your patience allows, keep at it for several hours.

Another thing good for itching is plain calamine lotion. You can also use nonprescription hydrocortisone-containing lotions such as **Cortaid, CaldeCort, Lanacort, Prepcort**, and **Dermtex HC**.

The only problem with hydrocortisone purchased over-the-counter is that it isn't terribly powerful. One dermatologist I know compared it to killing flies with a feather. He suggests that if you really want effective anti-itching power, you will need a prescription steroid ointment such as **Tridesilon** (desonide), **Aristocort** (triamcinolone), **Valisone** (betamethasone), or ultimately **Lidex** (fluocinonide).

These are strong steroids and should not be used indiscriminately over large portions of the body for long periods of time. But if you want fast relief for a day or two, such drugs are extremely effective. Of course, some docs would say that using such medications for bug bites is a little like killing flies with a hammer—overdoing it.

We've already covered insect-sting treatment in Chapter 4, but just as a reminder: A dab of meat tenderizer can be very effective at neutralizing the venom left behind by a bee or other stinging insect. Better yet, get your doctor to prescribe **Panafil Ointment**. This is a ready-to-use mixture containing papain, the enzyme found in papaya (and meat tenderizer).

Anyone who is severely allergic to insect stings probably knows it, and should be carrying an emergency kit which allows them to self-inject a dose of adrenalin. Such people face a life-threatening crisis when stung, and prompt treatment is absolutely vital.

## Fungus Infections: Athlete's Foot and Jock Itch

When traveling to warm, humid climes, even those who've never had a fungal infection can find it amazingly easy to become a breeding ground. What starts out as slightly reddened, slightly itching skin can in short order turn into a mass of white, soggy, macerated tissue that will itch more than you ever imagined anything can itch.

Fungal infections are notoriously difficult to combat. That's partly because of the way in which fungi live and reproduce, and partly because there just hasn't been as much research into drugs for fighting fungi as there has been on antibacterials.

For those who've suffered a lifetime of athlete's foot, forget the old names like **Desenex, Daliderm**, and **Quinsana Foot Powder**. There's a new, powerful antifungal available over-the-counter called miconazole, sold under the trade name **Micatin**. It's leagues ahead of any of the old antifungals, and even better than tolnaftate which (as **Tinactin**) was the newest and best OTC antifungal we could recommend when the first edition of *The People's Pharmacy* was written.

If things are really bad, it's possible you have not just a fungal infection, but a combined fungal/bacterial duet going on between your toes.

For a long time we assumed all athlete's foot was just a fungal infection. But diligent research established that very often the fungi colonize, but are then followed by bacteria that set up housekeeping in their own territory, adding to the problem.[6] One of the reasons some athlete's foot infections have been so treatment-resistant is that we've been trying to treat a fungal/bacterial infection with just an antifungal.

The answer may be to try aluminum chloride in a 20 percent to 30 percent solution. This is a nonprescription item any pharmacist should be able and willing to whip up in a jiffy. This common chemical has been used for years as an underarm deodorant or antiperspirant. It may also be helpful for resistant athlete's foot. By drying the skin, it makes the area between your toes inhospitable to the invading bacteria. Meanwhile, it kills the little devils at the same time.

Aluminum chloride should be applied once or twice a day until things start to look better. Never apply it after a shower or when feet are wet, since it will burn and sting. One other word of caution: Don't use aluminum chloride if your athlete's foot has open sores, since this could aggravate the irritation.

If you can't find a pharmacist who will brew up the aluminum chloride solution for you (some of them won't do anything but count pills out of big bottles into little ones) then talk to your doctor about a prescription product called **Drysol**, which is nothing more than a 20 percent solution of aluminum chloride in alcohol, sold for people who sweat excessively.

Once you've got the athlete's foot problem under control, you will want to keep those tootsies cool, calm, and dry to prevent flare-ups. A foot powder, cotton socks, and shoes that breathe are a good way to keep the fungi away. If you can wear sandals, so much the better.

## Jockstrap Itch

Jock itch (which is a misnomer, since it can affect women and men equally) is nothing more than the same type of fungal infection in a different location. Warm, moist areas provide great conditions from a fungus's point of view, and that's why the toes and pubic region are hot targets.

The same treatment here will work equally well. In fact, though you'll find **Micatin** filed at the pharmacy with the foot-care products, read the label: It says "Proven clinically effective in the treatment of athlete's foot (tinea pedis), jock itch (tinea cruris), and ringworm (tinea corporis)."

**Micatin** comes as an ointment, spray, and powder. Once the infection is controlled, an occasional dusting with the powder can help keep these normally moist areas dry while also killing off any fungal spores that might have notions of taking up residence.

You will also want to stick to light clothing, which prevents chafing. That rules out tight, form-fitting jeans or panty hose. Anything that soaks up sweat, like **Zeasorb Powder**, will help prevent the condition from starting in the first place.

## Cuts and Scratches

The idea that if it hurts, it must be good for you, has long been the mainstay of home remedies. The louder a kid hollers, the better it is. We have developed a ritual of pouring potent antiseptics that hurt like hell over our wounds and scratches. Killing germs is somehow associated with healing wounds. That is nonsense. Once again we have been convinced by companies that promote products like **Mercurochrome**. Minor cuts require absolutely no special attention. They should be washed carefully with plenty of mild soap and water, and that is all. By the way, if you have a choice between soggy bar soap and liquid soap, we'd pick the liquid soap. Dr. Jon Kabara, a pharmacologist at Michigan State University, has found that used bar soaps in public lavatories can harbor a wide variety of microbes. Dr. Kabara wrote to the *Journal of the American Medical Association:*

*To the Editor.* —Because my research findings have become a focal point of controversy in the choice of liquid soap *v* bar soap, I feel compelled to present further information for the followers of this saga. . . .

Others have talked on the dangers of bar soap: Steere and Mallison warned, "However, bars of soap frequently remain in pools of water that might support the growth of organisms"; two experts on infection control stated, "these bar soaps (multiuser) are frequently misused and stored carelessly in contact with moisture. The resulting jelly mass is unsightly, difficult to use effectively, and, in some cases, found to harbor live pathogenic bacteria of *Staphylococcus* and *Pseudomonas* genera, which may be transferred from one user to another"; still others affirm the potential danger of bar soap, "the frequent contamination of bars of soap suggests that organisms may be obtained during the very procedure performed to prevent transfer" and, finally a recent study has shown that "meticulous bathing with the bar soap issued by the hospital (containing triclocarbon) did not eliminate colonization and was frequently associated with the shifting of these bacteria to adjacent sites on the body."

Healthy people probably don't need to worry too much about the germs lurking on bar soap. But if you are washing out a cut or a scratch, it seems only good sense to avoid contamination if possible.[7] Remove any dirt that may have penetrated the wound but resist pouring special "degerming" junk on the tender skin.

Now I know that it is hard to resist temptation. If dear old Mom painted your scratches with **Merthiolate, Medi-Quik,** or **Unguentine,** you are going to want to do the same thing for your kid. If you can't fight the urge, then at least use something which is harmless and reasonably effective. Plain old alcohol is one of the best germ fighters we have. Do not pour the stuff directly over abraded tissue, because it will only make the kid scream bloody murder and do nothing for the healing process. Gently wipe the skin *around* the wound and then cover it with a bandage. If that is too simple, you could purchase some tincture of iodine. It is one of the oldest (first used in 1839) and most effective antiseptics available. It kills everything, including bacteria, fungi, and viruses. It also has a low tissue toxicity, so it can be applied around a scratch with little fear. If you take it on your trips, you can use it to purify water which may be suspect (iodine will even kill amoebas better than chlorine). Add three drops to one quart of water, and it will be safe to drink in fifteen minutes.

But what happens when the skin does become infected? Again,

the conservative approach is preferable. Hot water soaks or compresses will increase blood flow to the area and enable your own body to do the rest. A wet-oozy skin infection is also best treated by soaks or compresses. Dermatologists have long acknowledged that "wet-to-wet" treatment will paradoxically dry out the skin lesion.

Try to resist using a topical antibiotic cream. These agents have a tendency to produce an allergic sensitization of the skin which could aggravate an underlying infection. If you must use something, then it is best to use an antibiotic which has a low potential for allergic reactivity. **Achromycin Ointment** or **Terramycin Topical Ointment** (both are tetracycline derivatives) are relatively harmless and can be purchased without a prescription. **Polysporin Ointment** is another reasonable alternative. Since these antibiotics probably won't do you much harm, you can use them with a clear conscience, but don't expect them to do very much good, either. For a serious skin infection, see your doctor. He will prescribe an oral antibiotic that will be specific for the kind of infection that you have.

## Headache

Take two aspirin.

That's honestly the best possible prescription. Aspirin is really a wonder drug. It provides an incredible amount of pain relief, at a virtually invisible price if you buy only what you need—plain USP aspirin, no additives, no fancy brand name.

In the event of a genuine "my head is splitting open" episode, a good backup would be a few tablets of **Empirin with Codeine**. This is mighty high on the list of most frequently prescribed drugs. It's nothing more than good old aspirin with a bit of codeine. Both are excellent painkillers, and together they should do in almost any kind of pain you'd tolerate without going to the emergency room.

Lots of times people get headaches from nasal congestion, particularly when they've been on several flights with the numerous changes of cabin pressure. If the headache is a long-lasting one that seems to arise in the facial area, you may be more in need of a decongestant than anything else. If so, **Neo-Synephrine** or any one of the dozens of short-acting nasal-spray decongestants should do the job. Continued use, however, runs the risk of rebound nasal congestion. An oral decongestant like **Sudafed** is another alternative as long as you don't suffer from high blood pressure, heart trouble, diabetes, or thyroid disease.

## Colds and Allergies

Speaking of nasal congestion, suppose a common cold or an allergy rears its ugly head while you're away from home. Take solace, if you can, in the fact that being at home wouldn't help much. There's no cure, so access to the fanciest doctor in the world wouldn't help.

In an effort to reduce the misery, many people resort to cold pills of one sort or another such as **Contac, Comtrex, Dristan Ultra, CoTylenol Cold Formula**, or goodness-knows-what. These are shotgun preparations, containing a little bit of lots of different things, from decongestants and antihistamines to cough suppressants and pain relievers. Taking a combination pill always considerably ups the risk that *something* in there won't agree with you.

Far better to get exactly what you need. If you feel a decongestant is in order, buy it separately as **Sudafed**. If it's an allergy-like noseache, an antihistamine might provide relief until you can get away from whatever's bugging you. Try chlorpheniramine, in the form of **Chlor-Trimeton**.

If, on the other hand, that cold has produced a nasty cough that is really bothering you, you'd want something just for that. Sucking on a plain hard candy will often do the trick. If you don't get relief from a sucker, dextromethorphan all by itself can soothe the beast within. Products such as **Mediquell, Sucrets Cough Control, Hold 4 Hour, Romilar Children's Cough**, and **Extend-12** will all do the job.

If you are highly allergic or suffer from hay fever you may want to consider steroid nasal sprays such as **Beconase** or **Vancenase** (beclomethasone) or **Nasalide** (flunisolide). Such medications can provide considerable relief from allergies but will require a doctor's prescription. So will **Nasalcrom** (cromolyn), which prevents histamine from being released in the nose in the first place. If you anticipate going somewhere with a high pollen count you might want to plan ahead and take along lots of protection.

## Multipurpose Medicines

That takes care of the diseases and medical problems I'll discuss in this section, but before leaving the do-it-yourself topic I'd like to put in a good word for some drugs whose biggest virtue is that they will do several jobs. That makes them the ideal choice when you've got to travel light, yet want to be prepared to cope with as much as possible.

For example, we've already seen how the trimethoprim-sulfamethoxazole combination sold as **Bactrim** or **Septra** can be of help in fighting both traveler's diarrhea and urinary-tract infections. I'd have to say such double-duty capability could earn it a spot in any world traveler's kit.

Another must-take would be aspirin. Nothing else can give so much relief for so little cost. Not only will it relieve pain, but it is also effective in reducing fever and inflammation.

If sentenced to life on an island, and given one drug to tote, I'd probably opt for codeine. It's an excellent painkiller, relieving the agony of everything from a backache to a tooth with a cavity. Codeine is also effective against diarrhea at a dose of around 15 milligrams every four to six hours.

Codeine also is an excellent cough suppressent. In fact, codeine is the standard to which all other cough preparations are compared. If you have a really nasty, painful cough, codeine is your drug. A dose of 15 to 30 milligrams should do nicely.

On top of all that, codeine has a little sedative action, so it can

help put you to sleep if that cough, or painful tooth, is leading
to a loss of slumber time.

If codeine is so great, why isn't it used more often? Actually
it is. Compounds like **Tylenol with Codeine** or **Empirin with
Codeine** are very high on the list of most prescribed drugs. What
is surprising, however, is that codeine is rarely prescribed by
itself, even though it would be far cheaper generically than in a
brand-name preparation.

The FDA makes it harder for doctors to prescribe pure codeine than an aspirin-codeine combination. Apparently that is
because codeine by itself is seen as a drug with abuse potential,
and it's thus dispensed only by prescription and then often reluctantly. In reality, the abuse potential is minimal when the drug
is given in the small doses needed for the uses we're discussing
here.

You will have to ask the doctor for codeine. Ten tablets of
30-milligram potency will get you through most short-term medical emergencies. It would be very difficult to become much of
a big-time addict on that, so the doctor shouldn't be very reluctant. For diarrhea or cough, divide each 30-milligram tablet in
half and you'll have an adequate dose.

If that makes the doctor nervous, then just request his old
favorite **Empirin No. 3** (325 mg of aspirin and 30 mg codeine
phosphate) or **Tylenol No. 3** (300 mg acetaminophen and 30 mg
codeine phosphate). As long as the physician realizes that you
only need a small quantity to get you by during an emergency
he or she shouldn't have a problem providing such a prescription.

## Recommended Reference Material

Doctors always have lots of diplomas on their walls and lots of
books on their shelves. We can't help your doctoring with any
diplomas, but there are a few books the aspiring do-it-yourselfer
should have at hand, in sickness and in health.

First, of course, we do hope you'll take a look at the other books in The People's Pharmacy series: *The People's Pharmacy-2* and *The New People's Pharmacy-3*. Both contain additional information on a wide range of prescription and nonprescription medications. Each book is totally different from the others and hopefully will complement the book you are now reading.

Before purchasing anything else, you will probably want to invest a few bucks in a paperback medical dictionary. This will help in translating to English the remarkably complicated words medical people seem to favor for even the most straightforward of concepts. Don't get hung up trying to render every last word. A few of the big ones will usually be enough to help you figure out what they're trying to say to each other. One dictionary we can recommend is Robert Rothenberg's *The New American Medical Dictionary and Health Manual.*

The one book I would definitely take to that isolated island is *The Merck Manual of Diagnosis and Therapy,* which is now in its fourteenth edition. *The Merck Manual* is a phenomenon, a book originally published and intended for physicians which has grown to be a popular best-seller. Within its 2,500 tissue-paper pages you'll find a description of just about everything imaginable (and quite a few things unimaginable) that can go haywire with the human body, and what can and can't be done about each. The descriptions are concise, precise, and useful. The index alone is a virtual medical education, and it provides quick access to the material.

For drug information in a dictionary form I would recommend *The Pill Book* by Dr. Harold Silverman. It is available in paperback from Bantam Books for about four dollars. That makes it cheap and handy. A slightly larger and more expensive alternative is *The Essential Guide to Prescription Drugs* by Dr. James Long. Harper and Row publishes it for about nine dollars.

If you're particularly concerned about the problems of drug side effects and interactions, don't be without *Hazards of Medication: A Manual on Drug Interactions, Incompatibilities, Contraindications and Adverse Effects.* The title is a little less snappy than, say, *Gone with the Wind,* but the material is equally compelling to those who are interested. It's written by Eric Martin. The best part is the more than four hundred pages of tables charting drug interactions. The drawback is that the book is very expensive and is written in doctorspeak.

If you want a superb up-to-date guide to dangerous drug combinations, then seek *Drug Interaction Facts.* This is edited by Dr. Richard J. Mangini and is published by J. B. Lippincott. It too is expensive and written for health professionals but this is my bible when it comes to checking out which medicines don't mix.

No home medicine chest would be complete without a copy of *The Medicine Show.* It's an inexpensive and unbiased presentation by the editors of *Consumer Reports.* It's written for the consumer, so no problems here about understanding the medical terms. It aims at mostly nonprescription drugs, so don't look for answers on complicated medical questions in this one.

None of these books is perfect. For the money, *The Medicine Show, The Pill Book,* and *The Merck Manual* are best buys. Between them you can learn a lot about prescription and nonprescription drugs, and about what ails you.

You can undoubtedly find such reference books at the local library, so it's not necessary to plunk down a whole wad of dollars in order to get a reasonable amount of information into the house. Start with the basics, and expand the library as your interests and finances dictate.

## The Medicine Chest: A Practical Guide to Medications

The following is a list of what you might want in a reasonably well-equipped medicine chest. It's not necessary to stock the dispensary with everything that's recommended. Many of these drugs are alternates.

This formulary is meant only to serve as a guide in helping you build a supply of medications that will be useful in treating common, everyday medical problems. All drugs must be considered dangerous, and should not be left where children can get to them. Review the contents of the medicine chest on a regular basis, and properly discard drugs whose expiration dates have passed (see Chapter 3, p. 49).

If ever in doubt about your medical condition, consult a doctor. And by all means talk to your pharmacist. He or she is a highly trained health professional who should be more than willing to come out from behind the counter and make recommendations, offer instructions, and provide cautions. Never ever forget that all drugs can cause side effects in some people. The only way to use any medication wisely is to become informed about its dangers as well as its benefits.

And remember, whenever possible be patient and let the body heal itself. A little bit of restraint is the one drug I'd like to see in *everyone's* medicine chest, and it's always the first one I'd recommend using.

## ALLERGY

OTC = Over-the-Counter
Rx = Prescription Only

1. **Chlor-Trimeton** *(chlorpheniramine):* 4-milligram tablets                                                    OTC

   Usual adult dose: one tablet three or four times a day. (One-half tablet may work for some people.) Children's dose: six to twelve years old, one-half tablet every four to six hours. Never give more than 12 mg per day total dose.

   This antihistamine may be a little less likely to cause drowsiness than other antihistamines, but you should not drive or operate machinery after taking it. It can be used for sneezing, runny nose caused by allergy, itching, hives, and other skin allergies.

   Nonprescription compounds containing *chlorpheniramine* include: **Allerest, Alermine, Aller-Chlor, Chlorate, Chlor-Niramine, Coricidin**, and hundreds more.

2. **Beconase, Vancenase Nasal Inhaler**
   *(beclomethasone):* Each spritz of the inhaler provides 42 mcg of medication.                                          Rx

**Allergy** *cont.*

Usual dose: one spritz in each nostril two to four times a day. Children younger than twelve years old probably should not use such medication.

This steroid nasal spray provides medicine directly to the nose where it is needed. It is unlike cortisone-type medications, which are usually given orally and circulate throughout the body, often causing dangerous side effects. That does not mean, however, that such sprays can be taken for granted and used indiscriminately. If no improvement occurs within three weeks, this medication should be discontinued.

**CAUTION:** Do not use if you are pregnant. Do not use excessively. Do not use if you have an infection within the nose. The most common side effects are dryness, nasal irritation, and sneezing.

3. **Nasalide** *(flunisolide):* Each spritz of the inhaler provides 25 mcg of medication.                    *Rx*

Usual adult dose: initially two spritzes in each nostril two times a day. If necessary, this can be increased to two spritzes in each nostril three times a day. Children's dose: six to fourteen years old, one spritz in each nostril three times in a day. This can be changed to two spritzes in each nostril twice a day if necessary. Not for children under six years of age.

Once the allergy has been controlled, the dose can be reduced to the lowest amount possible to maintain relief. For some people that may be as little as one spritz per nostril each day.

This medication works very much the way *beclomethasone* does. One or the other should be considered, but not both. Much will depend on your physician's preference.

**CAUTION:** The same as above with *beclomethasone.*

4. **Nasalcrom** *(cromolyn sodium):* Each spritz of the inhaler provides 5.2 mg of medication.                    *Rx*

## Allergy *cont.*

Usual adult dose (and for children over six years old): one
spritz in each nostril evenly spaced from three to six times
during the day. You will require special instructions on
proper application from a physician or pharmacist, since it
can be complicated.

This medicine prevents histamine from being released in
the nose. It may take two to four weeks for the beneficial
effect to be noticed. The drug can cause stinging, sneezing,
irritation, and a burning sensation. The special Nasalmatic
pump must be replaced approximately every six months.


## ATHLETE'S FOOT/JOCK ITCH

1. **Micatin** *(miconazole):* cream, spray, powder.      OTC

   Far and away the most effective thing for treating basic athlete's-foot infections. Clean and dry the foot carefully. Apply
   twice a day. Fungal infections clear slowly, so keep at it for
   at least a couple of weeks, and then continue using powder
   to keep the area dry and infection free.


2. **Tinactin** *(tolnaftate):* cream, solution, or powder     OTC

   This is, I think, the second-best choice for treating mild athlete's foot and most other skin fungus infections. Because this
   medication is potent, it should be applied sparingly: two or
   three drops of solution suffice for the foot, including between-
   the-toe places. Application twice a day for two or three weeks
   should cure most infections. Powder can be used with the
   solution or after healing to help keep those moist areas from
   getting infected again. Dust **Tinactin Powder** on one or two
   times a day as a preventive measure.

   If the athlete's foot is still going strong after four weeks of
   treatment, it may not be athlete's foot. See a doctor.

   **CAUTION:** Keep out of eyes!

**Athlete's Foot/Jock Itch** *cont.*

3. Aluminum Chloride: 30 percent solution                    *OTC*

If your pharmacist cannot make up this product, it can be purchased with a prescription under the brand name **Drysol**. It should only be applied to dry skin, never after a bath or shower. Aluminum chloride will eliminate moderate to severe athlete's foot and should be used twice a day.

Once the worst part of the infections has been cleared up you can start using **Micatin** or **Tinactin** in order to clear up any residual fungus infection.

4. Potassium Permanganate: 300-milligram tablets
   (0.3 gm)                                                  *OTC*

Dissolve one tablet in three quarts of lukewarm or cool water to make a 1:10,000 concentrated solution. This beautiful purple liquid has astringent, germicidal, and antifungal action. It should be used as a wet compress. Undissolved crystals can burn the skin, and the solution should be made up fresh each time it is used—don't use leftovers.

A wet dressing of potassium permanganate 1:10,000 can be useful for many skin infections or inflammations, including poison ivy. It stains, but fingernails will come clean with a 3 percent hydrogen peroxide solution.


## BEE STINGS AND BEE-STING ALLERGIES

1. Meat Tenderizer (any brand with Papain)                  *OTC*

One-quarter teaspoon of tenderizer added to one to two teaspoons of water will make a paste which should be applied immediately to the sting. This should relieve the pain and reduce the inflammation.

Do not rely on this treatment if you are allergic to bee stings.

**Bee Stings and Bee-Sting Allergies** *cont.*

2. **Panafil Ointment, Papase** tablets                    *Rx*

Both of these prescription products contain papain as a major ingredient. **Panafil** is in a ready-to-use ointment form, while **Papase** tablets should be crushed and made into a wet paste. Both of these preparations should work as well as, if not better than, plain meat tenderizer in alleviating stings. **Panafil** can also be used for infected cuts or wounds which do not heal rapidly.

3. **Ana-kit** emergency insect sting treatment kit      *Rx*

If you are allergic to bee stings, you should not venture out without this excellent compact kit. It contains all of the necessary equipment for emergency treatment of serious allergic reactions, including a preloaded syringe containing adrenalin and easily understood precise instructions for its use.

Available with a prescription from Hollister-Stier Laboratories. Box 3145 T.A., Spokane, WA 99220.

**CAUTION:** Instructions on proper use, warnings, and adverse reactions must be obtained from a physician!

4. **EpiPen Auto-Injector** and **EpiPen Jr.**            *Rx*

This is an alternative to the **Ana-kit** and also provides adrenalin (epinephrine). If you are one of those people who says, "I could never give myself an injection," then **EpiPen** is for you. Unlike with the **Ana-kit** you do not need to give yourself a shot. The **EpiPen** auto-injector does it for you. It is activated by simply pushing the penlike device against the thigh. If that sounds complicated, the company will even provide a "reusable training device, with a harmless plastic prod in place of a needle and containing no drug product." You can practice under a doctor's supervision.

**EpiPen** and **EpiPen Jr.** (for children) are available by pre-

**Bee Stings and Bee-Sting Allergies** *cont.*

scription only from Center Laboratories, 35 Channel Drive, Port Washington, NY 11050.

CAUTION: Instructions on proper use, warnings, and adverse reactions must be obtained from a physician! Store in a cool dark place.


# BURNS


1. Cold Water

All burns, including chemical, electrical, and thermal, respond magnificently to cold water immersion or ice-cold moist towels. The faster the application the more complete the relief of pain and speed of recovery. Water should be kept between 41° and 55° Fahrenheit by adding a few ice cubes to a pan of tap water.

To be effective, cold treatment must be maintained until it is no longer painful to remove the affected part from the water. This may take anywhere from thirty minutes to five hours. Although this treatment requires patience, it will dramatically eliminate pain and will prevent damage and promote healing.

CAUTION: *All* second- and third-degree burns require immediate medical attention!


# CONSTIPATION


1. Proper diet, high in roughage with plenty of fresh fruits, vegetables, and whole grains, will help to avoid this problem. Two teaspoons of unprocessed bran can be taken with milk, water, or juice daily to increase roughage in the diet.

Large doses of Vitamin C (1-3 gm/day) may also help.

**Constipation** *cont.*

2. Mild, bulk-producing laxatives:                    *OTC*

   Nonprescription products containing methylcellulose: **Cellothyl, Cologel, Hydrolose, Serutan**

   Nonprescription products containing psyllium: **Effersyllium, Metamucil, Mucilose, Perdiem, Plova, Prompt, Syllamalt**

   Follow the instructions on the package. Try not to get into a laxative habit.


## COUGH

1. Coughs that are productive—bringing up mucus—should be treated conservatively by sucking on hard candy, drinking lots of fluids, and inhaling steam or mist. This type of cough will usually go away by itself, but if mucus changes color or if the cough persists see a doctor.

2. Codeine: 15-milligram tablets, 30-milligram tablets                    *Rx*

   Usual adult dose: one 15-milligram tablet or half a 30-milligram tablet every four to six hours. This treatment should be reserved for unproductive coughs.

   Follow the precautions for codeine listed under the heading *Pain.* If a nasty cough persists more than a few days, see a doctor.

3. Dextromethorphan-containing cough remedies:                    *OTC*

   **Benylin DM, Extend-12, Hold 4 Hour, Mediquell, Robitussin-DM, Robitussin Cough Calmers, Romilar Children's, St. Joseph's Cough for Children, Symptom 1.**

## Cough *cont.*

Although these nonnarcotic cough remedies offer no greater advantage than codeine, they can be purchased without a prescription. The products listed contain relatively few "extras" along with the cough suppressant dextromethorphan.

## CUTS AND SCRATCHES

1. Wash carefully with soap and water.
2. If necessary, alcohol or tincture of iodine may be applied around the edges of the wound.
3. Skin infections or infected scratches should be treated by soaking in hot water.
4. **Achromycin Ointment** *(tetracycline)*     OTC

   **Polysporin Ointment** *(Polymyxin and bacitracin)*   OTC

   **Terramycin Topical Ointment** *(oxytetracycline)*   OTC

   These ointments can be spread on the skin for antibiotic action. It is unlikely they will speed recovery, but they may help lower the risk of infection.

## DIARRHEA

1. Codeine: 15-milligram tablets; 30-milligram tablets     *Rx*

   Usual dose: one 15-milligram tablet or half a 30-milligram tablet every four to six hours. Maximum daily dose: 60 to 75 milligrams. Codeine should not be used casually, as it can be habit-forming, though this is extremely uncommon if used infrequently.

   **CAUTION:** Do not take codeine with alcohol, barbiturates, or tranquilizers.

**Diarrhea** *cont.*

2. **Mitrolan** *(calcium polycarbophil):* 500-mg.
   chewable tablets.                                    *OTC*

   Usual adult dose: two tablets four times a day. Children's
   dose: chew one tablet three times a day—six to twelve years;
   chew one tablet two times a day—three to six years.
   **CAUTION:** Do not take **Mitrolan** with tetracycline, or if
   intestinal obstruction is suspected.

3. **Pepto-Bismol:** liquid suspension                  *OTC*

   Usual adult dose: two tablespoons every one-half to one hour
   as needed until eight doses are taken. Suitable for children;
   check bottle.
   **CAUTION:** Do not combine **Pepto-Bismol** with aspirin,
   **Anturane, Benemid, Coumadin,** or methotrexate.

4. **Lomotil** *(diphenoxylate)* 2.5-milligram tablets  *Rx*

   Usual adult dose: two tablets four times a day. A smaller dose
   may work just as well.
   **Lomotil** is not safe for children, people with liver trouble,
   and people with glaucoma. **Lomotil** should not be used casually because it can be habit-forming, though this is extremely
   uncommon if used infrequently.
   **CAUTION:** Do not take **Lomotil** with alcohol, barbiturates, or tranquilizers.

5. **Kaopectate:** liquid suspension                    *OTC*

   Usual adult dose: four to eight tablespoons as needed. Children's dose: four tablespoons if older than twelve; six to
   twelve years: two to four tablespoons; three-six years: one to
   two tablespoons.

## INSECT BITES AND ITCHING (Prevention and Treatment)

1. DEET-containing insect repellents:                *OTC*

   **Ben's 100, Jungle Juice 100, Jungle Plus, Maximum Strength Deep Woods Off!, Muskol, Repel 100, Skram Insect Repellent, Space-Shield II Insect Repellant, Sportsmate II Premium Insect Repellent Cream**
   These insect repellents are among the most effective available. Apply liberally if the bugs are hungry.

2. Thiamine hydrochloride (Vitamin B₁): tablets     *OTC*

   Taking 150 milligrams to 300 milligrams of this vitamin has been reported to be of some value in keeping bugs from biting. Unfortunately, these reports have not been well verified, so this would have to be categorized as an unproven home remedy at this time. Nevertheless, I have received enough letters from readers to make me believe that it may work for some people at least some of the time.

3. Hot Water

   This is the fastest and most effective relief for minor itching. The water should be between 120° and 130° Fahrenheit (uncomfortably hot, but not hot enough to burn). Application for a few seconds should provide several hours' relief.

4. Hydrocortisone-containing creams and ointments:                *OTC*

   **Cortaid, CaldeCort, Clinicort, Delacort, Dermtex HC, Lanacort, Prepcort, Rhulicort, Sensacort, Ulcort, Wellcortin.**
   All of these topical creams contain hydrocortisone. They

## Insect Bites and Itching *cont.*

may be applied three to four times per day and will provide relief for the following skin problems:

| | |
|---|---|
| itching | eczema |
| allergy | hemorrhoids |
| dermatitis | general inflammation |
| rash | |

### 5. Aveeno Oatmeal                    *OTC*

Generalized itching over the entire body may be treated by soaking for ten to twenty minutes in a tub of lukewarm water to which one cup of colloidal oatmeal has been added.

**CAUTION:** Tub may become slippery. Place a bathtowel in the bottom of the tub to prevent slipping and sliding.

### 6. Cornstarch (Kitchen or **Linit** brand)                    *OTC*

One cup powder dissolved in four cups cool water added to a tub of lukewarm water will provide similar relief to the oatmeal bath.

### 7. Burow's Solution (Domeboro): tablets                    *OTC*

One tablet dissolved in a pint of water will make a solution which can be applied as a wet dressing to insect bites, poison ivy, or inflamed areas. The dressing should be kept moist for up to four hours.

### 8. Calamine lotion                    *OTC*

Apply as needed for relief of itching.

## LEG CRAMPS AND FATIGUE

1. Vitamin E                                                                  *OTC*

   It has been reported in the medical literature that a daily dose of four hundred to eight hundred International Units can reduce the discomfort of nighttime leg cramps or "restless legs." There has even been the suggestion that exercise cramps and poor leg circulation will benefit from this dose of Vitamin E.

2. **Quinamm** (quinine) tablets                                             *Rx*

   Usual adult dose: one tablet before bedtime. If necessary this dose can be increased to one tablet after supper and one tablet upon retiring.

   This drug may be useful in alleviating the symptoms of nighttime leg muscle cramps (including those related to diabetes, arthritis, thrombophlebitis, arteriosclerosis, varicose veins).

   **CAUTION:** Do not take **Quinamm** if you are pregnant or of child-bearing potential. If you are allergic to quinine or have the enzyme deficiency glucose-6-phosphate dehydrogenase, you must also avoid this medication.

   If the drug produces stomach cramps, take it with a small snack. If you notice ringing in the ears, skin rash, visual disturbances, or deafness discontinue the drug immediately.

## MOTION SICKNESS

1. Ginger                                                                    *OTC*

   For adults, approximately 900 mg of ground ginger in capsules has been reported to be helpful in reducing symptoms of motion sickness. For children a palatable alternative might be ginger-snap cookies with extra ginger.

**Motion Sickness** *cont.*

2. **Dramamine** (dimenhydrinate): 50-milligram
   tablets
                                                              *OTC*

   Usual adult dose for motion sickness: one tablet taken thirty
   minutes to one hour before departure. Children's dose: one-
   half tablet taken up to three times daily. The effect should last
   four hours.

   Young children should not take this medicine except with
   a physician's approval.

   Drowsiness may be severe when taking this drug. Never
   undertake any activity which requires attention or coordination. The sedative action of this drug can be put to good
   advantage as a sleeping pill.

   If possible, do not take **Dramamine** concomitantly with the
   following antibiotics: kanamycin, neomycin, ristocetin, streptomycin, and vancomycin. Damage to the ear is possible.

3. **Transderm-Scop** (scopolamine): transdermal skin patch;
   Contains 1.5 mg of scopolamine, which delivers 0.5 mg of
   the drug gradually over three days. Do not use for children!
                                                              *Rx*

   Carefully stick skin patch behind ear about four hours before
   exposure to motion.

   **CAUTION:** Scopolamine can cause sedation, confusion,
   and disorientation. Do not drive, operate machinery, or undertake any activity that requires concentration or coordination. DO NOT rub fingers in eyes after applying the patch.
   Wash fingers immediately! Side effects may include dry
   mouth, blurry vision, dilated pupils, memory disturbances,
   and drowsiness.

## PAIN (Headaches, Toothaches, Menstrual Cramps, ... )

1. Aspirin: 5-grain tablets (325 milligrams)                *OTC*

   Usual adult dose for mild pain: one or two tablets repeated
   every three to four hours. Aspirin is absorbed better and is
   less irritating to the stomach if it is crushed and "dissolved"
   or chewed with a mouthful of milk. Always take aspirin with
   a full glass of liquid. A pinch of baking soda at the same time
   will also counteract irritation if you are susceptible to this
   problem.

   Vitamin C taken at the same time will make the aspirin
   work harder and longer and could be advantageous if you
   want a bigger punch for pain.

   **CAUTION:** Do not take aspirin with alcohol, anticoagulants, antidepressants, arthritis medicines, or oral diabetes
   medicine.

2. Codeine: various doses; 30-milligram tablets
   preferred                                                *Rx*

   Usual adult dose: one tablet every four hours. Combined with
   two aspirin tablets, codeine is a powerful painkiller which is
   superior to anything else on the market, especially **Darvon**.
   One popular product, **Empirin #3,** combines aspirin and
   codeine and is a reasonable option.

   Codeine should not be used casually, as it can be habit-
   forming, though this problem has been somewhat exag-
   gerated.

   **CAUTION:** Do not take codeine with alcohol, barbiturates, or tranquilizers.

3. **Tylenol with Codeine:** tablets in various doses      *Rx*

   Usual adult dose: one or two tablets every four hours. These
   preparations contain acetaminophen instead of aspirin. They

## Pain *cont.*

can be used by people who are sensitive to aspirin or who for other reasons cannot take salicylates.

4. **Advil; Nuprin** (ibuprofen): 200-mg tablets.                    *OTC*

Usual adult dose is one to two tablets every four to six hours for garden-variety pain. For menstrual cramps the dose is 400 mg (two tablets) every four hours as necessary.

Until recently, ibuprofen was only available by prescription under the names **Motrin** or **Rufen.** It is now available over-the-counter for minor aches and pains associated with conditions like arthritis, tennis elbow, menstrual cramps, backaches, sprains, strains, toothaches, or whatever.

**CAUTIONS:** Stomach irritation, nausea, heartburn, diarrhea, vomiting, cramps, flatulence, and ulcers are not uncommon. Other side effects include dizziness, headache, nervousness, rash, ringing in the ears, anemias, and fluid retention. Kidney damage is rare but extremely serious. Any visual disturbances demand the drug be discontinued immediately. Do not take if you are allergic to aspirin.

## POISONING: CALL POISON CONTROL CENTER IMMEDIATELY!

1. Ipecac syrup: liquid                                            *OTC*

Usual dose: three teaspoonfuls

Usual dose for children under one year of age: one-half to one teaspoonful. This medicine will usually induce vomiting within fifteen to twenty minutes. Administer with a full glass of water and gently move child around either by walking or rocking. A second dose may be administered after twenty minutes if the first try was unsuccessful, but no more after that. Additional doses may be toxic.

## Poisoning *cont.*

**CAUTION:** Do not induce vomiting if the poison which was swallowed is corrosive: acid, alkali (lye), gasoline, kerosene, cleaning fluid, turpentine, or any other petroleum product. If the patient is unconscious, vomiting is extremely dangerous.

2. Activated charcoal (powder or liquid)                    *OTC*

   Usual dose: one large tablespoon of powder in a glass of water well mixed to form a soupy glop. If in liquid form: one ounce of a 25 percent suspension.

   Activated charcoal should follow vomiting in order to soak up any poison which is left in the stomach. Repeat the dose frequently.

3. Poison antidote kit: charcoal and ipecac                    *OTC*

   This excellent kit contains everything you need in case of an emergency in a handy, ready-to-use form. It is available from Bowman Pharmaceuticals, Inc., Canton, OH 44702.

4. In the case of corrosive or irritating poisons it is best to dilute the poison before rushing the patient to the emergency room of the nearest hospital. Demulcents such as milk, egg white, gelatin solution, aluminum hydroxide gel, flour and water, or oil may be of some benefit. DO NOT INDUCE VOMITING!

## STOMACH UPSET AND INDIGESTION

1. Aluminum and magnesium hydroxide: liquid
   suspension works best.                                       *OTC*

   Almost any of the dozens of combinations on pharmacy shelves will relieve excess acidity. Products that are best buys

## Stomach Upset and Indigestion *cont.*

include **Maalox TC, Mylanta II, Gelusil II, Delcid**, and **Simeco**.

**CAUTION:** People who are at risk of osteoporosis (weakened bones) should probably avoid large doses of aluminum-containing antacids. An acceptable alternative for such folks would be calcium-containing antacids such as **Tums, Tums E-X, Alka-2 Chewable, Alkets, Amitone, Chooz, Dicarbosil, Glycate, Gustalac, Pama, Ratio**, and **Titralac**.

No one should rely on antacids continuously to relieve symptoms. If indigestion and pain persist, medical supervision should be sought.

## SUNBURN

1. PABA and friends (para-aminobenzoic acid):
   suntan lotion                                              *OTC*

   Prevention is *always* the best medicine. To prevent a bad burn, use a sunscreen with an SPF (Sun Protection Factor) number greater than 10. If you are fair-skinned, blue-eyed, blond or red-haired, you will need an SPF of 15. Products that provide excellent protection include: **Block Out, Pabanol, Presun 15, Solbar Plus 15, Super Shade, Sundare 15, Sundown Sunblock Ultra Protection, Total Eclipse**, and many others.

2. In the event you blew it and did not get adequate sunscreen protection, there isn't much you can do to undo the damage. For the boiled-shrimp-look, you can take aspirin for the pain and soak in a cool tub of water.

   For severe burns see a dermatologist. He will probably prescribe prednisone or some other cortisonelike medication for several days to relieve the discomfort.

## URINARY-TRACT INFECTIONS (UTIs):

This is definitely NOT a self-help kind of problem. If you are within traveling distance of a physician, get moving. But if you are caught far from home without medical attention you may have to take independent action. If that is the case, here are some stopgap measures till you can obtain competent medical help.

1. Sulfisoxazole: Found in the following brand-name drugs: **Gantrisin, Azo-Gantrisin, Lipi Gantrisin, SK-Soxazole, Sulfagan, Sulfizin**, etc. Tablets generally come in 500-mg doses.                                              *Rx*

   This sulfa drug is one of the most commonly prescribed medications for uncomplicated cystitis and urinary-tract infections. Traditionally, the drug was prescribed for at least a week to ten days, but more recently doctors have taken to giving it for only one to three days with virtually comparable results. In fact, some physicians believe that just one big dose is all that's necessary for most simple UTIs. Two grams (four 500-mg tablets) taken as a single dose often does the trick.

   If symptoms are more severe (such as fever, chills, or flank pain) suggesting kidney involvement, then treatment should continue for ten to fourteen days and probably should involve amoxicillin or a trimethoprim-sulfamethoxazole combination product (**Bactrim** or **Septra**).

   To make sure the infection has been licked, the urine should be tested with a special strip such as **Microstix-3, Microstix-Nitrite**, or **N-Uristix**. These self-testing strips can be purchased in a pharmacy without a prescription and should go along on any trip. The urine should be checked periodically every couple of days after treatment to make sure the antibiotic has done the job.

   **CAUTION:** Side effects of short-term sulfa treatment are usually minimal. Nevertheless, such drugs should not be used

## Urinary-Tract Infections *cont.*

during pregnancy unless specifically recommended by a physician. Anyone allergic to sulfa drugs MUST NOT take any of these medications. Rash and itching are signs of an allergic reaction. These side effects are generally made worse by exposure to sunlight. NEVER take **Gantrisin**-like drugs and go out in the sun. If a rash or itching occurs, the drug should be discontinued. Other side effects may include digestive-tract upset, headache, fever, chills, and anemias. Fortunately, such problems are rare when the drug is only taken for a short period of time.

2. **Bactrim** or **Septra** (tablets usually contain 80 mg trimethoprim and 400 mg sulfamethoxazole; there is now a "DS" formulation which contains a double-strength dose).

*Rx*

The usual adult dose for treating urinary-tract infections is two regular-strength tablets (80 mg trimethoprim and 400 mg sulfamethoxazole) every twelve hours for ten to fourteen days. But here again some physicians believe that single-dose therapy can be almost as effective. Two regular-strength tablets or one "DS" (double-strength) tablet have been reported to do the job with fewer side effects. Patients with signs of kidney infection (fever, chills, flank pain, or other more serious symptoms) will need a two-week course of treatment.

Urine should be checked periodically after therapy with a strip test such as **Microstix-3, Microstix-Nitrite**, or **N-Uristix** to make sure the infection has been licked.

CAUTION: Such drugs should not be taken by pregnant women or people with kidney or liver damage. People with a history of allergy to sulfas should not take these medications. Side effects may include skin rash and itching. Both are aggravated by exposure to sunlight. At the first sign of rash or itching, the drug should be discontinued immediately. Other potential adverse reactions include anemias, digestive-

## Urinary-Tract Infections *cont.*

tract upset, headache, depression, fever, and chills. Fortunately, such side effects are rare when therapy is limited to a single-dose regimen.

# Recommended Medical Reference Books for Home Use

THE MERCK MANUAL OF DIAGNOSIS AND THERAPY
Editor, Robert Berkow
Merck & Co., Inc.
Rahway, NJ 07605

THE PEOPLE'S PHARMACY-2
By Joe Graedon with Teresa Graedon
Graedon Enterprises
P.O. Box 31788
Raleigh, NC 27622
Available in a mass-market paperback edition from St. Martin's Press, 175 Fifth Avenue, New York, NY 10010 in early 1986.

THE NEW PEOPLE'S PHARMACY #3
By Joe Graedon and Teresa Graedon
Bantam Books
666 Fifth Avenue
New York, NY 10103

THE MEDICINE SHOW
By the Editors of *Consumer Reports*
Consumers Union
Orangeburg, NY 10962

THE PILL BOOK
By Dr. Harold Silverman
Bantam Books
666 Fifth Avenue
New York, NY 10103

# References

1. Kluger, Matthew J., Ringler, Daniel H., and Anver, Miriam R. "Fever and Survival." *Science* 188:166–168, 1975.

2. Steffen, Robert, et al. "Epidemiology of Diarrhea in Travelers." *JAMA,* 249(9):1176–1180, 1983.

3. Cook, G. C. "Travellers' Diarrhoea—An Insoluble Problem." *Gut* 24:1105–1108, 1983.

4. Ibid.

5. Weiss, Barry. "Traveler's Diarrhea: Update 1983." *Am. Fam. Phys.* 27(4):193–195, 1983.

6. Leyden, J. L., and Kligman, A. M. "Aluminum Chloride in the Treatment of Symptomatic Athlete's Foot." *Arch. Dermatol.* 111:1004–1010, 1975.

7. Kabara, Jon J. "Bar Soap and Liquid Soap." *JAMA* 253:1560–1561, 1985.

# Afterword

We sure hope you enjoyed this book. Frankly, rewriting *The People's Pharmacy* was a lot more fun than we ever expected it to be. We have learned a lot from the thousands of letters we've received over the years from readers of the original *People's Pharmacy,* as well as *People's Pharmacy-2, The New People's Pharmacy,* and our syndicated newspaper column. They have made it clear that people really want to know more about the medications they use.

There have been a lot of changes in medicines and the pharmaceutical industry in the decade since the first edition of this book was published. There have been drug breakthroughs that have made people's lives better, but there have also been scandals that have killed people unnecessarily. We've tried to bring you up-to-date on these developments without getting sucked in by the drug companies' hired hypesters.

We take our readers' comments very seriously, whether they're commendations or criticisms. We cannot promise to answer every letter, because we sometimes get an awful lot of mail, but please let us know what you think. We'll try to answer as many questions as we can, and of course, we will definitely appreciate your ideas in the event we need to revise this book again sometime.

Address cards and letters to:

> Joe and Terry Graedon
> *The People's Pharmacy*
> c/o St. Martin's Press
> 175 Fifth Avenue
> New York, N.Y. 10010

# Appendix

# A Guide to Chain Store and Mail-Order Prices of Some Frequently Prescribed Drugs

The following price information was gathered in 1985 from a variety of sources, including chain stores and mail-order pharmacies. You may be surprised at how much prices can vary, especially between brand-name and generic products. Although you may not be able to match these prices in your area, we suggest you shop comparatively. But never forget that good information is worth paying for. If you have a pharmacist who takes the time to warn you about side effects, special precautions, and drug interactions as well as answer your questions, you'd do well to buy your drugs there.

The column headed "MG" gives milligrams per pill (or tablet or capsule), except where "gr" (grains), or "meq" (milliequivalent), or a percentage such as "1%" (liquid concentration) is listed.

## A Guide to Chain Store and Mail-Order Prices of Some Frequently Prescribed Drugs

| Brand Name | Generic Name | Mg | Price of 100 Branded Pills | Price of 100 Generic Pills |
|---|---|---|---|---|
| Achromycin V | tetracycline | 250 | $ 5.50 | $ 3.05 |
| Aldactazide | spironolactone | 25 | 20.10 | 9.20 |
| | hydrochlorothiazide | 25 | | |
| Aldactone | spironolactone | 25 | 28.05 | 9.35 |
| Aldomet | methyldopa | 250 | 15.10 | 9.95 |
| Aldoril-15 | methyldopa | 250 | 19.35 | N/A[1] |
| | hydrochlorothiazide | 15 | | |
| Amcill 250 | ampicillin | 250 | 17.89 | 8.93 |
| Amoxil | amoxicillin | 250 | 16.45 | 18.25 |
| Antivert | meclizine | 12.5 | 13.70 | 3.25 |
| Apresoline | hydralazine | 25 | 11.75 | 3.15 |
| Atarax | hydroxyzine | 50 | 45.49 | N/A |
| Aristocort | triamcinolone | 4 | 74.27 | 11.29 |

[1] "N/A" indicates generic price Not Applicable, or information not readily available. "n.y.a." has been used as an abbreviation for "not yet available." A generic form is expected to be marketed by 1986.

| | | | | |
|---|---|---|---|---|
| **Ativan** | lorazepam | 1 | 21.85 | n.y.a. |
| **Atromid-S** | clofibrate | 500 | 18.65 | (patent) |
| **Azulfidine** | sulfasalazine | 500 | 15.95 | 8.65 |
| **Bactrim** | sulfamethoxazole | 400 | 31.85 | 17.65 |
| | trimethoprim | 80 | | |
| **Bactrim DS** | sulfamethoxazole | 800 | 47.35 | 23.03 |
| | trimethoprim | 160 | | |
| **Benadryl Caps/Tabs** | diphenhydramine | 50 | 15.49 | 3.15 |
| **Benemid** | probenecid | 500 | 19.05 | 8.15 |
| **Brethine** | terbutaline | 2.5 | 12.60 | 11.55 |
| **Blocadren** | timolol | 10 | 23.80 | (patent) |
| **Cafergot** | ergotamine | 1 | 12.33 | N/A |
| | caffeine | 100 | | |
| **Calan** | verapamil | 80 | 18.30 | (patent) |
| **Capoten** | captopril | 25 | 26.95 | (patent) |
| **Carafate** | sucralfate | 1 | 37.57 | (patent) |
| **Cardizem** | diltiazem | 30 | 20.25 | (patent) |
| **Catapres** | clonidine | 0.1 | 16.85 | (patent) |

## A Guide to Chain Store and Mail-Order Prices of Some Frequently Prescribed Drugs *cont.*

| Brand Name | Generic Name | Mg | Price of 100 Branded Pills | Price of 100 Generic Pills |
|---|---|---|---|---|
| Ceclor | cefaclor | 250 | 102.37 | (patent) |
| Centrax | prazepam | 10 | 27.55 | (patent) |
| Chlor-Trimeton | chlorpheniramine | 4 | 8.19 | 2.10 |
| Choledyl | oxtriphylline | 200 | 15.05 | 12.19 |
| Clinoril | sulindac | 150 | 39.00 | (patent) |
| Compazine | prochlorperazine | 5 | 23.75 | (patent) |
| Corgard | nadolol | 40 | 34.60 | 14.20 |
| Coumadin Oral[2] | warfarin | 5 | 13.85 | (patent) |
| Dalmane | flurazepam | 30 | 21.90 | N/A |
| Darvocet-N 100 | propoxyphene napsylate | 100 | 22.20 | n.y.a. |
| | acetaminophen | 650 | | (patent) |
| Darvon | propoxyphene HCL | 65 | 19.49 | 6.95 |
| Darvon Compound-65 | propoxyphene HCL | 65 | 20.87 | 9.29 |
| | aspirin | 389 | | |
| | caffeine | 32.4 | | |

[2]Price is for 40 tablets.

| Brand | Generic | Strength | | |
|---|---|---|---|---|
| Deltasone | prednisone | 5 | 7.19 | 3.89 |
| Desyrel | trazodone | 50 | 30.45 | (patent) |
| Diabinese | chlorpropamide | 250 | 27.95 | 7.77 |
| Dilantin | phenytoin | 100 | 7.99 | 4.69 |
| Dimetapp Extentabs | brompheniramine | 12 | | |
| | phenylpropanolamine | 75 | | |
| Diuril | chlorothiazide | 250 | 6.00 | 3.65 |
| Donnatal | belladonna alkaloids | 5.09 | 1.99 | |
| | phenobarbital | 16.2 | | |
| Dyazide | triamterene | 50 | 16.20 | n.y.a. |
| | hydrochlorothiazide | 25 | | |
| E.E.S. | erythromycin ethylsuccinate | 400 | 24.19 | 11.40 |
| Elavil | amitriptyline | 25 | 16.99 | 4.95 |
| Empirin/Codeine #3 | aspirin | 325 | 16.45 | N/A |
| | codeine | 30 | | |
| E-Mycin | erythromycin | 250 | 20.15 | 15.75 |
| Endep | amitriptyline | 50 | 28.25 | 6.05 |
| Enduron | methyclothiazide | 5 | 18.55 | 10.95 |
| Equanil | meprobamate | 400 | 13.69 | 4.69 |
| Esidrix | hydrochlorothiazide | 50 | 13.95 | 3.89 |
| Feldene | piroxicam | 20 | 91.65 | (patent) |

## A Guide to Chain Store and Mail-Order Prices of Some Frequently Prescribed Drugs *cont.*

| Brand Name | Generic Name | Mg | Price of 100 Branded Pills | Price of 100 Generic Pills |
|---|---|---|---|---|
| Fiorinal | aspirin | 325 | | |
| | butalbital | 50 | 19.95 | 7.55 |
| | caffeine | 40 | | |
| Flagyl | metronidazole | 250 | 79.20 | 44.00 |
| Flexeril | cyclobenzaprine | 10 | 43.19 | (patent) |
| Gantrisin | sulfisoxazole | 500 | 13.25 | 6.69 |
| Garamycin | gentamicin | 15 gr | 10.85 | 7.19 |
| Halcion | triazolam | 0.25 | 27.55 | (patent) |
| Haldol | haloperidol | 1 | 28.75 | (patent) |
| Hydergine | ergoloid mesylates | 1 | 31.75 | 14.75 |
| HydroDIURIL | hydrochlorothiazide | 50 | 11.83 | 3.89 |
| Hygroton | chlorthalidone | 25 | 19.30 | 9.50 |
| Imodium | loperamide | 2 | 37.45 | (patent) |
| Inderal | propranolol | 40 | 16.50 | n.y.a. |
| Inderal LA | propranolol | 80 | 33.05 | (patent) |
| Inderide | hydrochlorothiazide | 40 | 24.40 | n.y.a. |
| | hydrochlorothiazide | 25 | | |

| Brand | Generic | Strength | | |
|---|---|---|---|---|
| **Indocin** | indomethacin | 25 | 28.05 | 16.95 |
| **Indocin SR** | indomethacin | 75 | 64.10 | (patent) |
| **Isoptin** | verapamil | 80 | 18.30 | (patent) |
| **Isordil** | isosorbide dinitrate | 10 | 13.63 | 3.69 |
| **K-Lor** | potassium Cl | 20meq | 26.10 | N/A |
| **K-Lyte** | potassium bicarb & citrate | 25 meq | 30.15 | N/A |
| **K-Tab** | potassium Cl | 10 meq | 9.45 | N/A |
| **Keflex** | cephalexin | 250 | 66.77 | (patent) |
| **Kenalog**[3] | triamcinolone | 0.1% | 8.89 | 3.29 |
| **Klotrix** | potassium Cl | 10 meq | 8.60 | N/A |
| **Lanoxin** | digoxin | 0.25 | 3.00 | 1.45 |
| **Lasix** | furosemide | 20 | 8.95 | 5.45 |
| **Librax** | chlordiazepoxide | 5 | 27.09 | 6.05 |
| | clidinium | 2.5 | | |
| **Librium** | chlordiazepoxide | 10 | 21.95 | 5.19 |
| **Limbitrol** | chlordiazepoxide | 10 | 47.34 | N/A |
| | amitriptyline | 25 | | |
| **Lomotil** | diphenoxylate | 2.5 | 30.69 | 6.79 |
| | atropine | .025 | | |

[3]Price is for a 5-gram tube.

## A Guide to Chain Store and Mail-Order Prices of Some Frequently Prescribed Drugs *cont.*

| Brand Name | Generic Name | Mg | Price of 100 Branded Pills | Price of 100 Generic Pills |
|---|---|---|---|---|
| Lopid | gemfibrozil | 300 | 25.75 | (patent) |
| Lopressor | metroprolol | 50 | 15.65 | (patent) |
| Lorelco[4] | probucol | 250 | 27.25 | (patent) |
| Lotrimin[5] | clotrimazole | 1% | 9.35 | 9.09 |
| Maxzide | triamterene | 75 | 26.00 | (patent) |
| | hydrochlorothiazide | 50 | | |
| Meclomen | meclofenamate | 100 | 31.45 | n.y.a. |
| Medrol Oral | methylprednisolone | 4 | 29.61 | 15.97 |
| Mellaril | thioridazine | 100 | 28.56 | 21.00 |
| Micro-K Extencaps | potassium Cl | 8 meq | 7.75 | (patent) |
| Miltown | meprobamate | 400 | 35.29 | 4.69 |
| Minipress | prazosin | 1 | 14.35 | (patent) |

[4]Lorelco price is for 120 tablets.
[5]Lotrimin price is for a 5-gram tube.

| Brand | Generic | Quantity | | |
|---|---|---|---|---|
| **Moduretic** | amiloride with hydrochlorothiazide | 50 5 | 23.30 | (patent) |
| **Motrin** | ibuprofen | 400 | 13.95 | 10.95 |
| **Mycostatin**[6] | nystatin | | 11.29 | 3.75 |
| **Mysoline** | primidone | 250 | 18.79 | 6.89 |
| **Nalfon** | fenoprofen | 600 | 31.20 | (patent) |
| **Naprosyn** | naproxen | 250 | 38.10 | (patent) |
| **Nembutal** | pentobarbital | 100 | 15.49 | 7.45 |
| **Nitro-Bid** | nitroglycerin TD | 2.5 | 15.10 | 4.25 |
| **Nitro-Dur** | nitroglycerin patch | 10 cm$^2$ | 25.35 for 28 patches | (patent) |
| **Nitrostat** | nitroglycerin | 0.15 | 2.35 | N/A |
| **Nolvadex** | tamoxifen | 10 | 68.95 | (patent) |
| **Normodyne** | labetolol | 200 | 29.95 | n.y.a. |
| **Norpace** | disopyramide | 100 | 26.10 | n.y.a. |
| **Oretic** | hydrochlorothiazide | 50 | 10.39 | 3.89 |
| **Orinase** | tolbutamide | 500 | 16.49 | 6.38 |
| **Ornade** | phenylpropanolamine chlorpheniramine | 75 12 | 35.18 | 9.80 |

[6]Price is for a 15-gram tube.

## A Guide to Chain Store and Mail-Order Prices of Some Frequently Prescribed Drugs cont.

| Brand Name | Generic Name | Mg | Price of 100 Branded Pills | Price of 100 Generic Pills |
|---|---|---|---|---|
| Parafon Forte | chlorzoxazone | 250 | 26.35 | 4.95 |
| | acetaminophen | 300 | | n.y.a. |
| Parlodel | bromocriptine | 2.5 | 24.10 | 4.05 |
| Pavabid | papaverine | 150 | 23.75 | 6.79 |
| Pentids | penicillin G | 250 | 11.66 | 5.95 |
| Pen-Vee K | penicillin V | 250 | 12.75 | 7.95 |
| Periactin | cyproheptadine | 4 | 18.05 | 13.19 |
| Peritrate SA | pentaerythritol tetranitrate | 80 | 26.03 | 10.86 |
| Persantine | dipyridamole | 25 | 18.10 | 8.93 |
| Polycillin | ampicillin | 250 | 20.96 | 8.45 |
| Premarin | conjugated estrogens | 1.25 | 15.95 | 7.00 |
| Pro-Banthine | propantheline | 15 | 26.49 | 16.95 |
| Procan-SR | procainamide-SR | 500 | 22.05 | (patent) |
| Procardia | nifedipine | 10 | 20.85 | 2.35 |
| Proloid | thyroid | 1 gr | 3.55 | 7.80 |
| Pronestyl | procainamide | 250 | 24.19 | 30.94 |
| Prostaphlin | oxacillin | 250 | 68.07 | n.y.a. |
| Proventil | albuterol | 2 | 19.25 | |

| Brand | Generic | Strength | | |
|---|---|---|---|---|
| Quinaglute Duratabs | quinidine gluconate-SR | 324 | 31.65 | 19.95 |
| Quinidex Extentabs | quinidine sulfate | 300 | 29.10 | N/A |
| Quinora | quinidine sulfate | 300 | 24.89 | 7.00 |
| Reglan | metoclopramide | 10 | 23.65 | (patent) |
| Restoril | temazepam | 15 | 25.35 | n.y.a. |
| Robaxin | methocarbamol | 500 | 15.85 | 4.95 |
| Robaxisal | methocarbamol | 400 | 18.99 | 9.30 |
|  | aspirin | 325 | | |
| Rufen | ibuprofen | 600 | 14.55 | n.y.a. |
| Salutensin | hydroflumethiazide | 50 | 41.09 | 23.29 |
|  | reserpine | 0.125 | | |
| Septra | sulfamethoxazole | 400 | 34.29 | 17.65 |
|  | trimethoprim | 80 | | |
| Septra DS | sulfamethoxazole | 800 | | |
|  | trimethoprim | 160 | 45.08 | 23.03 |
| Ser-Ap-Es | hydrochlorothiazide | 15 | | |
|  | hydralazine | 25 | 25.66 | 10.88 |
|  | reserpine | 0.1 | | |
| Serax | oxazepam | 15 | 31.65 | n.y.a. |
| Serpasil | reserpine | 0.25 | 5.25 | 2.45 |
| Sinemet | carbidopa | 25 | 32.00 | N/A |
|  | levodopa | 100 | | |

## A Guide to Chain Store and Mail-Order Prices of Some Frequently Prescribed Drugs cont.

| Brand Name | Generic Name | Mg | Price of 100 Branded Pills | Price of 100 Generic Pills |
|---|---|---|---|---|
| Sinequan | doxepin | 25 | 22.85 | N/A |
| Slow-K | potassium Cl | 600 | 8.20 | (patent) |
| Soma | carisoprodol | 350 | 43.19 | 11.49 |
| Sorbitrate | isosorbide oral | 5 | 8.95 | 2.75 |
| Stelazine | trifluoperazine | 2 | 27.50 | 16.50 |
| Symmetrel | amantadine | 100 | 31.70 | (patent) |
| Synthroid | levothyroxine | 0.2 | 7.95 | 2.45 |
| Tagamet | cimetidine | 200 | 28.95 | (patent) |
| Tegopen | cloxacillin | 250 | 83.98 | 32.78 |
| Tegretol | carbamazepine | 200 | 21.40 | (patent) |
| Tenormin | atenolol | 50 | 31.90 | (patent) |
| Terramycin | oxytetracycline | 250 | 37.17 | 10.83 |
| Tetracyn | tetracycline | 250 | 8.29 | 3.05 |
| Theo-Dur | theophylline | 300 | 13.95 | N/A |
| Timoptic[7] | timolol | 0.5% | 11.75 | (patent) |

[7]Price is for a bottle of ophthalmic solution.

| Brand | Generic | Strength | | |
|---|---|---|---|---|
| Tofranil | imipramine | 25 | 20.35 | 4.50 |
| Tolectin | tolmetin | 400 | 37.15 | (patent) |
| Tolinase | tolazamide | 250 | 27.95 | 19.95 |
| Trandate | labetolol | 200 | 29.95 | (patent) |
| Tranxene | clorazepate | 7.5 | 26.10 | (patent) |
| Triavil | amitriptyline | 25 | 28.00 | N/A |
| | perphenazine | 2 | | |
| Tylenol/Codeine | acetaminophen | 300 | 10.18 | 5.40 |
| | codeine | 30 | | |
| Urecholine | bethanecol | 10 | 27.70 | 5.50 |
| V-Cillin K | penicillin V | 250 | 17.59 | 5.95 |
| Valium | diazepam | 5 | 20.30 | (patent) |
| Vanceril | beclomethasone | 17 gr | 12.50 | (patent) |
| Vasodilan | isoxsuprine | 10 | 22.75 | 6.15 |
| Ventolin Inhaler | albuterol | 17 gr | 9.05 | (patent) |
| Visken | pindolol | 5 | 23.55 | (patent) |
| Wygesic | acetaminophen | 650 | 21.35 | 13.35 |
| | propoxyphene | 65 | | |
| Xanax | alprazolam | 0.5 | 27.29 | (patent) |
| Zantac | ranitidine | 150 | 70.65 | (patent) |
| Zyloprim | allopurinol | 500 | 23.75 | 16.75 |

# Index

Food and Drug Administration *cont.*
and **DMSO**, 27
drug expiration date, 49
drugs taken improperly, 2–3
and food additives, 297
on laxatives, 497
legal definition of a drug, 9
on menstrual products, 150
and methapyrilene, 110
on mouthwashes, 129, 132
New Drug Application and tests,
9, 29–30
OTC Drug Review, 57, 105, 107,
108, 129, 132, 147, 151, 152–53
Physician Package Insert, 37
*Physicians' Desk Reference*, 37
safety and effectiveness of drugs,
22–23, 26–32 *passim*
on sleep aids, 109
on sodium bicarbonate, 119
and starch blockers, 11–12
Sun Protection Factor, 498–99
and vaginal deodorants, 149
wart cures, 147–48
Food, Drug, and Cosmetic (FDC)
Act, 104–05
Yellow #5, 35, 203, 297, 328
foot problems: athlete's foot, 5,
144–45, 156, 503–504, 515–16
to warm feet, 89–91
warts, corns, and calluses, 102,
145–48, 162
**Formula 44-D**, 173
**Freezone**, 147, 162
Friedman, Marion, 175–76
frostbite, 95
**Fulvicin**, 188, 190
fungal infections: athlete's foot, 5,
144–45, 156, 503–504, 515–16
fingernails, 87–89
jock itch, 100, 502, 504–505,
515–16
vaginal, 145, 366
yeast (Candida), as side effect, 340,
386
**Furadantin**, 481
furosemide, 170, 242, 402, 481, 500,
541
**Furoxone**, 213, 241, 260–70

gallbladder, 354
**Gantanol**, 381, 410, 481, 500
drug interaction, 190, 203, 237

**Gantrisin**, 410, 481, 495, 530,
540
drug interaction, 190, 203, 237,
351
side effects, 381, 495, 500
**Garamycin**, 481, 540
gargles *see* mouthwash and gargles
**Gaviscon**, 116, 154, 254
**Gaviscon-2**, 116
**Gelusil**, 121, 125, 254, 285
**Gelusil II**, 121, 154, 529
gemfibrozil, 542
**Gemonil**, 188, 198–202, 225, 232,
258, 271–77
generic drugs *see* drugs, brand
name/generic name
gentamicin, 481, 540
**Geocillin**, 288
**Geritol**, 286
German measles vaccine, 235,
297–98, 406
**Gets-It Liquid**, 147, 162
ginger, 71, 90, 497, 524
**Gitaligin**, 246
glaucoma, 315, 521
glutethimide, 271–77, 480
**Glycate**, 125, 154, 529
glycopyrrolate, 483
Godfrey, R. C., 307, 309
goiter, 328, 405
**Goody's Headache Powder**, 36
gout, medication for, 29, 35, 179,
194, 224, 241
**Grapefruit Diet Plan with Diadax**,
165
**Grifulvin V**, 188
**Gris-Peg**, 188
**Grisactin**, 188
guanadrel, 210, 257
guanethidine, 47, 210, 257, 262, 351,
443
**Gustalac**, 125, 154, 529
**Gynergen**, 408

hair: dandruff, 101, 140–44, 157
growth, as side effect, 443–44
loss, as side effect, 42, 439
shampoo, 22, 101, 140–44, 157
halazepam, 271–77
**Halcion**, 170, 227, 258, 271–77, 282,
540
**Haldol**, 254–59, 402, 484, 540
**Haldrone**, 229–35

Noctec, 258, 271–77
Noludar, 258, 271–77
Nolvadex, 405, 543
nonprescription drugs *see* drugs,
    over-the-counter (OTC)
Nordette, 225–28, 234
norethindrone, 367
Norflex, 482
Norinyl, 225–28, 234, 352
Norisodrine, 329
Norlestrin, 225–28, 234, 352
Norman, Philip S., 299, 305
Normodyne, 171, 439, 543
Noroxine, 195, 215
Norpace, 543
Norpramin, 193, 208–15, 274, 351, 500
Nor-Q.D., 353
Norton, Lawrence, 87
nortriptyline, 208–15, 409, 500
Norwich-Eaton, 468
Novafed, 264
Novafed A Liquid, 373
Novahistine DH Liquid, 373
novobiocin, 409
Novrad, 408
Noxzema Sunburn Spray, 499
NP-27, 145
NP-27 Aerosol or Liquid, 156
NP-27 Powder, 156
Nubain, 484
Nuprin, 150, 159, 173, 189, 360, 527
N-Uristix, 530–31
nutrition *see* diet and food
*Nutrition & the M.D.*, 69
Nydrazid, 204, 230
nylidrin, 479
Nyquil, 101, 104, 173, 373, 375, 383
Nyquil Nighttime Colds Medicine Liquid, 373
nystatin, 482, 543
    and tetracycline, 283–88
Nytime Cold Medicine, 383
Nytol, 58, 109, 110
Nytol with DPH, 53, 110, 161, 312

Odara, 132, 160
Off!, 80
Off-Easy, 147, 148, 162
Old Spice Antiperspirant, 137
Old Time Woodsman's Liquid Fly Dope, 79

Omnipen, 288, 482
Oncovin, 405
One-a-Day Plus Iron, 286
Oraflex, 29, 30, 486
Oral Pentacresol, 132, 160
Oretic, 402, 432, 482, 543
Oreticyl, 402, 441
organic (definition and use), 12, 20–22
Orinase, 55, 404, 482, 543
    drug interaction, 220, 224, 236–41, 351
Ornade, 264, 489, 543
orphenadrine, 482
Ortho-Novum, 352
Ortho-Novum 7/7/7, 353
Os-Cal, 182, 184
osteoporosis, 123–25, 127–28, 154, 155, 529
Ovcon, 225–28, 234, 352
over-the-counter drugs *see* drugs, over-the-counter (OTC)
Ovral, 225–28, 234, 352, 485
Ovrette, 353
Ovulen, 225–28, 234, 352
oxacillin, 480, 482, 544
Oxalid, 409
oxazepam, 48, 227, 271–77, 483, 545
oxtriphylline, 226, 280, 480, 538
oxycodone, 482
oxyphenbutazone, 220, 409
oxytetracycline, 283–88, 483, 520, 546

PABA, 498, 529
Pabanol, 529
Pagitane, 255
pain relievers, 5, 17–18, 53, 86, 91, 150, 489, 508, 526–27
    drug interaction, 173, 186–87, 189–90, 219, 267–68
    no difference between them, 468–70
    use of, 102, 152
    *see also* anti-inflammatory drugs; aspirin
Pama, 125, 155, 529
Pamelor, 193, 208–15, 274, 500
Pamprin, 150, 159
Panadol, 150, 159, 189
Panafil Ointment, 75, 502, 517
pancreas, 67
Panmycin, 52, 381, 500

# About the Authors

Joe Graedon was born in 1945, and grew up in Bucks County, Pennsylvania. His interest in pharmacology developed while he was doing research on mental illness, sleep disorders, and brain physiology at the New Jersey Neuro-Psychiatric Institute in Princeton.

He went on to get a master's degree in pharmacology at the University of Michigan, Ann Arbor in 1971. He accompanied his anthropologist wife Teresa to Oaxaca, Mexico, where he taught pharmacology from 1973 to 1974 to medical students at the Universidad Autónoma "Benito Juarez" de Oaxaca. While he was there, he began work on *The People's Pharmacy,* which changed the direction of his career.

The surprising success of his first book showed Joe how interested people are in the medications they use, and encouraged him to begin writing a newspaper column, "The People's Pharmacy," which is syndicated by King Features to over a hundred newspapers around the country.

He and Teresa wrote *The People's Pharmacy-2* and *The New People's Pharmacy-3,* and he contributes regular columns to the magazine, *Medical Self-Care.* He also hosts a weekly call-in radio show for National Public Radio affiliate WUNC in Chapel Hill, North Carolina.

Joe guest-lectures frequently to civic organizations and health career students at Duke University and the University of North Carolina. He spent 1982–83 as Assistant Clinical Professor at the School of Pharmacy, University of California, San Francisco.

He was consultant to the Federal Trade Commission on non-prescription drug advertising from 1978 to 1983. He was a member of the editorial board of *Medical Communications,* the official journal of the American Medical Writers Association and is also a member of the advisory board of the Drug Studies Unit, University of California, San Francisco.

Joe belongs to the American Association for the Advancement of Science, the Society for Neuroscience, the Sleep Research Society, and the New York Academy of Science.

Teresa Graedon was born in 1947, and grew up in Cambridge, Massachusetts, and in northern New Jersey. She graduated magna cum laude from Bryn Mawr College in 1969, and went on to the University of Michigan, Ann Arbor, for graduate study in anthropology. Her doctoral research was on community health and nutrition in urban and rural Mexico.

After receiving her doctorate, Teresa taught as a medical anthropologist at Duke University School of Nursing from 1975 to 1979, and was an adjunct assistant professor in the Department of Anthropology.

When she left the Duke University faculty, she turned her attention to assisting Joe as coauthor of *The People's Pharmacy-2* and *The New People's Pharmacy-3.* She also collaborates with Joe on the newspaper column, and has contributed to the revised edition of *A Systems Approach to Community Health,* edited by Joanne Hall.

During 1982–83, Teresa was a postdoctoral fellow in the Medical Anthropology Program at University of California, San Francisco. She is a member of the American Public Health Association, the American Association for the Advancement of Science, the Society of Medical Anthropology and the American Anthropology Association.

Joe and Terry Graedon take readers' comments to heart, whether they be commendations or criticisms. They welcome reader response. If you would like to contact Joe and Terry, you can address your card or letter to:

Joe and Terry Graedon
*The People's Pharmacy*
c/o St. Martin's Press
175 Fifth Avenue
New York, NY 10010

Because they receive so many letters, they may not be able to answer each question individually, but they welcome comments, criticisms, suggestions, and recommendations.